The psychology of human thought

DATE DUE

MAY 3 0 1989		
JUL 1 1 1989		
DEC 0 5 1989		
APR 5 1990 JUN 2 1 03		

DEMCO 38-297

The psychology of human thought

Edited by

ROBERT J. STERNBERG
Yale University

EDWARD E. SMITH
University of Michigan

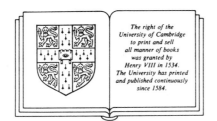

The right of the
University of Cambridge
to print and sell
all manner of books
was granted by
Henry VIII in 1534.
The University has printed
and published continuously
since 1584.

CAMBRIDGE UNIVERSITY PRESS

Cambridge
New York   New Rochelle   Melbourne   Sydney

Published by the Press Syndicate of the University of Cambridge
The Pitt Building, Trumpington Street, Cambridge CB2 1RP
32 East 57th Street, New York, NY 10022, USA
10 Stamford Road, Oakleigh, Melbourne 3166, Australia

First published 1988

Printed in the United States of America

Library of Congress Cataloging-in-Publication Data
The psychology of human thought.
Includes index.
1. Thought and thinking.   I. Sternberg, Robert J.
II. Smith, Edward E., 1940–   III. Title.
BF441.P82   1988   153.4   87–12075
ISBN 0 521 32229 4 hard covers
ISBN 0 521 31115 2 paperback

British Library Cataloguing in Publication applied for

Contents

v

Contributors

John D. Bransford
Vanderbilt University

M. Susan Burns
Tulane University

Victor R. Delclos
Vanderbilt University

Denise Dellarosa
Yale University

K. Anders Ericsson
Max Planck Institute

Baruch Fischhoff
Carnegie Mellon University

Bea Gattuso
Indiana University

Richard J. Gerrig
Yale University

Sam Glucksberg
Princeton University

Keith J. Holyoak
University of California, Los Angeles

P. N. Johnson-Laird
MRC Applied Psychology Unit

Alan Lesgold
University of Pittsburgh

Richard E. Nisbett
University of Michigan

William L. Oliver
University of Pittsburgh

D. N. Perkins
Harvard University

Lance J. Rips
University of Chicago

Miriam W. Schustack
University of California, San Diego

Maria Sera
Indiana University

Edward E. Smith
University of Michigan

Linda B. Smith
Indiana University

Robert J. Sternberg
Yale University

Nancy J. Vye
University of Western Ontario

Preface

The motivation for writing this textbook, like the incentive for writing so many others, was dissatisfaction with current texts in the area—in this case, the psychology of human thought. Both editors of this volume have taught undergraduate courses on thinking and related topics, and both have been unhappy with the available options. The books have never seemed up-to-date, or comprehensive with respect to the topics we wished to cover, or sufficiently free of the ax grinding that inevitably accompanies a textbook based on any one point of view, nor were they written in such a way as to evoke an enthusiastic response from undergraduates. We therefore decided to try our own hands at constructing a textbook on thinking. After initial consideration, we decided to edit rather than write the textbook. We made this decision for several reasons. The first was that the field has become exceedingly large and complex. Although each of us considers himself to be an expert in some areas, neither of us is an expert in all areas that concern thinking, nor did we believe that the two of us or any other set of individuals would collectively represent sufficient expertise in all areas of thinking research to write the best possible textbook. We therefore decided to ask those we considered to be foremost experts in each area to write individual chapters. We asked them to write on a level appropriate for undergraduates and to represent the state of the field, and not just their own work or point of view. We believe that a reading of the chapters will show that the authors fulfilled our request. Second, we hoped that by soliciting contributions from a number of authors we could convey to the students reading this book the excitement, challenge, and diversity of viewpoints currently permeating the field of thinking. When single or joint authors write textbooks, they frequently reveal their own enthusiasm or lack of enthusiasm. As a result, certain sections of their books have more sparkle than others, reflecting the authors' areas of greater and lesser interest. We believed that if experts wrote each of the chapters, the book would convey enthusiasm for each area of thinking, rather than just for those the editors happen to know best or to be most excited about. The chapters are quite even in their capacity to motivate students to pursue further reading and research in the wide variety of topics that constitute this field. Finally, one of us (R. J. S.) had previously edited a similar textbook on information-processing approaches to human abilities and had found that the edited format can result in a coherent, engaging, and wide-ranging text. On the basis of these considerations, we decided to give this edited textbook a try. We believe that it has met the goals we set for it.

All the areas of thinking that we believe worthy of inclusion in an introductory undergraduate (or graduate) course on the topic have been represented. Doubtless there will be those who will argue with our decisions to include one or another chapter, but most readers will find that all areas of thinking are well represented, and represented by distinguished contributors to the field. Because each of the editors has written on one topic, we decided that someone else should write the final, integrative chapter. We chose for this task Phil Johnson-Laird, who edited another textbook on thinking — also published by Cambridge University Press — and who is widely regarded as one of the most eminent individuals in the field of human thought. We were delighted that Professor Johnson-Laird agreed to write this chapter.

Although the book is intended to be an introductory text in thinking at the undergraduate or graduate level, broadly defined it can also be used in courses that are more narrowly focused, for example: reasoning, problem solving, thought and judgment, and decision making. Of course, not all courses on the psychology of human thought go by this name, and the book is eminently suitable for courses covering the same content but having a different name, such as "complex processes" or "higher processes." Moreover, teachers of cognate courses might wish to use the book as a supplementary text. For example, the book would be effective in courses on cognitive psychology, conceptual processes, or human information processing.

We have ordered the chapters in a way we believe makes conceptual and pedagogical sense. However, there is nothing sacred about the ordering we have chosen. Although there is cross-referencing, the chapters are written so as to be independent of one another, and teachers as well as students may read the chapters in any order that best suits their purposes. We would recommend, however, that the historical chapter be read first and the integrative chapter be read last in order to maximize the benefits obtained from the book.

As we read and edited the chapters, we found ourselves learning things we did not know, and our enthusiasm was rekindled even for areas of the field of thinking into which we have not delved deeply. We hope our readers share the learning and enthusiasm we have gained from the book and that they find the book to be an engaging and comprehensive overview of one of the most exciting fields of psychology, the psychology of human thought.

Robert J. Sternberg
Edward E. Smith

1   A history of thinking

Denise Dellarosa

> By ratiocination, I mean *computation*.
> —Hobbes, 1656

Questions concerning the nature of thought are as old as history itself. I do not pretend to present a complete history of this richly debated topic. Instead, I offer a brief history[1] that focuses on a particular question: Is thought a material process? This fundamental question has been hotly debated for centuries. René Descartes (1641/1951) held that the mind was a metaphysical entity that interacted with the material body and that thinking was a property of the mind, not the body. Thomas Hobbes (1656/1839), in contrast, held a mechanistic view of the nature of thought, believing it to be a wholly materialistic process. Thinking to Hobbes was like computing sums; rather than trafficking in numbers, however, thinking required trafficking in *ideas*. To Hobbes, thinking meant adding ideas together to form new ideas, subtracting ideas from each other, comparing ideas, and so on. He believed that thinking could be mechanized; in short, he believed that matter could think and that, in principle, machines could be built that were capable of thought.

It is this belief that thinking is a material process that fuels scientific investigation into the nature of thought. The rest of this chapter is devoted to describing the ways in which philosophers, mathematicians, psychologists, and computer scientists have attempted to investigate and explain the nature of thought since the early 1800s. In a sense, this work can be viewed as a serious attempt to make good on Hobbes's claim that thinking is a material, computational process.

Logical systems of thought

In 1854, George Boole, a mathematician, sought to determine the laws governing thinking and to describe them within a system of logic. According to Boole, thoughts were propositions or statements about the world that could be represented symbolically. These symbols could be combined in certain

1

ways to form other statements about the world. Thinking in Boole's system, then, was symbol manipulation.

To see how this system works, let us consider two propositions: "George is tall" and "Mary is tall." An important property of these and all propositions is their truth values. The proposition "George is tall" is true if George is in fact tall, and false otherwise. Boole proposed a number of connectives for combining single propositions like these into complex expressions, such as "George is tall AND Mary is tall." He also proposed truth tables, or rules, for determining the truth values of complex expressions. For example, the truth function for the connective "AND" states that the whole expression is true if and only if both propositions are true. So "George is tall AND Mary is tall" is true if both George and Mary are in fact tall; if either is short, the whole expression is false. More important, Boole proposed that propositions and complex expressions could be represented simply as binary truth values, a suggestion that would have great significance (as we shall see).

Following this syntactic approach to thinking, Gottlob Frege combined Boole's logic of truth functions with Aristotle's categorical logic. Under Frege's system, units smaller than propositions could be represented and combined in the same way as whole propositions in Boole's system. This move vastly increased the number and types of expressions and arguments that could be represented and evaluated. The system was formalized, axiomatized, and given a proof system by philosophers Bertrand Russell and Alfred North Whitehead. They called their compendium of human reasoning the "Principia Mathematica."

Physiological systems of thought

Whereas philosophers and mathematicians proposed logical systems of thought based on abstract propositions, scientists in other fields were concerned with deriving systems based on sensation and neural impulses. As intuitively obvious as this seems, there was some question at the time whether mental events such as thinking could be measured at all. Undaunted by such doubts, physiologist Ernst Weber and physicist Gustav Fechner began to study the relationship between external stimulation (e.g., light, sound) and internal sensations (brightness, loudness). They discovered that there existed lawlike relationships between changes in external stimulation and internal sensation. They then derived laws that captured these relationships and expressed them quantitatively.

Other scientists were interested in measuring the time it took to respond to stimuli and to carry out mental operations. Hermann von Helmholtz, a physicist and physiologist, measured the speed of neural transmission by requiring subjects to push a button whenever a stimulus was applied to their legs. E. C. Donders expanded this methodology to measure the time required to discriminate among stimuli (Gardner, 1985, p. 101). He did this by subtracting the time it took subjects to respond to a single event from the time it took them to respond to that same stimulus in the context of another, similar stimulus. The difference in time was attributed to the time required to perform the mental operation of discrimination. Together, this work on response latencies and sensation demonstrated that mental events could be scientifically studied. Thought was becoming a viable object of scientific investigation.

Structuralism and thought

While the nature of cognition was being studied in a variety of disciplines, scientists began to feel the need for a discipline devoted exclusively to its investigation. With this goal in mind, Wilhelm Wundt established the first laboratory of *experimental psychology* in Leipzig in 1879. A similar laboratory was later established in the United States at Cornell University by E. B. Titchener, an American who had studied in Wundt's laboratory.

The primary objective of this new discipline, as envisioned by Wundt and Titchener, was the scientific study of the *structure* of mind and its processes. In keeping with this objective, the *structuralists* (as they came to be known) were eager to explain consciousness in physical terms, employing the same types of explanatory models used in the natural sciences. The model they chose to guide their research was that of physical chemistry. Just as chemists had identified the fundamental elements of matter, the structuralists hoped to identify the fundamental elements of thought and the laws governing their combination. The idea was that by combining these simple elements in law-governed ways, the more complex forms of thought typically experienced by humans could be derived.

The structuralists were heavily influenced by British empiricists (e.g., Locke, Hume, and Berkeley) in defining their search for the elements of cognition. Like the empiricists, they believed that sensations were the foundation of all knowledge about the world and all mental activity. They rejected Cartesian mind–body dualism, adhering strictly to the doctrine that thinking is fundamentally a physical process, not a metaphysical phenomenon. As a result, most of their research focused on the identification of the physical sensations that underlie or accompany our everyday experiences. As Titchener (1910) put it:

When I am thinking about anything, my consciousness consists of a number of ideas. . . . But every idea can be resolved into elements . . . and these elements are sensations. (p. 33)

For Titchener, all mental events could be categorized as one of three types: images, affections (emotional responses), or pure sensations. Images and affections were themselves complex units that could be broken down into clusters of sensations. For example:

Thus the "taste" of lemonade is made up of a sweet taste, an acid taste, a scent (the fragrance of lemon), a sensation of temperature, and a pricking (cutaneous) sensation. (Titchener, 1910, p. 62)

Notice that a complex experience (the taste of lemonade) is decomposed into a conglomeration of several more elementary sensations. More complex reasoning processes were described in the same way. Chess playing, for example, was described in purely sensual terms:

The mental complexes involved in the game [of blindfold chess] consist of visual images, kinaesthetic images, and sensations . . . visual images predominate. From them arise the vertical board, and the pictures of past games. The kinaesthetic sensations and images . . . are centered in the heavy muscles and tendons of the shoulders. (Dallenbach, 1917, pp. 227–8)

For Titchener and his colleagues, then, thoughts were images – there was no such thing as "imageless thought." And since images were constructed from elementary sensations, all complex reasoning and thought processes could be broken down eventually into elementary sensations.

The method used to obtain reports like these was called *introspection,* a technique that required an observer to describe his or her own internal sensations while performing some task or attending to some stimulus. This was not as easy as it sounds, since the observer was required to describe his or her experiences in terms of elementary sensations. Novices often committed what Titchener termed the "stimulus error"; that is, they reported, for example, "seeing a book" rather than "experiencing the sensations of a certain color, intensity," and other qualities. To ensure the veridicality of introspective reports, therefore, observers were required to be well-trained in the discipline. Wundt required his observers to have no less than 10,000 supervised practice trials before they could participate in any experiment (Boring, 1953), leading William James to comment that Wundt's program "could hardly have arisen in a country whose natives could be bored" (James, 1890, p. 193). Using this methodology, the structuralists reported identifying more than 44,000 elementary sensations, sensations that, according to them, were the "atoms" of thought. They did not fare as well in detailing laws for combining these "atoms," relying exclusively on the principle of simple association: "Atoms" became associated, or linked together, not through any similarity of structure or content, but rather through the accident of temporal co-occurrence.

What brought about the downfall of the structuralist school was the use of introspection as an analytic technique. The procedure was doomed from the start, because it was based on the assumption that one could discern the elements in compounds just by reflecting on them. This is rather like attempting to discern the elements of water by looking at a drop of water. The perceived qualities of water are not anything like the (indirectly) perceived qualities of its components (i.e., hydrogen and oxygen). However, a more pragmatic difficulty presented itself: Despite the careful training that observers received, agreement among introspective reports was the exception rather than the rule. It was not unusual to obtain markedly different reports from two observers who were exposed to the same stimulus. Such disagreements could not be settled in any scientific fashion owing to the inherently private nature of internal events. In more technical terms, introspection failed as a bona fide scientific method because it violated a fundamental rule concerning scientific investigation: that of independent access to both causes and effects. Although the cause (i.e., stimulus) was open to public observation, the effect (i.e., internal sensation) was not. Without such independent observation of the internal sensation, it was impossible to tell which of two conflicting introspective reports was the correct one. The conflicting reports could have arisen because (a) Subject A was truly experiencing a different sensation than Subject B, or (b) Subject A was experiencing the same sensation as Subject B but was misreporting it, or (c) Subject A was simply lying (Cummins, 1983, p. 123). There was no scientific way to determine which of these three conditions was true.

While structuralism was beginning to topple under the weight of these rather fundamental difficulties, three other events occurred that hurried its journey downward. The first was Hermann Ebbinghaus's work on the mechanisms underlying learning and memory. Ebbinghaus (1913) proposed that learning consisted of simple associations among stimuli. He chose memorization of lists of nonsense syllables as a paradigm of simple learning, reasoning that the principles that govern the learning of novel, simple stimuli are the same ones that govern the learning of more complex stimuli, such as meaningful text. Using this methodology, Ebbinghaus carefully documented the quantitative relations between such variables as list length and study time, and repetitions and retention. His approach to questions about mental phenomena therefore differed dramatically from that of the structuralists, emphasizing the discovery of quantitative laws governing the forming of associations among stimuli rather than the discovery of the structure of the stimuli themselves.

The second and more dramatic event that changed the nature of psychology at this time was Pavlov's discovery of *stimulus substitution*: that pairing an arbitrary stimulus with a stimulus that naturally elicits some response will empower the arbitrary stimulus to elicit the same response.[2] This was a startling discovery, because it suggested that "reflexes" could be learned. More important for our discussion, however, it suggested that learning could be described without reference to associations among ideas, thoughts, or other mental constructs. Instead, learning could be described solely in terms of associations among stimuli and responses. Here was an answer to the independent access problem, since this methodology made it possible to observe publicly both cause and effect.

The third event that brought about structuralism's demise was the rise of pragmatism in academics and social policy (Cummins, 1983). Pragmatists stressed the relation between mental events and action. John Dewey, a leading pragmatist at the time, argued that thought could not be understood independently of its role as the antecedent to action. From this perspective, the structuralists appeared to be overemphasizing internal responses to stimuli (which could not be observed anyway) and ignoring action or external responses (which could). There was a revolution in the making, and a student of Dewey's, John B. Watson, brought it about.

Behaviorism and thought

Believing that the structuralists had swung the pendulum of psychological investigation too far in the direction of mental states and unobserved responses, J. B. Watson and his school of *behaviorism* gave it a vigorous shove in the other direction. It was a shove that would determine the nature of psychological investigation for the next 40 years, and it was based on the denial of the legitimacy of mental concepts, such as thinking.

The behaviorists overthrew the structuralist program by asserting that observable behavior was the true object of psychological study. They strove to eradicate such terms as *thought, belief,* and other intentional idioms from the whole of psychological theorizing, arguing that such mentalistic terms represented nothing more than fictitious constructs that clouded rather than clarified our understanding of human behavior. No reference to internal states was allowed, neither as effects of stimulation nor as causes of external behavior. Some behaviorists, such as Watson, went so far as to deny the existence of consciousness; others considered mental phenomena, such as thinking, to be epiphenomena, that is, side effects of external stimulation that could not themselves cause or explain behavior.

Behaviorists believed environmental influences to be the sole determinants of behavior and overt behavior to be the only legitimate object of scientific study. Within the behaviorist school, psychological investigation was devoted exclusively to the discovery of laws and principles governing the prediction and control of observable behavior. These laws and principles took the form of generalizations of observed relationships between environmental stimulation and organismic responses. An example of such a law is stimulus generalization. An organism exhibits stimulus generalization when it spontaneously responds to a stimulus in the same way it learned to respond to another stimulus without any pairing of the two stimuli.[3]

The phenomenon that most interested the behaviorists was that of learning, that is, how an organism's behavioral repertoire changed as a result of experience. They postulated two primary mechanisms for enacting these changes. The first was the simple associative learning discovered by Pavlov. This type of learning consisted of associating new stimuli with old responses through stimulus substitution. Moreover, the responses were primarily reflexive or visceral in nature, such as salivation in response to food, eye-blinking in response to sudden puffs of air, or emotional reactions to emotion-arousing stimuli. This type of learning is termed *respondent conditioning*.

The second mechanism of environmental shaping of behavior was reinforcement. The principle behind this mechanism is that, whenever a response terminates a noxious stimulus (negative reinforcement) or is followed by a "reward" (positive reinforcement), its probability of occurrence is increased.[4] The principle of positive reinforcement was proposed by Thorndike (1913), who called it the "Law of Effect." The notion of reinforcement in general was perfected by Skinner and his associates, who formulated various types and schedules of reinforcement and described their effects on behavior (Ferster & Skinner, 1957). Together, reinforcement and stimulus substitution constituted powerful mechanisms for shaping behavior.

If thinking was considered at all by the behaviorists, it was conceived as "laryngeal habits," that is, subvocal speech (Chaplin & Krawiec, 1974, p. 376). Such habits developed in early childhood out of spontaneous vocalizations. Through conditioning, these vocalizations become words; for example, *Da-da* becomes *Daddy* through reinforcement (response shaping). Social pressures inhibit spontaneous vocalizations, and they become subvocal. Now when seeing Daddy, the child can think *Daddy*. Thinking according to the behaviorists was quite simply talking to oneself.

Gestalt psychology and thought

Although behaviorism dominated most psychological circles following the demise of structuralism, it was by no means the only school bent on explaining psychological phenomena. In fact, just as behaviorism arose as a reaction against structuralism, a new school, called *Gestalt psychology,* grew out of a reaction against both structuralist and behaviorist doctrines. Unlike the behaviorists, however, the Gestaltists did not succeed in overthrowing their contemporaries' hold on psychological investigation. This lack of success was due largely to two factors. First, Gestalt psychology produced no cohesive, testable theory of behavior or cognition, nor was its work guided by any vision of what such a theory should be. Gestalt psychology tended instead to define itself in terms of objections to behaviorist and structuralist doctrines. As a result, the body of work the Gestaltists produced, though important and impressive, consists primarily of descriptions of phenomena that could not be explained through reductionist methods such as introspective analysis or by the simple associative principles of stimulus substitution and reinforcement. These phenomena were not taken as data upon which to build a model or theory of human psychology, but were presented simply as evidence of the inadequacy of the behaviorist and structuralist models. In contrast, both the behaviorists and the structuralists possessed very clear ideas of what a science of psychology should be and modeled their work after the physical sciences (i.e., physical chemistry and something akin to simple mechanics, respectively). When the behaviorists overthrew structuralism, they replaced one cohesive research program with another.

The second reason the Gestaltists did not succeed in overthrowing behaviorism is related to their failure to construct a comprehensive theory. They simply did not possess the tools and techniques for building models of the level of complexity they required. Unlike the behaviorists, who focused primarily on the prediction and control of simple response sequences, the Gestaltists attempted to explain complex behaviors, such as thinking, problem solving, and perception. The tools and techniques required to investigate these areas properly would be developed only much later, in the fields of cybernetics, information theory, and computer science. In a sense, the Gestalt school foreshadowed the cognitive revolution (see the next section), carving out the domains that would be explored later.

At the heart of the Gestaltists' investigations was the belief that higher-order psychological phenomena could not be *decomposed* into simple mental elements (structuralism) or simple stimulus–response chains (behaviorism). They argued that an adequate explanation of intelligent behavior required reference to internal states and highly integrated cognitive structures. Evidence for this belief came primarily from their work in the areas of perception, problem solving, and thinking.

Appreciating their arguments on the nature of perception requires a cognitive shift, which the following "thought experiment" might help us to achieve. Consider the difference between the way a human perceives the world and, for example, the way a frog does (to choose an organism sufficiently far down the phylogenetic scale). A frog's visual system (eyes and brain) responds only to very rudimentary stimulation, such as shadows and moving specks. In essence, this is all a frog can "see." The human visual system, of course, is capable of responding to a multitude of stimuli, including color, shape, and depth. The world we perceive bears very little resemblance to the world perceived by a frog because of the immense differences in the capacities of our visual systems. To put it another way, the nature of our internal states and architecture shapes our perceptual experience.

The Gestaltists presented even stronger evidence that our perceptual capacities shape our knowledge about the world. They showed that our visual system is capable of *augmenting and organizing* stimulation in reliable ways. A classic example is that of the phi phenomenon, an illusion produced by the sort of light display one sees around a movie marquee. If light bulbs are lined up in a row, and each one in succession is quickly turned on and off, one sees an illusion of movement down the line of bulbs. In fact, nothing in the physical environment is moving, but the pattern of light stimulation is "interpreted" by our visual system as movement. More important, the Gestaltists pointed out that the qualitative aspect of this illusion could not be decomposed or reduced to its components. The illusion was problematic for structuralists because it persists no matter how one tries to introspect the individual pieces separately. It was also problematic for behaviorists because they could not even talk about the illusion except in terms of differential responses. The question from this point of view is why the organism responds to the light display *as if it were movement*. Since this perception is spontaneous, there is no conditioning history to explain how successive light displays could become a substitution for genuine movement. Another example is that of melody transposition. If a melody is transposed into another key, it is still recognized as the same melody even though all of its elements are different.

Psychological phenomena such as these seemed to indicate that "the whole is greater than the sum of its parts," that is, that the wholeness of a perception cannot be found by analyzing any of its parts. The wholeness instead was probably a function of the internal organization of our perceptual−cognitive systems. The Gestaltists therefore believed perception to be an active, constructive process, not a passive, "reflexive" one (as envisioned by behaviorists). Essentially, this means that a type of organization is imposed on incoming stimulation by our internal states. (Bartlett, 1932, proposed the same thing about memory processes; that they were constructive.)

The Gestaltists believed thinking, like the process of perception, to be an active, constructive process. In fact, more than their predecessors or contemporaries, the Gestaltists concerned themselves with the nature of thinking and reasoning. Wertheimer (1945/1982) proposed a distinction between productive and reproductive thinking. Productive thinking involves a grasp of the structural relations in a problem or situation, followed by a grouping of those parts into a dynamic whole. Reproductive thinking is characterized by a failure to see relations among subparts. It instead involves blind repetition of learned responses to individual subparts. This type of thinking lacks insight, a phenomenon that Köhler (1925) characterized as a closure of the thinker's psychological field, where all elements come together into a whole structure.

Perhaps the most pragmatic and systematic approach to thinking among the Gestaltists was taken by Duncker (1945) in his work on problem solving:

A problem arises when a living creature has a goal but does not know how this goal is to be reached. Whenever one cannot go from the given situation to the desired situation simply by action, then there has to be recourse to thinking. (By action we here understand the performance of obvious operations.) Such thinking has the task of devising some action which may mediate between the existing and the desired situations. (p. 1)

Duncker studied human problem-solving behavior by requiring subjects to "think aloud" as they attempted to solve a problem. He used these "think-aloud" protocols to trace the reasoning processes, or cognitive states, that subjects generated on their way toward a solution. These verbal protocols differed from the structuralists' introspection reports in two important ways. First, they relied on the subject's existing skills rather than on any special training that could influence or bias the subject's reports. Second, the focus of the protocols was the task itself, not the observer. Subjects simply verbalized their plans and strategies, not the qualities of their sensations.

What these protocols revealed was that problem solving was better characterized as a top-down, goal-oriented process than as a bottom-up, stimulus-driven process of trial and error. Subjects typically recoded high-level goals into subgoals and searched for means to satisfy them. The steps generated by the subject while solving a problem, therefore, typically were not random or "blind," but highly purposive. In addition, there was a reliable relationship between the way subjects represented the problems to themselves (as evidenced by their protocols) and the accuracy of their solutions.

On the basis of these data, Duncker concluded that problem-solving behavior could be formalized as a search for means to resolve conflicts between current situations and desired goal situations. The process itself required an analysis of the differences, or conflicts, between the goal and current situations and an analysis of the means to reduce those differences. The outcome of this process was a collection of highly integrated internal representations that detailed the conflicting parts and subparts of the problem situation. Understanding and "insight" were characterized as internal states achieved by the problem solver, states that depended on the quality of the representation constructed by the subject (as evidenced in the concomitant verbal protocol).

This characterization of problem-solving behavior, with its reliance on internal representations and cognitive states, contrasted sharply with that of behaviorists. Since behaviorist doctrine would suffer no reference to internal states and processes (believing these to be "explanatory fictions"), its characterization of problem-solving behavior relied solely on trial-and-error learning. According to this view, responses were randomly emitted, or cued, by some aspect of the stimulus situation, and correct responses were reinforced through success. This model was simply not powerful enough to account for the observed data, particularly the goal-oriented purposiveness, or forward planning, of the problem solver. However, its attractiveness to the behaviorist is understandable because the goal of that school was the *prediction* and control of behavior. Conditioning histories, when they are observed, allow one to predict *which* response/strategy a subject will choose when solving a problem; that is, he or she is likely to choose one that met with success (reinforcement) in the past. However, the Gestaltists were not so much interested in the prediction as in the explanation of the phenomenon. At their level of analysis, it was much less important to predict which strategy a subject would choose than it was to derive an accurate characterization of the process itself. Verbal and written protocols clearly showed that, when solving a problem, subjects formed *plans*, generated *goals*, and developed *strategies* based on acquired *knowledge*. Removing these concepts from one's description of problem-solving behavior was tantamount to not describing the phenomenon at all.

However, such terms as *plans, goals, strategies,* and *thoughts* were troublesome to describe in any rigorous, non-question-begging manner. As a result, an uneasy tension arose in psychology between the behaviorists, who could see no way to characterize scientifically the existence of internal states, and the Gestaltists, who saw clearly the necessity of postulating them in order to explain cognition.

The cognitive revolution

What finally loosened behaviorism's grip on psychological investigation was a revolution that restored talk of internal states and processes to psychology, but in a scientifically rigorous manner. The discoveries that would form the bases of the revolution were made in a variety of disciplines during the 1940s and 1950s. It was not until the mid-1960s, however, that they came together (in rather scattershot fashion) to form a new psychology, one that Ulric Neisser dubbed *cognitive psychology*. The nature of these discoveries changed the way researchers in numerous other fields conceptualized the human mind. As a result, cognitive psychology became part of a larger discipline called *cognitive science*, which now includes researchers from such fields as philosophy, linguistics, psycholinguistics, computer science, and neuroscience. The common goal of these researchers is the explanation of higher mental processes.

One of the major foundations of cognitive science was mathematician Allen Turing's (1936, 1963) work on finite-state automata. Turing proposed a theoretical "machine" (mathematical abstraction) that could in principle carry out any recursive function. The "Turing machine," as it came to be called, is a very simple system. It consists of (a) a tape containing symbols, usually blanks and slashes; (b) a scanner to read the tape; and (c) four operations: move right, move left, write a slash, and erase a slash. What the scanner does at any given moment is fully determined by two factors: the symbol it reads on the tape (input) and its current internal state. This simple architecture comprises a machine of enormous computational power. It formed the theoretical basis on which the modern digital computer is built. And it was not long before researchers began wondering whether it represented a way to test Boole's (1854/1951) and Hobbes's (1656/1839) contention that thinking is *computation*.

One of the first researchers to test this idea was mathematician Claude Shannon (1948). Shannon's work was based on two major insights. The first was that information could be represented as binary choices among alternatives. The amount of information transmitted through a channel (e.g., a telephone wire) could be measured in bits, or binary digits, where one bit represents a choice between two equally probable alternatives. This perspective made it possible to quantify the concept of information. It also provided a means of representing information that was independent of its particular content or the nature of the device that carried it.

To appreciate the usefulness of this conceptualization of information, consider Shannon's second major insight: that electronic circuits could carry out Boole's operations of thought. Recall that, in Boole's system, propositions can be represented as binary truth values (true−false). Electromechanical relays also allow only two states: A circuit is either closed or open, on or off. Shannon demonstrated that, because of the binary nature of the two systems, electronic circuits could be used to simulate the logical operations of the propositional calculus. He had designed a machine that carried out the functions of thought in electronic circuitry.

This was a rather startling insight, for three reasons. First, it suggested that thinking (at least as proposed by Boole) could be automated. Machines could carry out reasoning processes. Second, it offered for the first time a means of describing the states and processes of mechanical systems in *information-processing* terms, that is, in terms of *what* information is represented and *how* it is processed. Third, it could be applied to the brain as well. In 1948, Warren McColloch and Walter Pitts proposed that, since neurons also operate as binary units (either they fire or they do not), they could be thought of as logical units carrying information.[5] They further demonstrated how communication among networks of neurons could simulate the logical operations of the propositional calculus, just as electromechanical circuitry can. Essentially, McColloch and Pitts had succeeded in "treating the brain as a Turing machine" (McColloch, as cited in Jeffress 1951, p. 32).

An implication of this neuronal model was that patterns of neuronal firing could be seen as statements about the world. This was a far cry from contemporary views of the human central nervous system, which was depicted as a predominantly quiescent, largely passive system that became active only in response to external stimulation − a view, incidentally, that fit well with behaviorist stimulus−response theories of organismic behavior. This view, however, was beginning to be questioned. Neurophysiologist Karl Lashley (1951), for example, pointed out that stimulus−response chains, even at the neuronal level, did not account for serially ordered behavior. He pointed out that the finger strokes of a pianist may reach 16 per second during complex passages. Sensory control of such rapid movements was impossible because there simply was not enough time for feedback from one finger movement to reach the brain in order to trigger the next movement. In fact, this speed exceeded visual recognition time. Complex piano skills, therefore, could not be made up of simple stimulus–response units. Lashley went on to argue that complex serial movements were products not of simple reflex arcs, but of an interaction among complex patterns of organization within the central nervous system. He proposed that complex movements were represented and activated as cohesive units. Control of such movements was therefore central rather than peripheral.

On the basis of observations and interpretations such as these, Lashley (1951) proposed a view of the central nervous system that closely resembles the characterization accepted today. He believed it to be "a dynamic, constantly active system, or rather, a composite of many interacting systems" (p. 135). This characterization was a far cry from the simple switching network conceptualization upon which behaviorist theory was built but entirely in line with the active, constructive processor proposed by the Gestaltists.

While neurophysiologists grappled with issues of feedback within the central nervous system, mathematician Norbert Wiener pursued similar questions concerning the use of feedback in mechanical systems. Wiener and his colleagues were concerned with servomechanisms, devices that kept airplanes and missiles on course. In order to perform this function, these devices had to correct themselves given feedback from the environment. Wiener argued that it was legitimate to describe the behavior of these machines as purposive, goal-directed activity (Rosenblueth, Wiener, & Bigelow, 1943). Wiener's servomechanisms worked by computing the difference between their goals and current states and employing operations to reduce those differences. This description of goal-directed, mechanized behavior is strikingly similar to Karl Duncker's description of problem-solving behavior in human subjects. Wiener's work clearly demonstrated that such terms as *plans* and *goals* could be precisely specified and instantiated in mechanical systems, contrary to behaviorist warnings.

Work in cybernetics, information theory, and automata theory had spawned a variety of rich concepts for researchers interested in explaining human cognitive capacities, and it was not long before the effects of these new resources were seen.[6] In the late 1950s and early 1960s, several models of cognition were put forth that capitalized on these concepts. In 1956, George Miller pointed out that peformance on a variety of cognitive tasks declined dramatically when they required maintaining more than seven items in memory at a time. This invariance in performance suggested that humans contained a processor with limits and that these limits shaped the nature of mental processes. For example, Bruner, Goodnow, and Austin (1956) observed that, when learning to classify objects, humans tend to employ *strategies* that, among other things, minimize storage requirements. A common strategy they observed was *successive scanning*: choosing a single hypothesis about a category description and choosing only those instances that directly test that hypothesis. Thus, the way we go about acquiring knowledge and thinking about the world is strongly influenced by the limitations of our "cognitive architecture."

Once it was demonstrated that rigorous answers could be obtained, more and more psychologists began to ask questions about our cognitive architecture. In 1958, Donald Broadbent proposed a model of the mind that consisted of a flow chart containing structures as well as processes. After Shannon, Broadbent conceived of the various sense organs as "channels" of information. These channels fed into a short-term memory, then through a filter, and finally into a limited-capacity channel. From there the information was stored in long-term memory and/or outputted as an external response. In retrospect, Broadbent's model was a curious blend of the past and the present. His limited-capacity channel was analogous to the structuralist's "unitary attention," or consciousness (p. 300); the probability of a stimulus getting through the processing filter was determined by behaviorist reinforcement (p. 301). Yet it was a fresh look at human cognition because it was one of the first models that described the flow of information *through* the organism.

In 1960, Miller, Galanter, and Pribram published a book in which they called for a cybernetic approach to behavior. The idea was that humans should be viewed as active *information processers*, not as passive recipients that respond "reflexively" to the pushes and pulls of the environment. (This shift was similar to the one proposed by Lashley about the central nervous system.) Miller et al. described cognitive architecture as a hierarchical organization of test−operate−test−exit (TOTE) units. A TOTE unit operated on some input, testing the outcome at each step, until some goal was met; then it stopped, or exited. Implicit in this idea was the notion of feedback, not as simple reinforcement, but as information to be used by the system to achieve some goal, as in Wiener's servomechanisms.

By the late 1960s, investigation into the nature of human cognition had become more the rule than the exception in psychology. Like the Gestaltists, researchers were interested in detailing *how* stimuli were "turned into" responses by the organism. Phenomena such as stimulus generalization were taken as capacities to be explained, not as explanations themselves. As Neisser (1967) put it:

The basic reason for studying cognitive processes has become as clear as the reason for studying anything else: because they are there. Our knowledge of the world must be somehow developed from stimulus input. . . . Cognitive processes surely exist, so it can hardly be unscientific to study them. (p. 5)

The influence of theories of computation on psychological theorizing was also apparent:

The task of a psychologist in trying to understand human cognition is analogous to that of a man trying to discover how a computer has been programmed. In particular, if the program seems to store and re-use information, he would like to know by what "routines" or "procedures" this is done. Given this purpose, he will not care much whether his particular computer stores information in magnetic cores or in thin films; he wants to understand the program, not the "hardware". By the same token, it would not help the psychologist to know that memory is carried by RNA as opposed to some other medium. He wants to understand its utilization, not its incarnation. (Neisser, 1967, p. 6)

While psychologists such as Broadbent and Neisser viewed the digital computer as a useful metaphor for conceptualizing issues about cognition, other researchers began to build actual computer models of cognition. One of the first was a program called Logic Theorist (Newell, Shaw, & Simon, 1958). Logic Theorist proved theorems from the Principia Mathematica. Moreover, it did so in ways that were similar to those employed by humans. Building on Logic Theorist's general architecture, Newell and Simon (1972) produced another program, General Problem Solver (GPS). GPS was constructed as a model, or theory, of human problem solving, and its performance paralleled quantitative and qualitative aspects of the performance of human novices. It is of some importance, then, to note that GPS analyzes and solves problems in the way described by Karl Duncker. GPS analyzes a problem into a list of differences, or conflicts, between a current state description and a goal state description. A table of connections is used to resolve these differences, working backward from the goal. The table of connections is essentially a production system (body of rules) containing descriptions of possible differences between states and actions that will reduce those differences. This procedure for solving problems is called *means–ends analysis*, and it is a procedure often employed by human novices. Duncker's model of problem-solving behavior had been scientifically instantiated and tested.

Subsequent work on computer modeling has fallen into two general categories. The first contains programs that, like GPS, are intended to be viable models of human cognition. These models contain aspects of human processing, such as a limited-capacity working memory, and are based on and tested using data on human subjects. (Included in this category is John Anderson's (1983) ACT* system, a system that includes operations for producing the behaviorist processes of discrimination, generalization, and strengthening, or reinforcement.) The second category contains programs called *expert systems*, programs that generate expert levels of performance in circumscribed domains. The focus of these programs is to perform a task as efficiently and error free as possible. No human-like constraints are placed on their execution. Nonetheless, these systems carry out the processes of thought when performing their assigned tasks.

It would be misleading to give the impression that all current work on thinking is done by computer simulation. In fact, many investigators complain that computer models suffer from a certain rigidity that is uncharacteristic of human performance. Some argue that the face of psychological

investigation is being shaped too closely to fit the limitations and characteristics of digital computers:

Unlike men, "artificially intelligent" programs tend to be single-minded, undistract-
able, and unemotional. . . . in my opinion, none of [these programs] does even
remote justice to the complexity of human mental processes. (Neisser, 1967, p. 9)

Ironically, Gestalt psychologists are among the strongest critics. They hold
that the most important aspects of human reasoning have not been explained or even exhibited by computer simulation models:

Missing in such work is the crucial step of *understanding*, that is, grasping both what
is crucial in any given problem and why it is crucial. (Wertheimer, 1985)

Nonetheless, the influence of theories of computation can be found in the
majority of psychological investigation. Computational concepts, such as
memory buffers, encoding, search, and retrieval, are standard components
of modern theories of cognition. The fundamental idea underlying most psychological theories today is that the human brain *processes* information in
order to produce our percepts, memories, and other experiences. This idea
has spawned such diverse psychological theories as Marr's (1982) computational theory of perception, Kintsch and van Dijk's (1978) process model of
text comprehension, and Raaijmakers and Shiffrin's (1981) computational
model of associative memory search. From the perspective of these theories,
a percept or memory is the *outcome* of a (computational) process.

Many of the chapters in this book describe work on various aspects of
cognition that are not embodied in computer models. However, the influence of the computer revolution on the cognitive revolution will still be
found in these approaches. Theories and models that contain references to
internal states, processes and structures are the intellectual progeny of theories of computation.

Notes

1 Although the information reported here was gathered from a variety of sources, my choice of
historical perspective was influenced by Gardner's (1985) *The Mind's New Science,*
Cummins's (1983) *The Nature of Psychological Explanation,* and Haugeland's (1985) *Artificial
Intelligence: The Very Idea.* These three volumes are recommended to the reader who wishes
more information.

2 For example, dogs normally salivate when food is placed in their mouths; if a bell is paired
with food placement several times in a row, the dogs will come to salivate in response to the
bell alone.

3 In our earlier example, dogs came to salivate in response to a bell if the bell were paired with
food. If the dogs then spontaneously salivated in response to a musical tone (without any
pairing of stimuli), this would be an instance of stimulus generalization. The same response
generalized to the new stimulus.

4 An example of negative reinforcement is stopping a television from flickering by turning a
knob. One's "knob-turning behavior" has been reinforced by the cessation of the flicker. An
example of positive reinforcement is arriving at home by following a certain route. One's
"route-following behavior" has been reinforced by arriving home.

5 This should not to be taken to mean that the brain is necessarily a digital machine. Although neurons fire in an all-or-none manner, neural coding occurs through continuous changes in the *rate* of firing. Moreover, there is good evidence that the brain operates in a massively parallel fashion, with numerous interactions among its neurons. The point of this early neuronal model was to show how thinking could be automated in a process that was simple enough for neuronal networks in principle to execute.

6 In fact, automata theory did more than this. It revealed the inadequacy of the behaviorist model or explaining behavior. Briefly, it showed that predictions of a system's behavior – behaviorism's goal – were not possible without information concerning its internal states. A rather crude approximation of this proof follows. The interested reader should consult Nelson (1969, 1975) for a more complete exposition of the following proof:

A system's response is a function of its input and its internal state,

$$r_i = f(s_i, \sigma_i)$$

The internal state is in turn a function of past inputs and past internal states,

$$\sigma_i = g(s_{i-1}, \sigma_{i-1})$$

Since we are trying to compute *r*, we need information about at least one internal state somewhere along the way (or some way to reduce it to zero), or else we will continue to have one more unknown than we have equations, making *r* uncomputable.

References

Anderson, J. A. (1983). *The architecture of cognition.* Cambridge, MA: Harvard University Press.

Bartlett, F. C. (1932). *Remembering: An experimental and social study.* Cambridge University Press.

Boole, G. (1951). *An investigation of the laws of thought.* New York: Dover. (Original work published 1854.)

Boring, E. G. (1953). A history of introspection. *Psychological Bulletin, 50,* 169–89.

Broadbent, D. E. (1958). *Perception and communication.* Elmsford, NY: Pergamon.

Bruner, J. S., Goodnow, J., & Austin, G. (1956). *A study of thinking.* New York: Wiley.

Chaplin, J. P., & Krawiec, T. S. (1974). *Systems and theories of psychology.* New York: Holt, Rhinehart & Winston.

Cummins, R. C. (1983). *The nature of psychological explanation.* Cambridge, MA: Bradford/ MIT Press.

Dallenbach, K. M. (1917). Blindfold chess: The single game. In *Studies in psychology: Titchener commemorative volume* (pp. 214–30). Worcester, MA: Wilson.

Descartes, R. (1951) *Meditation on first philosophy.* New York: Library on Liberal Arts, Liberal Arts Press. (Original work published 1641.)

Duncker K. (1945) On problem solving. *Psychological Monographs, 58,* 1–110.

Ebbinghaus, H. (1913). *Memory: A contribution to experimental psychology.* New York: Teachers College.

Ferster, C. S., & Skinner, B. F. (1957). *Schedules of reinforcement.* New York: Appleton-Century-Crofts.

Gardner, H. (1985). *The mind's new science: A history of cognitive revolution.* New York: Basic.

Haugeland, J. (1985). *Artificial intelligence: The very idea.* Cambridge, MA: Bradford/MIT Press.

Hobbes, T. (1839). *Elements of philosophy* (Vol. 1). London: Molesworth. (Original work published 1656.)

James, W. (1890). *Principles of psychology.* New York: Holt.

Jeffress, L. A. (Ed.) (1951). *Cerebral mechanisms in behavior: The Hixon Symposium.* New York: Wiley.

Kintsch, W., & van Dijk, W. (1978). Toward a model of text comprehension and production. *Psychological Review, 85,* 363–94.

Köhler, W. (1925). *The mentality of apes.* New York: Harcourt, Brace.

Lashley, K. (1951). The problem of serial order in behavior. In L. A. Jeffress (Ed.), *Cerebral mechanisms in behavior: The Hixon Symposium* (pp. 112–35). New York: Wiley.

Marr, D. (1982). *Vision: A computational investigation into the human representation and processing of visual information.* New York: Freeman.

McColloch, W., & Pitts, W. (1948). The statistical organization of nervous activity. *Journal of the American Statistical Association, 4,* 91–9.

Miller, G. A. (1956). The magical number seven, plus or minus two: Some limits on our capacity for processing information. *Psychological Review, 63,* 81–97.

Miller, G. A., Galanter, E., & Pribram, K. (1960). *Plans and the structure of behavior.* New York: Holt, Rinehart & Winston.

Neisser, U. (1967). *Cognitive psychology.* Englewood Cliffs, NJ: Prentice-Hall.

Nelson, R. J. (1969). Behaviorism is false. *Journal of Philosophy, 66,* 417–52.

(1975). Behaviorism, finite automata, and stimulus response theory. *Theory and Decision 6,* 249–67.

Newell, A., Shaw, J. C, & Simon, H. A. (1958). Elements of a theory of human problem solving. *Psychological Review, 65,* 151–66.

Newell, A., & Simon, H. A. (1972). *Human problem solving.* Englewood Cliffs, NJ: Prentice-Hall.

Raaijmakers, J. G. W., & Shiffrin, R. M. (1981). Search of associative memory. *Psychological Review, 88,* 93–134.

Rosenblueth, A., Wiener, N., & Bigelow, J. (1943). Behavior, purpose, and teleology. *Philosophy of Science, 10,* 18–24.

Shannon, C. E. (1948). A mathematical theory of communication. *Bell Systems Technical Journal, 27,* 379–423, 623–56.

Thorndike, E. L. (1913). *Educational psychology: The psychology of learning.* New York: Teachers College.

Titchener, E. B. (1910). *A textbook of psychology.* New York: Macmillan.

Turing, A. M. (1936). On computable numbers, with an application to the Entscheidungs problem. *Proceedings of the London Mathematical Society,* Ser. 2, *42,* 230–65.

(1963). Computing machinery and intelligence. In E. A. Feigenbaum & J. Feldman (Eds.), *Computers and Thought.* New York: McGraw-Hill.

Wertheimer, M. (1982). *Productive thinking.* Chicago University Press. (Original work published 1945.)

Wertheimer, M. (1985). A Gestalt perspective on computer simulations of cognitive processes. *Computers in Human Behavior, 1,* 19–33.

2 Concepts and thought

Edward E. Smith

Introduction

The notion of a *concept* is essential for understanding thought and behavior. If we want to understand, say, how a child learns through experience that stoves can burn, we assume that the child uses the concepts *stove* and *burn*; without this assumption, it is not clear why a child's experience with one particular stove and one particular burn will be related to his or her experience with another stove and another possible burn. It is only when we treat the objects and events of a situation as instances of concepts that we see what there is to learn. And just as it is hard to think about learning without concepts, it is hard to think about communication and reasoning without concepts. In short, concepts reflect the way that we divide the world into classes, and much of what we learn, communicate, and reason about involves relations among these classes.

Functions of a concept

The preceding paragraph suggests that concepts are worth knowing about because they serve important functions in mental life. This argument deserves to be spelled out in detail because it provides the basic rationale for the psychological study of concepts.

From a psychological perspective, concepts are mental representations of classes (e.g., one's beliefs about the class of dogs or tables), and their most salient function is to promote *cognitive economy* (Rosch, 1978). By partitioning the world into classes, we decrease the amount of information we must perceive, learn, remember, communicate, and reason about. Thus, if we had no concepts, we would have to refer to each individual entity by its own name; every different table, for example, would be denoted by a different word. The mental lexicon required would be so enormous that communication as we know it might be impossible. Other mental functions might

Preparation of this chapter was supported by U.S. Public Health Service Grant MH37208 and by the National Institute of Education under Contract US-HEW-C-400-82-0030.

19

collapse under the sheer number of entities we would have to keep track of.

Another important function of concepts is that they enable us to *go beyond the information given* (Bruner, Goodnow, & Austin, 1956). When we come across an object, say a wolf, we have direct knowledge only of its appearance. It is essential that we go beyond appearances and bring to bear other knowledge that we have, such as our belief that wolves can bite and inflict severe injury. Concepts are our means of linking perceptual and non-perceptual information. We use a perceptual description of the creature in front of us to access the concept *wolf* and then use our nonperceptual beliefs about wolves to direct our behavior, that is, run. Concepts, then, are recognition devices; they serve as entry points into our knowledge stores and provide us with expectations that we can use to guide our actions.

A third important function of concepts is that they can be *combined to form complex concepts and thoughts* (e.g., Osherson & Smith, 1981). *Stoves* and *burn* are two simple concepts; *Stoves can burn* is a full-fledged thought. Presumably our understanding of this thought, and of complex concepts in general, is based on our understanding of the constituent concepts.

Although concepts no doubt have other functions, cognitive economy, going beyond the information given, and conceptual combination seem the most important. Moreover, because these functions impose constraints on the structure of concepts (just as the functions of physical objects constrain their structure), we shall return to these functions throughout our discussion.

Agenda

Our discussion is organized as follows. First, we consider the *contents* of concepts. If concepts are representations of classes, exactly *what* is being represented? Are the contents restricted to properties that are true of all instances of a concept, or are the contents restricted in some other fashion—say, that the properties are perceptually salient and useful in recognizing concept instances. In the second section we discuss the *organization* of concepts, specifically organization by levels. We consider taxonomies of concepts (e.g., *poodle, dog,* and *animal*) and ask whether one level of the taxonomy provides a uniquely useful way of partitioning the world into classes. The third section focuses on the *combinational function* of concepts. We discuss, for example, how adjective and noun concepts can be combined into conjunctions, and how verb and noun concepts can be combined into units that correspond to thoughts. In the final section, we briefly discuss two remaining issues. One concerns the *format* of a concept: Must a concept always be an abstraction, or can it instead be a collection of exemplars? The other issue concerns whether the principles that apply to simple object concepts hold for other kinds of concepts. Throughout the chapter, our emphasis is on natural concepts and their use by adults.

Contents of concepts

To have a concept of *X* is to know something about the properties of *X's* instances. Hence, the knowledge contained in a concept describes properties. The nature of these properties is our concern in this section.

Definitions

The classical view. An old and influential idea is that the properties contained in a concept are *singly necessary* and *jointly sufficient* to define that concept. For a property to be singly necessary, every instance of the concept must have that property; for a set of properties to be jointly sufficient, every entity having that set must be an instance of the concept. We can illustrate this with the concept *bachelor*. For many of us, this concept has three critical properties: (a) male, (b) adult, and (c) unmarried. Each of these properties is necessary — one cannot literally be a bachelor if one is a woman, or if one is a young child, or if one is married. And these three properties are jointly sufficient — if one is male, adult, and unmarried, one must be a bachelor. Such properties are referred to as *defining*, for collectively they constitute a definition. The position that concepts consist of definitions is called the *classical view*; according to this view, an object will be categorized as an instance of a concept if and only if it contains the defining properties of the concept (Smith & Medin, 1981).

The classical view of concepts dominated the psychology of thought for many years. (Every major historical figure, including Freud, Piaget, and Skinner, seems to have endorsed it.) Since the early 1970s, however, the classical view has been seriously undermined by the collective work of linguists, philosophers, and psychologists. This work is discussed in detail by Schwartz (1979), Fodor, Garrett, Walker, and Parkes (1980), and Smith and Medin (1981). In what follows, we summarize a few of the major criticisms of the classical view, emphasizing those points that have led to the development of alternative views.

Failure to specify defining properties. The greatest shortcoming of the classical view is that decades of analysis by linguists, philosophers, and psychologists have failed to turn up definitions of most everyday concepts. Everyday concepts include "natural kinds," like animal and plant concepts, as well as common artifacts. *Bird, tiger, daisy, fruit, furniture, car, spoon,* and *jacket* are all everyday concepts, and in all of these cases (and endless more) there is no accepted, fixed definition. Consider *tiger*. For most people, its properties include "striped" and "carnivorous." If we came across a tiger, however, whose stripes had been painted over and whose digestive system had been altered surgically so that it could eat only vegetables, most likely we would still want to call it a tiger. Hence, "striped" and "carnivorous" cannot be defining properties. But if they cannot, what can? Arguments like this have led scholars to conclude that many natural concepts are not mentally represented as definitions.

Typicality effects. A number of experimental findings about the way in which people use concepts have also challenged the classical view. The starting point for these findings is that people can reliably order the instances of any concept in terms of the extent to which the instances are "typical" or "representative" of the concept. Table 2.1 presents some typicality ratings for the concepts *fruit* and *bird*. (The ratings were made on a 7-point scale, 7 corresponding to the highest typicality.) As can be seen, *apple* and *peach* are considered typical fruits, *raisin* and *fig* less typical, and *pumpkin* and *olive* atypical. There are similar variations among the instances of *bird*. Ratings like these have been obtained for numerous concepts and have been shown to be relatively uncorrelated with simple frequency or familiarity (Mervis, Catlin, & Rosch, 1976; Rosch, 1975).

What is most important about these ratings is that they predict performance on a wide variety of tasks. One such task is categorization. If people are asked to decide as quickly as possible if an item is an instance of a concept (e.g., "Is a fig a fruit?"), their responses are faster for more typical instances than for less typical instances. When *fruit* is the target concept, for example, *apple* and *peach* are categorized more quickly than *raisin* and *fig*, which in turn are categorized more rapidly than *pumpkin* and *olive* (e.g., Smith, Shoben, & Rips, 1974). If people are asked to generate from memory all instances of a concept, they retrieve typical instances before atypical ones (e.g., Rosch, 1978). And children learning to name concept members master the typical instances before the atypical ones (e.g., Rosch, 1978). In addition to its effects on categorization, memory, and naming, typicality influences a number of other psychological processes, including deductive and inductive reasoning (e.g., Cherniak, 1984; Rips, 1975; Tversky & Kahneman, 1983).

What are the implications of these typicality effects for the classical view? The findings seem inhospitable to the view − they show that not all instances of a concept are equal, yet equality is what we would expect if every instance met the same definition. This by itself is not a very convincing argument. The argument is considerably strengthened, however, by the additional finding that typicality effects are due to nonnecessary properties. In an important study by Rosch and Mervis (1975), subjects listed properties of instances of a number of everyday concepts (e.g., *furniture*). Virtually all of the properties listed for each concept were nonnecessary ones (e.g., the property "has a back" for *furniture*). Some instances had properties that many other instances also had (e.g., "has a back"), whereas other instances had properties that occurred less frequently in the concept (e.g., "made of

Prototypes

Fuzzy concepts. The typicality findings discussed above have led to a new view of concepts. Instead of offering defining conditions, the properties of a fuzzy concept are assumed to occur in some instances, not all, and to be perceptually salient. A collection of such properties is called a *prototype*, for it accurately describes only the "best examples" of a concept. According to this prototype view, the content of a concept is its prototype; an object will be categorized as an instance of a concept if it is sufficiently similar to the prototype, similarity being determined in part by the number of properties that the object and prototype share (Smith & Medin, 1981).

Figure 2.1 contains parts of the prototypes for the concepts *bird* and *fruit*. Each representation contains a set of relevant attributes − for example, for *bird*, external covering, locomotion, and size − and, for each attribute, the most likely *value* that instances of the concept will have − for example, feathered, flies, and small. (The reason for including attributes as well as values will become evident later in the chapter.) For *bird*, we have taken the six values that we considered previously; we chose these values because they occurred relatively frequently and seem salient. This method of determining a prototype is indirect in that we use properties listed for instances of a concept rather than properties listed for the concept itself. The prototype for *fruit* was determined more directly − the values in Figure 2.1 are those properties listed most frequently for *fruit* (as determined by the ratings of Smith, Osherson, Rips, & Keane, 1987). The *fruit* and *bird* prototypes in Figure 2.1 are not anywhere near complete, but they will suffice for our purposes.

The prototype view is tailored to explain the findings that embarrassed the classical view. Obviously, the prototype view is comfortable with the lack of definitions of everyday concepts, for this view does not require definitions. Indeed, almost all of the values in Figure 2.1 are nonnecessary ones. The prototype view is also compatible with typicality effects. The critical assumption is that the typicality of an instance is a measure of the instance's similarity to the prototype. Thus, typical instances should be categorized more rapidly than atypical ones, because the more similar an instance is to its prototype the faster one can tell that it exceeds a threshold level of similarity. (Analogously, one is faster at deciding that two objects have at least three features in common if they in fact share five rather than three features.) There is a comparable explanation of why people retrieve typical instances before atypical ones in a memory task. When they are asked to retrieve instances of *fruit*, for example, *fruit* is effectively a retrieval probe, and it is well known that items similar to a probe are retrieved earlier than those dissimilar to the probe (e.g., Tulving, 1974).

The findings pertaining to family resemblance are also compatible with

Bird		Fruit	
External Covering	– feathered	Color	– red
Locomotion	– flies	Shape	– round
Size	– small	Size	– small
Food	– insects	Taste	– sweet
Communication	– sings	Texture	– smooth
Habitat	– trees	Juiciness	– juicy

Figure 2.1. Parts of the prototypes for the concepts *bird* and *fruit*.

concepts being prototypes. Of course, people use nonnecessary properties in categorization because that is mainly what prototypes are made of. And since the nonnecessary properties that occur most frequently in a concept's instances are the ones most likely to be values in the concept's prototype, instances with frequent properties should be judged most typical of the prototype. For example, the properties of *robin* – flies, small, eats insects, and so on – characterize numerous other instances of *bird*; hence, these properties are likely to be values in the prototype for *bird*, which means that *robin* should be typical of *bird*.

There is, then, a direct correspondence between an instance's family resemblance score and its similarity to a prototype. This claim is amplified in Figure 2.2. The figure includes the prototoype for *bird* (taken from the previous figure) as well as the representations of *robin* and *chicken* (taken from our earlier illustration of family resemblance but now in attribute–value form). Recall that the family resemblance scores of *robin* were among the highest, and those of *chicken* among the lowest. Let us now determine the similarity of *robin* to *bird*, and of *chicken* to *bird*; we count the number of values each pair has in common, subtracting from this the number of values that the prototype has but the instance does not. (This is a simplification of Tversky's, 1977, model of similarity.) For *robin–bird* there are six common values and zero distinctive ones, yielding a similarity score of 6; for *chicken–bird* there is only one common value and five distinctive ones, yielding a similarity score of −4. Hence, family resemblance scores are highly correlated with similarity scores.

In addition to its capacity to accommodate experimental findings, the idea of concepts as prototypes fits with the common intuition that we often think more concretely than a situation demands. If a friend says that she had to see a dentist, we may conjure up a representation of a specific dentist, that representation being our prototype for *dentist*. Why do we do this? Perhaps there are certain mental operations that can be performed only on concrete representations, and one purpose of prototypes is to foster these operations.

Classical concepts. Even classical concepts have prototypes. This is often the case because the definitions of many classical concepts do not contain per-

Bird		Robin		Chicken	
External Covering	– feathered	External Covering	– feathered	External Covering	– feathered
Locomotion	– flies	Locomotion	– flies	Locomotion	– walks
Size	– small	Size	– small	Size	– medium
Food	– insects	Food	– insects	Food	– grain
Communication	– sings	Communication	– sings	Communication	– squawks
Habitat	– trees	Habitat	– trees	Habitat	– farms
		Sim. = 6 – 0 = 6		Sim. = 1 – 5 = – 4	

Figure 2.2. Part of the prototype for the concept *bird*, along with partial representations of *robin* and *chicken*.

ceptual properties whereas the prototypes do. Consider the concept *grand-mother*. It clearly has defining properties, namely female and parent of a parent, but the latter property is not visible. Because one cannot be a parent of a parent without reaching a certain mature age, the property "being older" is a more perceptible indicator of *grandmother*. Hence, being older and being female become part of the *grandmother* prototype. Other properties of the prototype are also relatively perceptual, though they may lack a clear-cut relation to a defining property; for example, grandmothers are kindly and sweet. Such prototypes for classical concepts may be learned early in life, and children may continue to rely on them even after they have learned the definitions of concepts (Landau, 1982).

Even classical concepts with relatively perceptual definitions appear to have prototypes. The most striking examples have been reported by Armstrong, Gleitman, and Gleitman (1983). They studied four classical concepts: *even number, odd number, plane geometric figure,* and *female.* In each case, Armstrong et al. showed that subjects could reliably order the instances of the concept according to typicality. For *even number,* 8 and 22 are typical whereas 30 and 18 are not; for *odd number,* 7 and 13 are typical whereas 15 and 23 are not; for *plane geometry figure,* rectangle and triangle are typical whereas ellipse and trapezoid are not; and for *female,* aunt and ballerina are typical, whereas widow and waitress are not. Armstrong et al. further showed that when subjects had to make rapid categorizations (e.g., "Is 30 an even number?") their responses were faster for typical than for atypical instances. Given that results like these were used to argue for prototypes with fuzzy concepts, it seems we must conclude that concepts as clear as *even number* also have prototypes.

This conclusion may be too hasty, however. For one thing, the typicality variations cited above may be qualitatively different from the ones observed with fuzzy concepts. With fuzzy concepts, an instance is typical to the extent that its properties occur frequently in the concept. There is no reason to believe that property frequency is the basis of typicality variations in concepts like *even number*; indeed, there is evidence that typical instances like 4 and

8 have less frequent properties than atypical instances like 30 and 18 (Smith, 1984). Furthermore, the typicality effects with concepts like *even number* may not reflect a prototype at all, but rather may be due to the ease of determining whether the definition applies. For example, if the way people determine whether a number is even is to see if it can be divided by 2 without a remainder, then less processing is probably required for 22 than for 30, which may be why the former is judged to be more typical than the latter.

In short, some classical concepts clearly have prototypes, namely, those whose definitions are removed from perception. Other classical concepts, namely, those whose definitions are relatively perceptual, manifest "typicality" effects but they may not have true prototypes.

Prototypes plus cores

Fuzzy concepts. The proposal that a natural-kind concept includes only a prototype turns out to be too simple. A more defensible claim is that a natural-kind concept contains two components: a prototype and a *core*. As we have seen, prototype properties tend to be perceptually salient though not perfectly diagnostic of concept membership; in contrast, the properties that comprise the core are more diagnostic of concept membership but tend to be relatively hidden. Consider again the concept *bird*. Our prototype might include the properties "winged," "flying," "chirping," and "nesting in trees." Our core includes those properties that are most diagnostic of being a bird, for example, that it has bird genes (or that it was born of bird parents if we are not that sophisticated), that it is made of skin and bones, and other crucial biological facts (see Carey, 1985). Because only the prototype properties are accessible, we use them for categorization even though they are less diagnostic than core properties. A prototype, then, is a categorization heuristic, a "quick and dirty" means of getting beyond the information given.

Note that the cores of fuzzy concepts are not definitions. For one thing, cores need not be fixed. One's core for many animal concepts may involve some notion of genes; but scientists may change their theories, and genes may be out and something else in. For another thing, cores are often too sketchy to qualify as definitions. One's core for *bird* may involve some notion of genes, but it is likely to be very vague. Rather than define *bird* precisely, most of us are content to have some vague biological knowledge plus the assurance that there are experts somewhere who can fill in that knowledge (Medin & Smith, 1984).

If cores are not used for rapid categorizations, what purposes do they serve? For one thing, we may appeal to them as the ultimate arbiter of categorization decisions in special cases. For example, if one wants to know whether the expensive pet dog one is thinking of buying is truly a terrier, one will inquire about its parentage rather than rely exclusively on prototype features like its coloring. A more important function of cores is their role in reasoning. If I know something is a tiger, for example, I can infer that it is more closely related (biologically) to cats than to dogs, that it has a digestive system, and that it will bleed if its skin is pierced. These inferences, and others like them, follow from my core knowledge about *tiger* (for further discussion of the function of cores, see Armstrong et al., 1983; Carey, 1985; Osherson & Smith, 1981).

Classical concepts. We have already seen evidence that some classical concepts fit the "core plus prototype" format, with definitions being the cores. What we wish to emphasize here is that the prototypes of classical concepts are learned before their cores.

A number of lines of developmental research indicate that until a certain age children base their categorizations on prototypes rather than cores. We can illustrate this point with a study by Keil and Batterman (1984). Children aged 5 to 10 were presented descriptions of items and asked to decide whether the items were instances of particular concepts. For example, one description for the concept *robber* concerned a person who matched its prototype but not its core: "a smelly, mean old man with a gun in his pocket who came to your house and takes your TV set because your parents didn't want it anymore and told him he could have it." Another description for *robber* concerned a person who matched its core but not its prototype: "a very friendly and cheerful woman who gave you a hug, but then disconnected your toilet bowl and took it away without permission and no intention to return it."

The younger children often thought the prototypical description was a more likely instance of the concept than was the core description. Not until age 10 did children show a clear shift from the prototype to the core as the final arbiter of concept decisions. But although we may know by age 10 that the core is decisive, we may hold onto the prototypes we learned earlier, which may be why as adults we have prototypes even for clearly defined concepts.

Organization of concepts

Concepts do not exist in our minds in isolation; rather, they are organized into larger mental structures. Some of these structures correspond to dimensions; for example, the concepts *red, blue* and *green*, are organized into the color dimension. Other structures are more "factorial"; for example, kin concepts like *mother* and *uncle* can be seen as the combination of specific values of the dimensions "gender," "generation," and "lineage." But the most common structures seem to be hierarchies. In particular, many object concepts are structured into a *taxonomy*, a type of hierarchy in which successive levels refer to increasingly more specific concepts. In the taxonomy of animals, for example, an upper level would include the concepts *mammal* and *fish*, whereas a lower level would include the more specific concepts *dog* and *shark*.

The existence of such complex mental structures raises new questions about concepts, questions related to the basic functions of concepts mentioned at the outset. Given that concepts function as recognition devices, is one level of a taxonomy more useful than others for recognition purposes? To put it another way, in our effort to go beyond the information given, what level of a taxonomy offers the most useful "entry point"? Another important question concerns the cognitive-economy function of concepts: Do we distribute the information in our hierarchies so as to minimize the total amount stored? These two questions are our chief concerns in this section, which focuses almost exclusively on fuzzy concepts.

Basic levels

Distinctive properties. Figure 2.3 presents a portion of a taxonomy of fruits and vegetables (for the purpose of simplicity, we have omitted the attributes and included only the values). Assuming that this taxonomy corresponds to people's mental structure, a particular object, say a McIntosh apple, may be correctly categorized at different levels, including *McIntosh apple, apple, fruit,* and *plant.* In a seminal paper, Rosch and her colleagues argued that one of these levels is the preferred or "basic" one, that being the level that includes *apple* and *watermelon* (Rosch, Mervis, Gray, Johnson, & Boyes-Braehm, 1976). Rosch et al. defined the basic level as that level at which concepts have the maximal number of "distinctive properties," a concept's property being distinctive to the extent that other concepts at that level do not share it. To illustrate, in Figure 2.3 the high-level concept *fruit* has only one property − sweet − that is distinctive (*vegetable* does not have it); the medium-level concept *apple* has numerous properties, and many of them are relatively distinctive (like "red," "round," "grows on trees," and "has a stem"); the low-level concept *McIntosh apple* has the most properties of all, but hardly any of them are distinctive (*Delicious apple* shares all of them but one). Because *apple* has the most distinctive properties, it is said to be basic, whereas *fruit* is superordinate and *McIntosh apple* is subordinate. Note that many of the properties involved are prototypical ones; this fact will figure in our subsequent discussion.[1]

Now that we have a means of defining the basic level, we can consider the evidence that this level is the preferred one for recognition and categorization. In one of Rosch et al.'s studies, subjects were presented with a concept

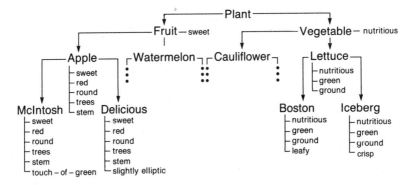

Figure 2.3. Part of a taxonomy of fruits and vegetables.

name followed by a picture of an object; the subjects' task was to decide as quickly as possible whether the pictured object was an instance of the named concept, the concept being either subordinate, basic, or superordinate. Subjects responded faster for basic concepts than for either subordinate or superordinate ones. In another of Rosch et al.'s experiments, subjects were presented pictures of common objects and simply had to name them. Subjects overwhelmingly named the objects with basic names rather than subordinate or superordinate ones. In a follow-up study by Smith, Balzano, and Walker (1978), subjects were required to name objects at a particular level; they were faster when naming at the basic level than at the superordinate level. All of these results strongly suggest that objects are first recognized as instances of basic concepts; membership in superordinate concepts is then inferred ("If the object is an apple, it must also be a fruit"), and membership in subordinate concepts is decided by observation of additional properties ("If the object is an apple, and is green and round, it is probably a Pippin apple").

Why do we enter our mental taxonomies at the basic level? Presumably we do so because this level permits us to infer a substantial number of properties without much perceptual effort. That is, the fact that basic concepts have numerous properties, including nonperceptual ones, enables us to go substantially beyond the information given, and because so many of the perceptual properties are distinctive, the decision as to which concept is the appropriate one is relatively easy to make. In contrast, superordinate concepts have relatively few properties and hence cannot move us far beyond the information given. And although subordinate concepts have many properties and consequently can move us far beyond the information given, they have so few distinctive properties that it is difficult to decide perceptually which concept is the appropriate one. Categorization at the basic level thus maximizes the number of low-cost inferences that we can draw.

Some restrictions on basic levels. Thus far we have assumed that, if one concept at a particular level is basic, then all concepts at that level are basic. If *apple* is basic, then so are *watermelon* and *olive*; if *cauliflower* is basic, then so are *lettuce* and *seaweed*. To put it another way, we have assumed that "basicness" – or "subordinateness" or "superordinateness" – is a property of levels, not of individual concepts. This assumption is violated in many cases. Consider *bird* one more time. Rosch et al. found that, for American college students, *bird* is generally basic whereas *robin*, *bluebird*, and other typical species are subordinates. Thus, a pictured robin can be categorized more rapidly as *bird* than *robin* and is more likely to be named "bird" than "robin." However, things are different when we consider atypical instances of *bird*, like *penguin*. A pictured penguin is categorized more rapidly as *penguin* than *bird*, suggesting that *penguin* is basic whereas *bird* is now superordinate (Jolicoeur, Gluck, & Kosslyn, 1984; Murphy & Brownell 1985). Similar reversals occur in other cases. For typical fish like trout, *fish* is basic whereas *trout* is subordinate; for atypical instances like sharks, *shark* is basic and *fish* superordinate.

These reversals make sense when we consider the role of distinctive properties in determining basic levels. *Bird* has many distinctive properties, but they tend to be part of its prototype and hence do not characterize atypical instances like *penguin*. Indeed, the number of distinctive *bird* properties that actually apply to any particular penguin is probably lower than the number of distinctive *penguin* properties that apply to it; therefore, the basic level should move down from *bird* to *penguin*. The same logic accounts for other cases in which the basic level for atypical instances is lower than that for typical instances.

Hence, basicness – or subordinateness or superordinateness – is not a property of an entire level. However, treating basicness as a property of individual concepts is problematic as well. In the preceding discussion, *bird* was sometimes basic (relative to robins) and other times superordinate (relative to penguins). It seems, however, that we will simply have to live with the ambiguity of the basicness of *bird*. It is the prototype of *bird* that is at issue here, and the prototype of *bird* is basic for typical instances but not for atypical ones. In sum, when we talk about basic levels, we are usually talking about prototypes, and the level of a prototype depends on the typicality of the instances under discussion.

There is another kind of restriction on the notion of basic levels. With increasing expertise, subordinate concepts may become basic. For American urbanites, *bird* may be basic (vis-à-vis typical instances), whereas *robin* and *blue jay* are subordinate; in rural cultures, however, where people are knowledgeable about wild life, *robin* and *bluejay* are basic whereas *bird* is superordinate (Berlin, 1972; Rosch et al., 1976). Similar shifts in the basic level occur in other cases of expertise. For an apple farmer, *McIntosh* is probably basic whereas *apple* is superordinate; for a person who sells clothing, *sports jacket* may be basic, whereas *jacket* is superordinate.

Again, this variation can be interpreted in terms of the dependency of basic levels on distinctive properties. Part of what is involved in becoming an expert about a domain is learning more distinctive properties about objects in the domain. Apple farmers know many properties of McIntosh and Pippin apples, clothing sales people know many properties of sports jackets and suit jackets, and experts in general know many distinctive properties of lower-level concepts in their domain, so many in fact that such concepts become basic.

Hierarchiacal storage and cognitive economy

A glance at Figure 2.3 reveals that each property is associated with every concept to which it applies. The property "sweet," for example, is listed with *fruit, apple, McIntosh apple,* and *Delicious apple.* An alternative way to store properties in a taxonomy was proposed by Collins and Quillian (1969), and it is illustrated in Figure 2.4. In this kind of "hierarchical storage," a property is stored only with the most general concept to which it applies; "sweet," for example, is stored only with *fruit,* and "round" only with *apple.* Then one must infer whether a property applies to a concept that is less general than that with which it is stored. Thus, one deduces that an apple is sweet from the stored facts that an apple is a fruit and that fruit is sweet. We refer to such inferences as *deductive retrieval.*

Do we in fact represent taxonomic knowledge in the way illustrated in Figure 2.4? Given that one purpose of concepts is to promote cognitive economy and that hierarchical storage in some sense maximizes such economy, we might expect hierarchical storage to be the rule. A consideration of various cases suggests that, although hierarchical storage is often used, by no means is it always used. Consider first those cases in which intuition alone suffices to establish that hierachical storage is used. When people answer questions like "Did Spinoza have an elbow?" or "Does Ronald Reagan have a four-chambered heart?" they deduce the answer from the stored facts that Spinoza (Reagan) is a person and People have elbows (four-chambered hearts). What makes these cases clear-cut is that the property relation of interest has probably never been encoded. You probably have never thought about Spinoza having an elbow before, nor heard about it, nor seen it. The same is true for Reagan's four-chambered heart. Since the critical property relation has never been encoded, hierarchical storage and deductive retrieval must be used (Anderson & Bower, 1973).

Let us move on to the case in which we cannot decide by intuition alone whether hierarchical storage is involved. Consider the questions "Do robins have wings?" and "Does a bird have skin?" Do people answer the latter

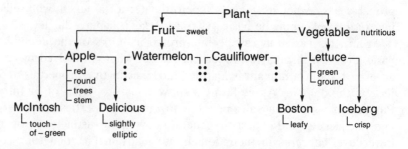

Figure 2.4. Part of a taxonomy of fruits and vegetables in which a property is stored only with the most general concept to which it applies.

question by deduction from the stored facts that a bird is an animal and an animal has skin? Experiments on such questions have yielded mixed conclusions. Collins and Quillian (1969) reported that it takes longer to answer questions like the preceding ones than questions in which the property would presumably be stored directly with the concept (e.g., "Does a robin have a red breast?"); such findings indicate hierarchical storage. Conrad (1972), however, pointed out a problem in interpreting the Collins and Quillian findings: Questions that presumably required deductive retrieval may in fact have required only direct retrieval, but the property involved was only weakly associated with the concept. To illustrate, it may have taken relatively long to answer "Does a bird have skin?" not because the property is stored only with *animal* and hence must be deduced, but rather because the property "skin" is stored directly with *bird* but is a relatively weak associate of it.

Some of these in between cases most likely reflect true hierarchical storage, whereas others do not. What factors determine whether hierarchical storage is involved? One is clearly the frequency with which the property relation has been presented. (Collins & Loftus, 1975; Smith, Haviland, Buckley, & Sack, 1972). The more one hears propositions about robins having wings, for example, the more likely it is that "wings" will be directly stored with *robin* even if initially it was learned as a property of *bird*. A second factor concerns the levels of the concepts involved. Because basic concepts are learned before subordinates or superordinates (Anglin, 1977), any property of a basic concept may be stored directly with it even though it may be true of the relevant superordinate. For example, because *apple* was learned before *fruit*, the property "has seeds" may be stored directly with *apple* even though it applies to all *fruit*. (The property may eventually also be stored with *fruit*, but it is unlikely to be erased from its starting concept.) Thus, "Do apples have seeds?" might not require deductive retrieval. In contrast, the property "has seeds" may not be stored with *McIntosh apple* because this subordinate was learned after *apple*. Thus, "Does a McIntosh apple have seeds?" might require deductive retrieval. All of this is quite speculative. It remains a task for future research to determine whether the use of hierarchical storage and deductive retrieval can be determined by factors like frequency of expression and levels of the relevant concepts.

Combining concepts

Thus far we have focused on "simple" concepts, roughly those that are denoted by single words, such as *apple, fruit, bird,* and *jacket.* We have proposed, among other things, that each such concept is represented by a prototype plus core. Simple concepts, however, make up only a small fraction of our conceptual repertoire. Most of our concepts are "composite"; that is, they are denoted by more than one word, such as *red fruit* or *very large bird.* Such concepts also seem to have prototypes and cores, but unlike the case of simple concepts, the prototypes and cores of composite concepts often cannot be learned from experience with exemplars. This is because many composite concepts are novel combinations and hence unfamiliar (e.g., *smiling Canadian Mountie*). We must therefore have some means, or principles, for composing a composite concept from its simple constituents − for example, some way of composing *red fruit* from *red* and *fruit,* or *Stoves burn* from *stove* and *burn.* Such combinatorial activities comprise the third function of concepts.

In this section we emphasize conceptual combination with prototypes of fuzzy concepts. Research on this topic is relatively recent, and only a few cases have been examined. We shall discuss three of these cases. One involves adjective−noun conjunctions like *red fruit* and *large bird*; in such cases, the adjective concept seems to modify the noun concept. The second case of conceptual combination concerns adverb−adjective−noun conjunctions like *very red fruit* and *slightly large bird*; in such cases, the adverb concept appears to intensify aspects of the adjective−noun conjunction. The third case of combination involves noun−verb combinations like *Birds eat insects*; in such cases, the noun concepts seem to fill slots in, or *instantiate,* the verb concept.

Modification: adjective−noun conjunctions

There have been a number of recent proposals about the way in which people combine the prototypes of adjective and noun concepts into the prototypes of conjunctions (e.g., Cohen & Murphy, 1984; Hampton, 1986; Smith & Osherson, 1984; Smith et al., 1987; Thagard, 1984). Since some of these proposals are similar in spirt, we focus on only one of them, that of Smith et al. (1987).

Smith et al. start with a prototype representation for simple noun concepts; that for *fruit* is illustrated in the leftmost panel of Figure 2.5. Like the prototype representation we considered earlier, the representation in Figure

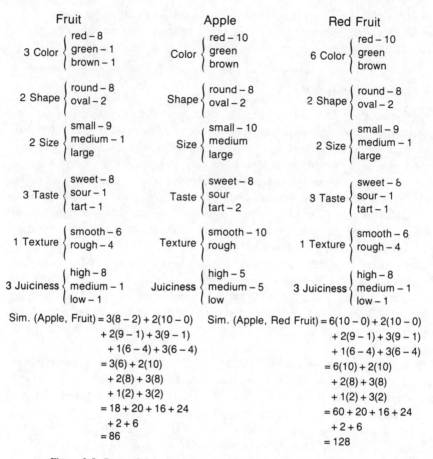

Figure 2.5. Parts of the prototypes for the concepts *fruit* and *red fruit*, along with a partial representation of *apple*.

2.5 has an attribute−value format. However, for each attribute, we now specify a set of possible values that instances of the concept can assume (e.g., for color, the values include red, green, and brown). This prototype representation also has two additional new aspects: (a) It specifies the salience of each value of an attribute (which presumably reflects the value's perceptibility and subjective likelihood of appearing in any instance), as indicated by the number to the right of the value (this number represents the "votes" for the value), and (b) it specifies the diagnosticity of each attribute for the concept as indicated by the number to the left of the attribute. Thus, the value "red" is quite salient (it has a large number of votes), presumably because red is easily perceived and a common color of many fruits, and the attribute "color" has a relatively high diagnosticity because it can be used to distinguish *fruit* from similar concepts like *vegetable*.

The center panel of Figure 2.5 illustrates a representation of an instance of *fruit*, namely, *apple*. It has the same aspects as those listed for *fruit*, except that it lacks diagnosticity weights. As described earlier, the typicality of an instance in a concept is determined by the similarity of the instance to the concept's prototype, similarity being measured by the number of votes on each attribute that is common to the prototype and instance minus the number of votes on each attribute that is distinct to the prototype. In computing the similarity between the *apple* and *fruit* representations in Figure 2.5, we compute the number of common and distinctive votes for an attribute (see Figure 2.5); then we weight the difference between the common and distinctive votes by the diagnosticity of the attribute and sum the results over all attributes.

With this as a background, we can ask how prototypes for simple concepts like *fruit* are modified by adjective concepts like *red*. The basic idea is that the adjective concept does three things: (a) It selects the relevant attribute in the noun ("color" in the example of *red fruit*); (b) it shifts all votes on that attribute into the value named by the adjective (e.g., "red"); and (c) it increases the diagnosticity of the attribute. The effects of these modification procedures are illustrated in the rightmost panel of Figure 2.5, which presents the prototype for *red fruit*. The only differences between this representation and that of *fruit* involves the "color" attribute. Now, all votes are on "red," and the diagnosticity of "color" has increased substantially. These differences have implications for typicality. When we calculate the similarity of *apple* to the prototype *red fruit*, there are now more common features and fewer distinctive ones, and the common features are worth more because they are more diagnostic (see Figure 2.5). The upshot is that this model predicts that, if an object is an instance of a noun concept and an adjective–noun conjunction, it should be judged more typical of the conjunction than of the noun concept. This prediction has been verified by a number of experiments (e.g., Smith & Osherson, 1984; Smith et al., 1987).

The basic idea behind modification is that the adjective and noun concepts play different roles, the noun being the frame to be operated on and the adjective being the operator. This fundamental asymmetry in the roles is revealed by the fact that, when an adjective–noun conjunction is reversed, its meaning changes. Consider *bird house* and *house bird*. A *bird house* is a kind of dwelling, one whose "occupancy" attribute has most of its votes on "small birds"; in contrast, a *house bird* is a kind of *bird*, one whose "habitat" attribute has most of its votes on "house."

Intensification: adverb–adjective combinations

When certain adverbs are applied to adjective–noun conjunctions, they seem to intensify aspects of the prototypes on which they operate (e.g.,

Clark & Clark, 1977; Cliff, 1959). Such *intensifying* adverbs include *very,* *slightly*, and *non*. Thus, in *very red fruit, very* appears to augment the redness in *red fruit*, whereas in *slightly red fruit* or *non-red fruit*, the adverbs diminish the redness in *red fruit*.

These intuitions about the effects of *very, slightly*, and *non* can be incorporated into the approach we took with adjective–noun conjunctions.

1. Assume that *very* augments the modified value in a conjunction (e.g., the *red* in *red fruit*) by multiplying the votes on that value by some number greater than 1. Suppose, for example, that the number of red votes on *red fruit* is 10 and the multiplier is 2; when *very* is applied to *red fruit*, the number of red votes increases to 20.
2. Assume that *slightly* diminishes the modified value in a conjunction by multiplying the votes on that value by some number between 0 and 1. This means that there will be a decrease in the votes on the value, but some votes will be left. If, for example, the number of red votes on *red fruit* is 10 and the multiplier is .5, then when *slighlty* is applied to *red fruit* the number of red votes decreases to 5.
3. Assume that *non* diminishes the modified value in a conjunction by multiplying the votes on that value by a number less than or equal to 0. This means that there will be no votes left on the value. If, for example, the number of red votes on *red fruit* is 10 and the multiplier is 0, then when *non* is applied to *red fruit* the number of red votes is 0.

These proposals are adapted from Smith et al. (1987). In a partial test of the proposals, Smith et al. asked subjects to rate the typicality of various instances in a number of complex concepts. Some concepts were adjective–noun conjunctions like *red fruit*; others were adverb–adjective–noun constructions formed by adding *very* or *non* to an adjective–noun conjunction (e.g., *very red fruit, non-red fruit*). The same set of instances was used with all of the concepts. Some results are presented in Table 2.3. The first column lists the 15 fruit instances ordered by the number of their red votes (which was determined by the number of times "red" was mentioned when another group of subjects were asked to list properties of *fruit*). The second, third, and fourth columns give the typicality ratings of each instance in three conjunctions: *red fruit, non-red fruit*, and *very red fruit*. (Typicality was rated on a 10-point scale, 10 being the highest typicality.) The ratings for instances in *red fruit* increase roughly monotonically with the number of red votes in the instance. (*Watermelon* does not fit this problem, presumably because some subjects mistakenly rated inside rather than outside color.) More important for our purposes, the ordering of the instances in *non-red fruit* is essentially the reverse of that in *red fruit*. This reversal is in line with our assumption that *non* multiplies the votes on "red" by a number less than or equal to 0, because instances that are typical of *red fruit* (because the instances have many red votes and so does the concept) are likely to become atypical of *non-red fruit* (because the instances still have many red votes but the concept no longer has any), and vice versa. Turning to *very red fruit*, the

Table 2.3. *Typicality ratings for three kinds of conjunction*

Instance	Red fruit	Non-red fruit	Very red fruit
Tomato	6.37	0.07	9.24
Strawberry	8.57	0.34	9.40
Apple	9.37	1.03	9.14
Pomegranate	6.07	3.34	6.60
Grape	3.60	5.24	4.20
Peach	3.33	5.60	3.37
Pear[a]	1.37	8.03	1.70
Fig[a]	1.07	7.07	1.17
Raisin[a]	0.77	7.14	1.67
Coconut[a]	0.24	8.64	0.07
Avocado[a]	0.44	8.70	0.47
Watermelon[a]	5.44	2.84	6.90
Pickle[a]	0.27	7.77	0.30
Lemon[a]	0.30	9.44	0.27
Blueberry[a]	0.47	9.00	0.37

[a]Instance had zero red votes.
*Source:*After Smith, Osherson, Rips and Keane (1987).

ratings are again roughly monotonic with the number of red votes in the instance. This is compatible with our assumption that *very* multiplies the votes on "red" by a number greater than 1, for then instances with more votes on "red" will be more typical of *very red fruit*.

Instantiation: verb—noun combinations

Ideas about the way in which verb, or action, concepts are combined with noun concepts are plentiful in linguistics, psycholinguistics, and artificial intelligence. One idea that cuts across these disciplines is that a verb concept can be thought of as a frame whose slots or attributes must be filled, or instantiated, by noun concepts (e.g., Fillmore, 1968; Norman & Rumelhart, 1975; Schank, 1972). Consider the verb concept *eat*. It contains a slot for an agent – the one who eats – as well as a slot for the object – that which is eaten. Moreover, the values that can fill these slots (or attributes) are restricted; for example, the agent slot can be instantiated only by something animate, the object slot only by something ingestible. When this concept is combined with noun concepts, as in *Birds eat insects*, the agent slot is instantiated by the concept *birds*, and the object slot is instantiated by *insects*. (More realistically, the slots are filled by "pointers" to the relevant noun concepts, since it is most unlikely that every attribute—value of the noun enters into the combinatorial process.)

Perhaps the best evidence for the validity of this instantiation approach is the fact that it explains some basic aspects of language understanding. In the work of Norman and Rumelhart (1975), for example, verb concepts play a pivotal role in the understanding of sentences. Upon hearing the sentence "John gives Mary the book," for example, presumably one builds a representation like that in the top half of Figure 2.6. At the center of the representation is the concept *give*, with *John* instantiating the agent slot, *Mary* instantiating the recipient slot, and *book* instantiating the object slot. Such a representation enables one to answer questions like "Who gives the book to Mary?" or "What does John give to Mary?" The latter question, for example, could be represented as shown in the bottom half of Figure 2.6 and then matched to the representation in the top half to determine the information that is being sought. Hence, the approach accounts well for our ability to answer questions.

Summary

Our three cases of conceptual combinations reveal two important commonalities. The first is that all cases require framelike representations, that is, representations that include a distinction between a slot or attribute, on the one hand, and a slot filler or attribute—value, on the other. This distinction is critical in combining adjectives and noun prototypes, for the effect of the adjective is to select the relevant attribute and "operate" on its values (i.e., collapse all votes into the value named by the adjective). The distinction between attributes and values is as important in combining adverb concepts and adjective—noun conjunctions. To appreciate this, consider what is involved in deciding whether an object is typical of the concept *non-red fruit*; to know that *blueberry* is a good example of this concept, one must know that "blue" and "red" are mutually exclusive values, which suggests that one must know that they are values of the same attribute. And, of course, a frame representation is essential for combining noun and verb concepts, for the critical idea is that of instantiating a frame.

The second commonality is that the concepts involved do not play symmetric roles. In the case of adjective—noun conjunctions, the noun concept is the basic frame being operated on and the adjective is the operator. In adverb—adjective—noun combinations, the representation that results from the adjective—noun combination plays the role of the frame being operated on whereas the adverb is the operator. In the case of noun—verb combinations, the verb is the basic frame being operated on and the noun plays the role of filler. Asymmetry, then, seems to be a hallmark of conceptual combination.

Our discussion of conceptual combination would not be complete without some mention of the core—prototype distinction. Although our treatment of adjective—noun conjunctions concerned only prototypes, our discussion of adverb concepts and noun—verb combinations involves cores as well. That

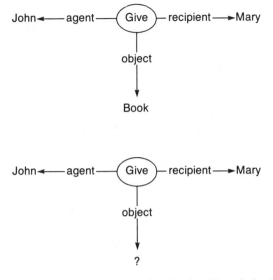

Figure 2.6. Representations of "John gives Mary the book" (top) and of "What does John give to Mary?" (bottom).

is, adverbs like *very slightly* and *not* may intensify both core and prototype properties, and our description of the instantiation process for noun–verb combinations applies not just to prototypes, but to cores as well. The only case, then, in which we are left without a proposal for cores is that of adjective–noun conjunctions. In this case, Osherson and Smith (1981, 1982) have proposed that the traditional approach to conceptual combination – intersection of the adjective and noun properties – may be tenable. Thus, the core of *red fruit* would consist of just those properties that are in the core of *red* and in the core of *fruit*.

Remaining issues

Our discussion of the contents, organization, and combination of concepts has covered some of the critical issues in this area, but we have not by any means touched on all the important problems. In this final section, we briefly discuss two issues. The first concerns the *format* of concepts, specifically whether the representation is an abstraction or a collection of exemplars. The second issue concerns the extension of principles that apply to simple object concepts to other kinds of concepts.

Format of concepts

It seems natural to think of a concept as an abstraction, that is, as a summary of the properties of instances. This notion has held sway for eons, but lately a new idea about the format of concepts has been advanced, namely, that a concept, particularly a fuzzy concept, is represented by its exemplars. Here, *exemplar* refers either to a specific instance of a concept or to a subset of the concept. An exemplar representation of the concept *pants*, for example, might include the exemplars "a favorite pair of faded blue jeans" or the subset of pants that corresponds to blue jeans in general.

Evidence for the validity of exemplar representations. Exemplar representations are compatible with the basic findings about typicality (e.g., Mervis, 1980; Smith & Medin, 1981). Suppose that a person's representation of the concept *bird* consisted of its best examples, such as *robin* and *blue jay*. The typicality of any other instance could then be determined by its similarity to the best examples, and categorization would be a matter of ascertaining whether an item had some critical level of similarity to the best examples. Furthermore, an exemplar representation provides the most straightforward explanation of why we often think of concrete cases when dealing with concepts – a concept is simply a set of concrete cases.

These findings, however, are hardly strong evidence for the validity of exemplar representation. (Earlier we showed that these findings are also compatible with an abstract-prototype representation.) More decisive evidence has been provided by Medin (e.g., Medin & Schaffer, 1978; Medin & Smith, 1981) and Nosofsky (e.g., 1986) in their studies with artificial concepts. These studies show that the ease of learning an instance–category relation is better predicted by the similarity of the instance to other category exemplars than by the similarity of the instance to an abstract representation. Furthermore, research by Estes (e.g., 1986) has shown that the learning of instances of artifical concepts is best predicted by a model based on exemplars, even when the categories contain numerous instances and each instance has values on numerous attributes. Thus, there is evidence for exemplar-based representations with artificial concepts whose complexity and structure approach that of natural concepts.

Related evidence for exemplar representations comes from studies of the strategies people use in learning artificial categories (e.g., Brooks, 1978). In a typical study, subjects are induced to adopt a strategy that promotes either analysis (e.g., searching for properties common to most instances) or memorization of individual instances. If the analytic strategy is used, presumably the subject's representation of a concept is an abstraction; if a nonanalytic strategy is used, presumably the subject's representation of a concept is a set of memorized exemplars. Surprisingly, nonanalytic strategies sometimes lead to more accurate categorizations than analytic strategies. For example, Brooks (1983) showed that, when a subject does not know the form of the "rule," or set of conditions, that describes whether an item belongs in a concept, often the most efficient strategy is to respond on the basis of the similarity of the to-be-categorized item to exemplars in the subject's memory. This is true even when the conditions are defining ones, as long as their form is unknown. Exemplar representation, then, may be highly adaptive.

The usefulness of nonanalytic strategies (and the exemplar representations they result in) is particularly evident in young children. Because it is often difficult for them to attack problems analytically, young children should be most likely to acquire concepts by memorizing typical exemplars. Indeed, left to their own devices, children generally learn artificial categories by a nonanalytic exemplar strategy, and encouraging them to be more analytic can lead to poorer performance (e.g., Kemler Nelson, 1984; Kossan, 1981). Kemler Nelson (1984) argued persuasively that exemplar representation may underly our early prototypes of natural concepts.

Some limits to exemplar representations. The work described so far leaves little doubt that people sometimes represent concepts by their exemplars. This fact seems incompatible with one of the major functions of concepts, that of cognitive economy. That is, at the beginning of this chapter we claimed that the major reason for employing concepts is to avoid treating each instance as a separate mental entity, yet now we seem to be accepting concept representations that in some sense treat each instance as a separate mental entity. This apparent conflict can be resolved, or at least alleviated, by three considerations.

First, to the extent that natural concepts are represented by exemplars, they may be represented by a few typical instances (see Smith & Medin, 1981, chap. 7); hence, exemplar-based concepts still afford ample cognitive economy. Second, even if exemplar-based concepts involve many exemplars, the only loss in cognitive economy may involve storage; for purposes of perception and thought, we may select, and use for processing, only one or a few of the exemplars. For example, even if we store a thousand *bird* exemplars, when we have to decide whether a novel object is a *bird* we may sample only three of our exemplars, determine their similarities to the novel object, and base our decision on the greatest of these similarities. Third, it is extremly unlikely that any natural concept is represented *only* by exemplars. There is simply too much evidence that concepts are at least partly abstractions. For example, we frequently learn facts about a general class rather than about specific instances, such as "All birds lay eggs," and we probably store such facts as summary information.

Other kinds of concepts

Our final concern is with whether the principles and findings about simple object concepts apply to other kinds of concepts, including goal-derived, social, and situation concepts.

Goal-derived concepts. Some complex concepts are created during our efforts to achieve certain goals. For example, a goal to lose weight can lead to the concept *foods not to eat on a diet*; a goal to escape a fire can lead to the concept *things to save in the event of a fire.* The question of interest is whether these "goal-derived" concepts obey the same principles as do simple object concepts.

Most of the work on this question is due to Barsalou (e.g., 1985). Barsalou has shown that goal-derived concepts give rise to typicality effects; for example, people consider chocolate to be a better example of the concept *foods not to eat on a diet* than is bread. However, the basis for these typicality effects is qualitatively different from that with fuzzy object concepts. Recall that, in the latter case, family resemblance predicts typicality; that is, the higher the frequency of an instance's properties among concept members, the more typical is the instance. Barsalou (1985) has shown that family resemblance does not predict typicality for goal-derived concepts. Rather, the typicality of an item in a goal-derived concept is determined by (a) its value, or amount, on the dimension(s) relevant to the concept (e.g., for *foods not to eat on a diet*, "amount of calories" is the relevant dimension, and chocolate clearly has a higher value than bread), and (b) the frequency with which that item has been used as an instance of the concept in the past (e.g., chocolate frequently arises as an instance of *foods not to eat on a diet*).

These typicality effects may therefore be explicable in terms of only the cores of goal-derived concepts. The core of *foods not to eat on a diet* includes the property "low in calories," and so-called typical instances may be those that can be readily determined to satisfy the critical property. (This is similar to our earlier account of typicality effects with concepts like *even number.*) According to this account, goal-derived concepts do not even contain prototypes, which makes them very much unlike most object concepts. This account may be too extreme, however. Perhaps goal-derived concepts contain some nonnecessary properties (e.g., the property "tastes sweet" for *foods not to eat on a diet*), and those properties affect typicality ratings. If this is the case, then goal-derived concepts, like object concepts, have a core–prototype structure, but typicality effects in goal-derived concepts, unlike those in object concepts, are at least partly due to the core.

With regard to other principles of object concepts, the status of goal-derived concepts remains open. It is not entirely clear whether goal-derived concepts are fuzzy or classical. (The property "low in calories" may constitute a definition of *foods not to eat on a diet.*) Furthermore, we know little about the organization of goal-derived concepts and how they stack up on questions about basic levels and cognitive economy. There has also been little discussion of the format of such concepts. It seems obvious, however, that most goal-derived concepts are represented as abstractions, because the origin of the concept often lies not in induction from experienced instances but rather in abstract thought (e.g., "I have to lose weight; what are the *foods not to eat on a diet?*")

Social concepts. As Brown (1980) points out, people are most commonly classified according to concepts pertaining to occupation (e.g., *doctor, teacher*), race (e.g., *black, white*), religion (e.g., *Jew, Catholic*), and nationality (e.g., *German, Italian*). All of these concepts have a core—prototype structure. Thus, part of the core of *doctor* is having medical training and being involved in the treatment of the ill, whereas the prototype includes properties like being male and middle-aged. Similarly, part of the core of *German* is being of German descent, whereas the prototype includes properties like being serious and meticulous. Furthermore, the cores of these concepts seem to constitute definitions; for example, having a medical degree and being involved in the treatment of the ill are necessary and sufficient conditions for being a doctor.

Social concepts, then, like some object concepts we considered earlier, are classical but contain prototypes. Clearly, these prototypes give rise to typicality variations, because there is some consensus about who is a typical doctor or a typical German and so on. Furthermore, there is some evidence that these typicality variations rest on the same processes as typicality effects in object concepts; Dahlgren (1985) has shown that family resemblance predicts typicality for occupation concepts.

There is, of course, a major difference between the prototypes of social concepts and those of object concepts. Whereas the prototype properties of object concepts are true of most instances (e.g., most birds fly), the prototype properties of many social concepts are true of only a few instances (e.g., how many Germans are really meticulous?). To mark this distinction, social prototypes are usually referred to as *stereotypes*. Stereotypes may be an overextension of what is usually an adaptive process − prototype formation − an aberration of our desire to go beyond the information given.

These social concepts have other features in common with object concepts. Clearly, profession and nationality concepts can be structured into hierarchies (e.g., *professional, doctor, surgeon*), and observation suggests that one level is basic (that corresponding to *doctor*) (Brown, 1980; Dahlgren, 1985). Moreover, social concepts, like object concepts, are probably represented by both abstractions and exemplars.

Profession, race, religion, and nationality are not the only social concepts that have been studied. Personality-oriented concepts like *extrovert, introvert,* and *cultured person* have also been scrutinized. Again there is evidence for a core−prototype structure in which the prototype gives rise to typicality variations. For example, Cantor and Mischel (1979) showed that the extent to which an "instance," that is, a description of an individual, was judged typical of *extrovert* increased with the number of properties the individual shared with extroverts in general. This suggests that typicality effects with such concepts have the same basis − family resemblance − as typicality effects with object concepts.

These personality-oriented concepts may differ from object concepts in other respects. Object concepts have a tight hierarchical structure; concepts at the same level are mutually exclusive. In contrast, personality-oriented concepts need not have a tight hierarchical structure since concepts at the same level can apply to the same person; for example, someone can be both an extrovert and a cultured person (see Medin & Smith, 1984). Furthermore, the properties underlying personality-oriented concepts may be far more complex and perhaps even qualitatively different from those underlying object concepts. Consider a property of *extrovert*, that of being outgoing. This property is not only far more abstract than the typical object property (e.g., "red"); it also may have a different kind of internal structure. To decide whether "outgoing" applies to a person, we must consider not only the person's behavior but also the situation: a person's making jokes at a party is evidence that he or she is outgoing; a person's making jokes at a funeral is not. Thus, we should not be too quick to treat personality concepts as another instance of fuzzy concepts.

Situation concepts: scripts. Representations of stereotyped situations, such as going to a restaurant, are called *scripts* (Schank & Abelson, 1977). Though usually thought of as components of story understanding, scripts can also be viewed as concepts (Abelson, 1981). The properties of a script as concept would include the actions that unfold in a situation. For example, some properties of the *restaurant* script include entering the restaurant, finding a table, reading the menu, eating a meal, and paying for it. Given this characterization, scripts seem to have a core−prototype structure; in this case, the paying for a meal that is prepared by someone else might be part of the core, whereas finding a table and reading the menu might be part of the prototype. Specific stories based on the script could be construed as instances of the concept, and presumably they would be judged typical of the script to the extent they shared properties with it.

As usual, however, we should be cautious about assuming that complex concepts follow all the principles of simple object concepts. Work by Abbott, Black, and Smith (1985) suggests that, rather than being akin to an object concept, a script may be more like an entire hierarchy of object concepts. At the top level is the general goal (e.g., eating at a restaurant), at the intermediate level are "scenes," or sets of actions (e.g., entering the restaurant, ordering, eating, and leaving), and at the lowest level are the actions themselves. However, the hierarchy is not a taxonomy, but a *partonomy*; that is, the entities at one level, like reading a menu, are *part* of the entities at the next higher level, like ordering. (For further discussion of the similarities and differences between object concepts and scripts, see Barsalou & Sewell, 1985.)

In sum, the principles that govern simple object concepts have taught us something about situation concepts – but only something. As is the case with goal-derived and social concepts, some aspects of concepts may differ for different conceptual domains.

Note

1 In determining the basic level, not all distinctive properties may be equally important. Murphy and Smith (1982) argue that perceptual properties are more important than non-perceptual ones, and Tversky and Hemenway (1984) have evidence that part properties (e.g., the stem of an apple) are more important than global attributes (e.g., the color of an apple).

References

Abbott, V., Black, J., & Smith, E. E. (1985). The representation of scripts in memory. *Journal of Memory and Language, 24,* 179–99.

Abelson, R. P. (1981). Psychological status of the script concept. *American Psychology, 36,* 715–29.

Anderson, J. R. & Bower, G. H. (1973). *Human associative memory.* New York: Winston.

Anglin, J. M. (1977). *Word, object and conceptual development.* New York: Norton.

Armstrong, S. L., Gleitman, L. R., & Gleitman, H. (1983). What some concepts might not be. *Cognition, 13,* 263–308.

Barsalou, L. W. (1985). Ideals, central tendency, and frequency of instantiation as determinants of graded structure in categories. *Journal of Experimental Psychology: Learning, Memory, and Cognition, 11,* 629–54.

Barsalou, L. W., & Sewell, D. R. (1985). Contrasting the representation of scripts and categories. *Journal of Memory and Language, 24,* 646–65.

Berlin, B. (1972). Speculations on the growth of ethnobotanical nomenclature. *Language in Society 1,* 51–86.

Brooks, L. R. (1978). Nonanalytic concept formation and memory for instances. In E. Rosch & B. B. Lloyd (Eds.), *Cognition and categorization* (pp. 169–211). Hillsdale, NJ: Erlbaum.

   (1983). *On the insufficiency of analysis.* Unpublished manuscript, McMaster University, Hamilton, Ontario.

Brown, R. (1980). *Natural categories and basic objects in the domain of persons.* Katz–Newcomb Lectures. Ann Arbor: University of Michigan.

Bruner, J. S., Goodnow, J., & Austin, G. (1956). *A study of thinking.* New York: Wiley.

Cantor, N., & Mischel, W. (1979). Prototypes in person perception. In L. Berkowitz (Ed.), *Advances in experimental social pscyhology* (Vol. 12, pp. 3–52), New York: Academic Press.

Carey, S. (1985). *Conceptual change in childhood.* Cambridge, MA: Bradford/MIT Press.

Cherniak, C. (1984). Prototypicality and deductive reasoning. *Journal of Verbal Learning and Verbal Behavior, 23,* 625–42.

Clark, H. H., & Clark, E. V. (1977). *Psychology and language: An introduction to psycholinguistics.* San Diego, CA: Harcourt Brace Jovanovich.

Cliff, N. (1959). Adverbs as multipliers. *Psychological Review, 66,* 27–44.

Cohen, B., & Murphy, G. L. (1984). Models of concepts. *Cognitive Science, 8,* 27–60.

Collins, A. M., & Loftus, E. F. (1975). A spreading activation theory of semantic processing. *Psychological Review, 82,* 407–28.

Collins, A. M., & Quillian, M. R. (1969). Retrieval time from semantic memory. *Journal of Verbal Learning and Verbal Behavior, 8*, 240−7.

Conrad, C. (1972). Cognitive economy in semantic memory. *Journal of Experimental Psychology, 92*, 149−54.

Dahlgren, K. (1985). The cognitive structure of social categories. *Cognitive Science, 9*, 379−98.

Estes, W. K. (1986). Array models for category learning. *Cognitive Psychology, 18*, 500−49.

Fillmore, C. J. (1968). The case for case. In E. Bach & R. T. Harms (Eds.), *Universals in linguistic theory* (pp. 1−88). New York: Holt, Rinehart & Winston.

Fodor, J. A., Garrett, M. F., Walker, E. C. T., & Parkes, C. M. (1980). Against definitions. *Cognition, 8*, 263−367.

Hampton, J. A. (1986). *Overextension of conjunctive concepts: Evidence for a unitary model of concept typicality and class inclusion.* Unpublished manuscript, City University, London.

Jolicoeur, P., Gluck, M., & Kosslyn, S. M. (1984). Pictures and names: Making the connection. *Cognitive Psychology, 16*, 243−75.

Keil, F. C., & Batterman, N. (1984). A characteristic-to-defining shift in the development of word meaning. *Journal of Verbal Learning and Verbal Behavior, 23*, 221−36.

Kemler Nelson, D. G. (1984). The effect of intention on what concepts are acquired. *Journal of Verbal Learning and Verbal Behavior, 23*, 734−59.

Kossan, N. E. (1981). Developmental differences in concept acquisition strategies. *Child Development, 52*, 290−8.

Landau, B. (1982). Will the real grandmother please stand up? The psychological reality of dual meaning representations. *Journal of Psycholinguistic Research, 11*, 47−62.

Malt, B. C., & Smith, E. E. (1984). Correlated properties in natural categories. *Journal of Verbal Learning and Verbal Behavior, 23*, 250−69.

Medin, D. L., Schaeffer, M. M. (1978). Context theory of classification learning. *Psychological Review, 85*, 207−38.

Medin, D. L., & Smith, E. E. (1981). Strategies and classification learning. *Journal of Experimental Psychology: Human Learning and Memory, 7*, 241−53.

  (1984). Concepts and concept formation. In M. R. Rosenzweig (Ed.), *Annual Review of Psychology* (Vol. 35, pp. 113−38). Palo Alto, CA: Annual Reviews.

Mervis, C. B. (1980). Category structure and the development of categorization. In R. Spiro, B. C. Bruce, & W. F. Brewer (Eds.), *Theoretical issues in reading comprehension.* Hillsdale, NJ: Erlbaum.

Mervis, C. B., Catlin, J., & Rosch, E. (1976). Relationships among goodness-of-example, category norms and word frequency. *Bulletin of the Psychonomic Society, 7*, 268−84.

Murphy, G. L., & Brownell, H. H. (1985). Category differentiation in object recognition: Typicality constraints on the basic category advantage. *Journal of Experimental Psychology: Learning, Memory, & Cognition, 11*, 70−84.

Murphy, G. L., & Smith, E. E. (1982). Basic-level superiority in picture categorization. *Journal of Verbal Learning and Verbal Behavior, 21*, 1−20.

Norman, D. A., & Rumelhart, D. E. (1975). *Explorations in cognition.* New York: Freeman.

Nosofsky, R. M. (1986). Attention, similarity, and the identification−categorization relationship. *Journal of Experimental Psychology: General, 115*, 39−57.

Osherson, D. N., & Smith, E. E. (1981). On the adequacy of prototype theory as a theory of concepts. *Cognition 9*, 35−58.

  (1982). Gradeness and conceptual combination. *Cognition, 12*, 299−318.

Rips, L. J. (1975). Inductive judgements about natural categories. *Journal of Verbal Learning and Verbal Behavior, 14*, 665−81.

Rosch, E. (1975). Cognitive representations of semantic categories. *Journal of Experimental Psychology: General, 104*, 192−233.

  (1978). Principles of categorization. In E. Rosch & B. B. Lloyd (Eds.), *Cognition and categorization* (pp. 27−48). Hillsdale, NJ: Erlbaum.

Rosch, E. & Mervis, C. B. (1975). Family resemblances. Studies in the internal structure of categories. *Cognitive Psychology, 7*, 573−605.

Rosch, E., Mervis, C. B., Gray, W., Johnson, D. & Boyes-Braem, P. (1976). Basic objects in natural categories. *Cognitive Psychology, 3*, 382–439.

Schank, R. (1972). *Conceptual information processing.* New York: Elsvier.

Schank, R., & Abelson, R. P. (1977). *Scripts, plans, goals, and understanding.* Hillsdale, NJ: Erlbaum.

Schwartz, S. P. (1979). Natural kind terms. *Cognition, 7,* 301–15.

Smith, E. E. (1984). *Comments on "What some concepts might not be."* Unpublished manuscript.

Smith, E. E., Balzano, G. J., & Walker, J. H. (1978). Nominal, perceptual, and semantic codes in picture categorization. In J. W. Cotton & R. L. Klatzky (Eds.), *Semantic factors in cognition* (pp. 137–68). Hillsdale, NJ: Erlbaum.

Smith, E. E., Haviland, S. E., Buckley, P. B., & Sack, M. (1972). Retrieval of artificial facts from long-term memory. *Journal of Verbal Learning and Verbal Behavior, 11,* 583–93.

Smith, E. E., & Medin, D. L. (1981). *Categories and concepts.* Cambridge, MA: Harvard University Press.

Smith, E. E. & Osherson, D. N. (1984). Conceptual combination with prototype concepts. *Cognitive Science, 8,* 337–61.

Smith, E. E., Osherson, D. N., Rips, L. J., & Keane, M. (1987). *Combining prototypes: A modification model.* Cognitive Science and Machine Intelligence Laboratory Report 1. Ann Arbor: University of Michigan.

Smith, E. E., Shoben, E. J., & Rips, L. J. (1974). Structure and process in semantic memory: A featural model for semantic decisions. *Psychological Review, 81,* 214–41.

Thagard, P. (1984). Conceptual combination and scientific discovery. In P. Asquith & P. Kitcher (Eds.) *PSA 1984,* (Vol. 1). East Lansing, MI: Philosophy of Science Association.

Tulving, E. (1974). Cue dependent forgetting. *American Scientist, 62,* 74–82.

Tversky, A. (1977). Features of similarity. *Psychological Review, 84,* 327–52.

Tversky, A., & Kahneman, D. (1983). Extensional versus intuitive reasoning. The conjunction fallacy in probability judgment. *Psychological Review, 90*(4), 293–315.

Tversky, B., & Hemenway, K. (1984). Objects, parts, and categories. *Journal of Experimental Psychology: General, 113,* 169–93.

3   Induction

Keith J. Holyoak and Richard E. Nisbett

Introduction

A child who has never heard verbs rendered incorrectly into the past tense exclaims, "I goed to bed." A stock analyst, observing that for several years market prices for petroleum stocks have risen steadily in the final two months of the year and then dropped in January, urges her clients to buy petroleum stocks this year at the end of October and sell in late December. A physicist, observing the patterns formed by light as it undergoes refraction and diffraction, hypothesizes that light is propagated as waves. These are examples of induction, or, as Holland, Holyoak, Nisbett, and Thagard (1986) put it, of inferential processes that expand knowledge in the face of uncertainty.

Induction is a very broad concept indeed, one that interrelates most of the basic topics in the psychology of thinking. Induction typically involves categorization (see Chapter 2). Thus, the child who has heard verbs the past tense of which is formed by the addition of *-ed* behaves as if he has established a hypothesis about how to form the past tense of *all* verbs (see Brown, 1973). Such a hypothesis requires the formation of the category *verb*, as well as the category *past tense*.

Induction also involves reasoning – drawing inferences in order to generate hypotheses that extend one's knowledge. Often the purpose of reasoning is to provide an explanation for tentative inferences. For example, the stock analyst may infer that the pattern of petroleum stock prices is cyclic because people buy petroleum stocks for tax purposes near the end of the year, causing a short-term increase in demand that disappears in January. Finding a satisfactory explanation will increase the stock analyst's confidence that the pattern will recur in future situations in which the same causal factors are present. If the tax laws were changed, the analyst might alter her recommendation rather than blithely assume that the pattern observed in past years will recur.

Reasoning involves the use of both rules about events in particular domains (e.g., rules about the behavior of stocks) and higher-order, more ab-

Preparation of this chapter was supported by NSF Grants BNS-8216068 to Holyoak, SES-8507342 to Nisbett, and BNS-8409198 to Holyoak and Nisbett. Holyoak was also supported by an NIMH Research Scientist Development Award, 1-K02-MH00342-05. While writing the chapter Holyoak was a Visiting Scholar at the Learning Research and Development Center, University of Pittsburgh. Many of the ideas described in this chapter were developed in collaboration with our colleagues John Holland and Paul Thagard.

stract rules termed *inferential rules*. These rules include what Kelley (1972, 1973) has called *causal schemas*, or very general rules about causal relations having to do with patterns of evidence suggesting "necessariness" or "sufficiency," multiple versus single causation, and so on. Inferential rules also include *heuristics*, or problem-solving strategies. Examples are the representativeness heuristic, which suggests that outcomes should resemble their generating mechanisms, and the availability heuristic, which suggests that the ease with which events come to mind is a guide to their likelihood. Other inferential rules are closer to the scientist's formal principles and include *statistical heuristics* (Nisbett, Krantz, Jepson, & Kunda, 1983), which are intuitive, rule-of-thumb versions of such statistical principles as the law of large numbers.

Induction is also closely tied to problem solving (see Chapter 7). This is true in several respects. First, induction is often used to solve a problem. Second, the basic theoretical framework for problem solving, in which the process is viewed as a search in some space of possible solution attempts (Newell & Simon, 1972), can be applied to induction as well. A person (or other cognitive system, such as an artificial intelligence program) can be viewed as searching for generalizations that allow successful predictions to be made about future events. Third, many problems in everyday life are probably solved by analogy to other problems and their corresponding solutions. Analogy is generally considered to be one of the major means by which inductive reasoning is carried out.

Induction is a major component of the topic of learning. As Winston (1978) has pointed out, different forms of learning fall along an approximate continuum of autonomy, from direct instruction by a teacher (least autonomous), through "guided discovery," to learning by experience and observation in the absence of guidance from a teacher (most autonomous). Induction is autonomous, inference-guided learning, which to some degree is involved in all but the most rote forms of instruction. Underlying all considerations of induction is the fact that it is a risky business, as each of our introductory examples shows. A very good guess about the way to render a verb into the past tense is simply that one adds *-ed*. But this solution works only some of the time. Fortunes are made by shrewd hypotheses like our stockbroker's guess about the behavior of petroleum stocks − and fortunes are lost on the basis of guesses that appear to be as well justified. For many purposes the notion that light propagates in waves provides good predictions and explanations, but for others the notion is misleading. Inductive processes, as we shall emphasize at many points, must deal with uncertainty in two major ways. First, any mental representation of knowledge must take into account the variability that exists in the world. Second, this knowledge of variability must be exploited in order to reduce uncertainty. The inductive processes that achieve these goals are best understood as mechanisms for generalization and specialization. Processes that produce generalization increase the range of examples that are covered by some category or rule. Processes that produce specialization do the opposite. Procedures for dealing with uncertainty do not guarantee that an inductive inference will be correct or useful in any given instance, but they increase the odds. In the remainder of this chapter, we amplify the themes we have just introduced. We examine the heuristics and constraints that underlie reasoning and learning, we investigate the role of categorization and category formation in expanding knowledge about the world, we explore the ways in which generalization and specialization take place, we discuss the basis for the view that people (and other organisms) possess inferential rules, and we consider the ways in which people use analogies to solve problems. First, however, we discuss briefly how knowledge is represented. Before knowledge can be extended, it must be coded in such a way that a person can use it both to understand events and to make predictions about future events.

Induction and knowledge representation

In order to understand induction, it is helpful to consider the way in which knowledge is represented in the mind. What are the cognitive units in which knowledge is expressed, and how can these be modified by experience? We begin by describing the growth of knowledge in very general terms and then consider more specific ideas about the types of knowledge that are actually induced by humans.

Building blocks for inductive mechanisms

The growth of knowledge in the mind of an individual, like the growth of an embryo in the womb, is mysterious. How does complexity arise out of simple beginnings? Why is the complex emerging form generally highly adapted to its environment rather than a monstrous product of compounded errors? These questions are perhaps more difficult to answer with respect to knowledge than with respect to an embryo, because in the latter case we know that development, although certainly influenced by environmental factors, is highly constrained by an innate genetic "blueprint." An individual's knowledge, however, is influenced enormously by experience. Although innate constraints on induction surely exist, ideas do not simply arise in accord with some prewired genetic plan. Whether a person arrives at such concepts as *tractor, privacy,* and *witchcraft* will depend jointly on learning mechanisms and experience.

Although the explanations cognitive psychology has to offer about induction are much less precise than those biologists provide about physical development, we can at least see how knowledge grows. Knowledge develops from simple innate cognitive units that serve as "building blocks"; these are combined through the operation of innate inductive mechanisms to form more complex units. These higher-order units may themselves be transformed and recombined (as may the inductive mechanisms), so that knowledge grows in a "bootstrapping" fashion, ever more responsive to the environment and less dependent on innate units.

Concepts and procedures

Two basic types of knowledge are modified by induction: concepts and procedures. Concepts are representations of general categories, such as *number, elephant,* and *greenness,* and of more specific categories and instances, such as *5, Jumbo,* and *the greenness of my living-room chair*. Procedures are operations that are adapted to achieve particular goals. Examples include multiplication, training a circus elephant, and changing the upholstery on a living-room chair. Concepts and procedures are closely interrelated. Thus, arithmetic operations and procedures are defined in part by the concepts to which they apply, such as *number*. Concepts and procedures are often learned together; new concepts enable one to construct new procedures that apply to these concepts (Riley, Greeno, & Heller, 1983). This link is important for providing pragmatic constraints on induction: If, in attempting to solve a problem, one reaches an impasse, one might attempt to construct a new procedure, which may require the formulation of new concepts. Thus, people do not usually induce utterly useless concepts, such as *living-room chairs for green elephants doing multiplication*, or useless procedures, such as *multiplying the number of elephants by the number of green living-room chairs*. Rather, they typically learn new cognitive units in the context of a perceived need for new knowledge in order to achieve a pragmatically important goal.

Rules and mental models

How can concepts and procedures be represented? One general proposal is that knowledge is encoded in *condition−action rules*, "if−then" rules of the form "If Condition 1, Condition 2, . . ., Condition N, then Action 1, Action 2, . . ., Action N" (Anderson, 1983; Newell, 1973). The following statements are examples of condition−action rules (also called *production rules*): "If something is gray, large, and has a long trunk, then it is an elephant," and "If something is an elephant, then it can be trained for a circus." Rules can be used to represent knowledge about both concepts and procedures. The first example above represents knowledge that can be used to classify an object as an instance of the concept *elephant*. The second rule suggests a procedure that might be applied to an elephant to achieve a certain goal. In more general terms, rules can be used to place instances in categories and to make predictions about the way in which category members will change over time in response to actions. A pragmatically important concept will typically play a role in a number of procedures, just as an important procedure will apply to a range of concepts. Both concepts and procedures, therefore, are often represented not by a single rule but by interrelated clusters of rules with overlapping conditions or actions. Sometimes rule clusters represent the kind of organized knowledge often referred to as a *schema* for a concept or procedure.

Holland et al. (1986, chap. 2) describe how rules and rule clusters operate as "mental models" that mentally "simulate" the effects of possible actions in the world. The induction of rules that form effective mental models is crucial to planning and prediction.

An important property of rule-based mental models is that the rules can be useful even if they are fallible. For example, we might have the general rule "If something is an animal, then it does not fly." However, we would also like to have the more specific rule "If something is a bird, then it can fly." This rule must in turn be supplemented by more specific rules, such as "If something is a penguin, then it does not fly." More general rules generate fallible but useful "default expectations," which can nonetheless be overridden by more specific rules that capture exceptional conditions under which the default does not hold. Note that atypical category members, such as *penguin*, are more likely to require exception rules, whereas more typical members, such as *robin*, can be quite accurately modeled by default rules for the superordinate category (see Chapter 2). A mental model represented by layers of default and exception rules is termed a *default hierarchy* (Fahlman, 1979). Default hierarchies make the work of the inductive mechanisms easier, since even imperfect default rules may serve a useful role if they are supplemented by appropriate exception rules.

Default hierarchies are a useful way of thinking both about how people represent variability and about how they change their store of knowledge by generalizing and specializing. Animals are variable with respect to the property "capable of flying." We can represent this variability by partitioning animal concepts with respect to whether or not they *generally* have the property "can fly." These concepts are only generally correct with respect to that property and others, and the exceptions are represented as such (e.g., as exceptions to a rule about mammals or birds in general). When we learn that some bird cannot fly, we specialize the concept for that kind of bird by noting that fact. In general, people tend to work with whatever level of the default hierarchy is adequate for the purpose at hand. Sometimes this becomes problematic, of course, but the costs are outweighed by the great economies afforded by the rules-plus-exceptions approach as opposed to the much more cumbersome representation systems that would be required to maintain exceptionless rules.

Some rules in the cognitive repertoire are of particular significance because they specify general procedures that guide thinking itself. Holland et al. (1986) refer to rules of such broad scope as *inferential rules*. Inferential rules are used to make inferences, to direct the course of problem solving, and to control inductive mechanisms. For example, the use of analogies in problem solving might be controlled by an inferential rule such as "If you are at an impasse and a concept corresponding to a different problem is activated in memory, then try to draw an analogy between the activated problem and the one with which you are having trouble." Inferential rules, as we shall see in the next section, constitute the most general kind of heuristics.

Heuristics and constraints

The central puzzle of induction was posed by the nineteenth-century philosopher Charles Peirce, who wrote the following almost a century ago (published in 1931–58):

Suppose a being from some remote part of the universe, where the conditions of existence are inconceivably different from ours, to be presented with a United States Census Report which is for us a mine of valuable inductions. . . . He begins, perhaps, by comparing the ratio of indebtedness to deaths by consumption in counties whose names begin with different letters of the alphabet. It is safe to say that he would find the ratio everywhere the same, and thus his inquiry would lead to nothing. The stranger to this planet might go on for some time asking inductive questions that the Census would faithfully answer without learning anything except that certain conditions were independent of others. . . . Nature is a far vaster and less clearly arranged repertoire of facts than a census report; and if men had not come to it with special aptitudes for guessing right, it may well be doubted whether in the ten or twenty thousand years that they may have existed their greatest mind would have attained the amount of knowledge which is actually possessed by the lowest idiot. (Vol. 1, p. 121)

In this paragraph, Peirce raises the fundamental question of how induction can be constrained. How do people avoid generating innumerable fruitless hypotheses in their search for useful generalizations? Peirce's reference to "special aptitudes for guessing right" reflects his belief that constraints on induction are based on innate knowledge. Whether this is so need not concern us. What is clear is that people have some means, whether innate or learned, of sharply confining the hypotheses they generate to some reasonably sized, and reasonably plausible, subset of possible ones.

Peirce's point can be restated in terms of search. Like problem solving per se, induction involves a generate–test cycle: New hypotheses are generated and then tested with respect to their accuracy and utility in making predictions. But the space of potential hypotheses is essentially infinite; without some constraints on generation, useful hypotheses will rarely be proposed by the generation mechanism. A cognitive system that passed its time wandering aimlessly in the enormous space of possible inductive generalizations would be no more likely to hypothesize that stoves cause burns than to hypothesize that ice cures baldness. Needless to say, such a system would have a very limited life expectancy if exposed to the everyday environment of our planet.

A realistic inductive system, therefore, must impose constraints on the generation and testing of hypotheses. In general terms, the system must be "biased" to generate hypotheses that are plausibly useful and also be equipped to test efficiently the hypotheses generated so as to select those that are actually useful. An important trade-off can be identified here: The more efficient the generation mechanism in proposing only useful hypotheses, the less work that need be done by the test mechanism. In the limit, if only "correct" hypotheses were generated, no testing would be needed at all. It is important to realize, however, that such an ideal generation mechanism is unattainable in an open, changing environment. No matter how many confirming instances have been encountered, it is possible that new cases will be found that violate expectations based on current hypotheses. On some grim morning in the next few billion years, the sun will fail to rise. And to the extent that creativity depends on the capacity to generate bold new conjectures that go far beyond the immediate evidence, it is necessary to have ways of recovering from the inevitable errors that result.

The "biases" that constrain human induction are of two general types. First, there are adaptive heuristics, akin to heuristics for search in problem solving, that tend to favor certain classes of hypotheses over others. As we shall see, these generation heuristics govern both when induction is performed and what is induced when appropriate occasions arise. The second type of bias involves cognitive limitations. A variety of limitations constrain induction. These include the fact that only events that occur relatively close together in time are likely to be associatable, the fact that events must be attended to and encoded properly in order to be candidates for incorporation into an inductive inference, and the fact that associations between events in the world may be too weak in a statistical sense to allow us to induce a linkage. These biases limit the number of useless hypotheses that people generate, but they also prevent people from generating hypotheses that would have been useful to them. Induction is inevitably a matter of trade-offs.

Heuristics

The representativeness and availability heuristics. One set of heuristics that is important in problem solving and induction has been identified by Kahneman and Tversky in their work on judgment (for reviews of this work, see Einhorn & Hogarth, 1981; Kahneman, Slovic, & Tversky, 1982; Nisbett & Ross, 1980; see also Chapter 6). Those investigators found that when estimating the frequency or likelihood of events, people relied on the representativeness and availability of those events, propensities termed the *representativeness heuristic* and the *availability heuristic*, respectively.

One event may be said to be representative of another to the degree that the first event resembles the second. Events may resemble one another because their surface features are similar (water and alcohol look and feel alike, although they do not taste alike) or because one event is often associated with the other (pretzels and beer) or because one event seems likely to generate the other (randomly tossing a coin six times seems likely to result in three heads and three tails and seems more likely to result in the sequence HTTHHT than in the sequence HTHTHT).

Although the representativeness heuristic is sometimes a good basis for prediction and explanation − indeed, sometimes the only one − it can be misleading or worse. For example, the sequence HTTHHT seems more likely than the sequence HTHTHT because the former seems more representative of the outcomes generated by random processes. But in fact both sequences are equally likely. As another example, suppose we told you that we know a student who likes to write poetry, is rather shy, and is small in stature. Then suppose we asked you whether you thought it was more likely that the student was majoring in Chinese studies or in psychology. If you are like most people, you would probably be more inclined to guess the former than the latter. It seems clear that the basis of this inclination is the greater similarity of the person we described to the stereotype for students in humanistic fields such as Asian studies than for those in behavioral science fields such as psychology. But now consider how many people on most campuses are psychology majors rather than Chinese studies majors. Next consider the proportion of psychology majors who might be expected to fit the description versus the proportion of Chinese studies majors who might be expected to fit the description. Since there are very many more psychology majors than Chinese studies majors, you are obligated to guess that the person we described is a psychology major − *unless* you think that virtually no psychology students could be expected to fit the description *and* a high proportion of Chinese studies students could be expected to fit the description. Technically, the error here is a failure to take into account the statistical consideration of differential *base rates* in the population of Chinese studies majors versus psychology majors.

The representativeness heuristic is useful as far as it goes: Prediction usually has to take into consideration the similarity of known events to those that are predicted. The problem is that people often use it as the exclusive basis for making an inference and often ignore other information that is logically necessary, in this case, the base rates for the categories in question.

The same point can be made about people's use of the availability heuristic. When making a guess about the frequency or likelihood of events, people often rely on the salience or availability of the events in memory. For example, when asked to guess whether words in the English language with the letter R in the first position or words with R in the third position have the higher frequency, people generally guess the first. Of course, it is very easy to think of words beginning with R, apparently because one basis for organizing words in memory is organization by first letter. In contrast, it is hard to think of words with the letter R in the third position because we do not store words in that way. Because of the greater ease of recalling words with R in the first position, people guess that such words are more common than words with R in the third position. This is a mistake, however, since the latter are, in fact, more common.

Causal analysis often makes use of a similar version of the availability heuristic. People attribute events to other events because they are salient perceptually or in memory. For example, people are likely to remember one participant in a conversation as having been more influential than the other if that participant was wearing a brightly colored shirt, was rocking in a rocking chair, or is a member of a minority group − a black in a group of whites, a white in a group of blacks, a woman in a group of men, and so on (McArthur & Post, 1977; Taylor & Fiske, 1978). It is easy to show how heuristics also aid judgment and reasoning. Our point in discussing them here is to remind the reader that their use is ubiquitous in reasoning of all types and to show their continuity with other types of heuristics in inductive reasoning.

The unusualness heuristic. A very general heuristic that people and organisms use for generating causal hypotheses is termed the *unusualness heuristic* (Holland et al., 1986). When an unusual event occurs, people "mark" it and hold it in memory. If another unusual event occurs within some reasonably short time, people attribute the second event to the first, or at any rate assume some connection between the two events, such that, if the first event is encountered again, people expect the second one to occur also. People induce this rule because events often occur in this pattern. Of course, it is not an infallible guide to correct expectations or solid causal analysis, but as a source of hypotheses it is invaluable.

A variation of the unusualness heuristic was termed the *specialization rule* by Holland et al. (1986). If a prediction based on a strong rule fails, people tend to create a more specialized rule that includes a novel property associated with the failure. Thus, if a child were to chase a chunky bird that failed to take to the air, the child would be prepared to infer that chunkiness in birds is associated with flightlessness. Again, the heuristic is hardly infallible, but it is a useful source of hypotheses.

Statistical heuristics. Although Kahneman and Tversky demonstrated that people often violate statistical considerations in preference to simpler heuristics such as the representativeness and availability heuristics, people are not completely uncomprehending of statistical principles. On the contrary, as we shall see in later sections, people are often well aware of the need to obtain more evidence before reaching a conclusion. People often make use of an inferential rule that might be termed the *law of large numbers heuristic.* The law of large numbers holds that sample values of parameters approach population values as a function of the size of the sample. No one would reach very strong conclusions about the height of Trobriand Islanders from observing a single Trobriander and finding him to be five feet six inches tall. If, however, one were greeted on arrival at the island by a delegation of 20 or so Trobriand males who were an average of five feet six inches tall and showed the normal variation in height, one would be inclined to draw fairly strong conclusions about the average height of Trobrianders (Nisbett et al. 1983). People show this kind of inferential behavior because they have an intuitive appreciation of the law of large numbers.

In subsequent sections we provide more evidence that people make use of the law of large numbers heuristic and other statistical heuristics when categorizing, generalizing, and predicting.

Reasoning schemata. In addition to the relatively simple rules described so far, which can be expressed as simple sentences and which we probably share with lower animals, people have more complicated sets of interrelated rules that can produce a large number of inferences. Holland et al. (1986) refer to these rule sets as *reasoning schemas.* An example is the causal schemata discussed by Kelley (1972, 1973). Kelley proposed that people distinguish among some kinds of very general causal patterns and use these distinctions when searching for causes of effects that they observe. For example, people are aware that certain classes of effects have any of a number of causes, any one of which, under normal conditions, is *sufficient* to produce the effect. Some causes are in addition *necessary.* That is, unless the causal factor is present, the effect will not occur. People are also aware that certain kinds of effects have many different causes, whereas other kinds of effects have only one cause.

According to Kelley, when reasoning about an effect, people apply the causal schemata that they take to hold for that effect. Thus, if they are trying to determine why a particular physical effect occurred, they are more likely to assume that a single cause was responsible than if they are trying to determine why a particular social effect occurred. Similarly, when reasoning in a "forward" direction, people will not assume that the effect has occurred if they know that a cause they take to be necessary is absent. In contrast, they will assume that the effect may have occurred if the absent cause is merely sufficient; this is because other factors may have been present that were capable of producing the result.

Cheng and her colleagues (Cheng & Holyoak, 1985; Cheng, Holyoak,

Nisbett, & Oliver, 1986) have identified another class of reasoning schemata that apply very broadly in the social domain. They term these *regulation schemata*. An example is the *permission schema*: If you wish to do X, then you must first do Y (e.g., "If you wish to drink, then you must be 21"). Another example is the *obligation schema*: If X occurs, then you must do Y (e.g., "If an employee is injured, then you must pay him or her a pension"). Such schemata are induced because they describe common regularities in relationships among events and because they enable us to reason about events with substantial economy. For example, if people can characterize a situation as falling under the rubric of the permission schema, they can readily tell whether certain events constitute a violation of a rule. One might think that people do this easily anyway, but that would be a mistake. In fact, people make many errors when trying to determine the sorts of events that constitute violations of a rule. Cheng and her colleagues argue that it is primarily when people invoke a well-rehearsed reasoning schema that they normally avoid errors.

Many investigators would include the rules of logic – the laws of the conditional and the rules governing syllogistic reasoning – in our list of reasoning schemata (see, e.g., Braine, 1978). In fact, however, a great deal of work by Wason (1966, 1983), Johnson-Laird (1975, 1983), Cheng and her colleagues (Cheng & Holyoak, 1985; Cheng et al., 1986), and many others suggest that this is not the case. There is substantial evidence that people do not possess, or at any rate rarely use, such extremely general rules as the purely syntactic ones that govern logicians' use of conditional and syllogistic reasoning.

Constraints

It should be clear that heuristics are a kind of constraint, in the sense that Peirce showed that induction must be constrained to forego all possible inferences if people are ever to learn the most useful things. But heuristics are more than a constraint. They are guides in the realm of inference – not infallible guides, but guides nevertheless. Induction is also subject to constraints of a more restrictive kind, however – constraints that literally prevent inferences from being made or that curtail the number and range of inferences that are made. Like heuristics, these constraints are only partially benign. They prevent us from making an infinite number of useless inferences, but they also prevent us from making (a much smaller number of) useful inferences.

Triggering conditions. Perhaps the most pervasive constraint on induction is that not even that most curious of organisms, the human, constantly makes inferences. No one infers anything at all from the fact that there is a beige, oblong pebble next to a dead leaf on the sidewalk. For the most part, inductions are limited to problem-solving contexts. A problem arises when a person does not know what to do next or when a prediction has failed. Under those circumstances, mental work takes place, including all the range of processes that we group under the heading of induction. People make no inference from the observation of a pebble next to a leaf because they probably have no expectations that were disconfirmed by the observation and because the conjunction thwarts no goals.

In more general terms, we may say that people make inferences only when there is some *triggering condition*. An event or relationship must be problematic, unexpected, or at least interesting, before people begin to make inferences. This fact alone spares them from the unbearable tedium of Peirce's statistician from space, endlessly calculating relations among events whose conjunction is of no interest.

Temporal and statistical impediments to induction. There are a number of impediments to learning and inference that protect people from making many useless inferences at the cost of preventing them from discovering some useful ones. The literature on animal conditioning shows that animals (and people) usually fail to make a connection between events that are separated by more than a few seconds in time. A bell that signals the presentation of meat powder to a dog will come to produce salivation in the dog only if the gap between the sound of the bell and the appearance of meat powder is a few seconds long. If it is many seconds long, the connection may never be made. If it is minutes long, the connection will certainly never be made.

A second type of barrier is related to the degree of statistical association between events. If events are related only slightly, if the bell predicts the meat powder at only somewhat better than chance levels, the association may never be learned. Work on humans shows that events that are correlated at less than moderately high levels (.6 or lower) may never be perceived to be associated (Chapman & Chapman, 1967, 1969; Jennings, Amabile, & Ross, 1982).

Conversely, events that are not related in a statistical sense at all may be perceived to be associated, by animals as well as humans, if the organism has a strong enough sense that the events are linked. For example, rats who have been poisoned (by X-irradiation) several hours after eating a distinctive-tasting food will avoid that food forever (Garcia, McGowan, Ervin, & Koelling, 1968). In contrast, pigeons will starve to death before they will learn that *not* pecking at a lighted key will bring them food. Nature has seen to it that rats have a very strong presumption that gastrointestinal illness is caused by something unusual they have eaten in the relatively recent past. Similarly, nature has seen to it that pigeons believe that pecking, not not-pecking, is an activity that brings relief from hunger. In Seligman's (1970) terms, animals are "prepared" to see associations between certain kinds of stimuli and "counterprepared" to see other kinds of associations. The same is true of people, as we shall see in the section on covariation detection, although the genetic basis is not as clear.

Encoding. Perhaps the most fundamental barrier to induction concerns the way in which inputs are initially encoded. If some property of the input is not coded in the appropriate mental representation, it will be impossible to make any inductions involving that property. Some encoding failures result from lack of attention to properties that are readily perceptible. A good illustration is provided by the work of Siegler (1983), who found that five-year-old children generally failed to solve balance-beam problems that eight-year-olds could usually solve quite readily. The five-year-olds understood that the weight on each side of the fulcrum was important but seemed to lack a rule relating the distance of the weight from the fulcrum to movement of the beam (see Figure 3.1). Even those eight-year-olds who initially had trouble were able to induce an appropriate distance rule when given feedback about the accuracy of their estimates of the way the beam would move, whereas such feedback was of little use to the five-year-olds. Siegler hypothesized that this was because the younger children generally failed to attend to and encode the distance dimension, so that they lacked a prerequisite for forming a distance rule.

To test the encoding hypothesis, Siegler gave subjects of both ages practice in attending to the distance of weights from the fulcrum. The children were simply asked to count the weights on each side of the fulcrum and to count the number of pegs that lay between each weight and the center. Three days later, the children were given the kind of feedback that had previously improved the performance of only the older subjects. After the attention-training session, the five-year-olds were able to benefit from the feedback almost as well as were the trained eight-year-olds. Siegler's results thus support the important general point that changes in the basic encoding of inputs may be crucial in the successful induction of useful rules.

Now that we have considered some of the basic heuristics and constraints that influence induction, let us examine some important inductive tasks and the mechanisms of induction used to accomplish them. We shall encounter many more illustrations of the role of heuristics and constraints as we proceed. In the remainder of this chapter we survey the major topics that are central to induction. The mechanisms involved in different tasks are highly interrelated, so that any division is necessarily somewhat arbitrary. However, it will be useful to organize our discussion around four major topics: covariation detection, category and concept formation, generalization and

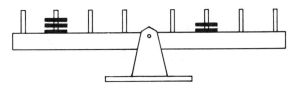

Figure 3.1. Balance beam of the type used by Siegler (1983) in his study of encoding and rule learning.

specialization, and analogy. We close with a brief discussion of whether people's inductive procedures can be improved by education.

Covariation detection

Conditioning and learning in animals

The heuristics and constraints just described may be seen to operate even in the simplest form of induction – simple rule learning, or covariation detection. We have already alluded to the role that constraints play in conditioning. (*Conditioning*, or more precisely *classical conditioning*, is the process by which an organism comes to behave toward a neutral stimulus in the same way that it behaves toward a motivationally relevant one. For example, an animal may salivate and appear excited when it hears a bell that has been associated with meat powder.) Animals will not learn a rule that they are "counterprepared" to learn by virtue of heredity or overwhelming experience. Similarly, animals will "learn" even rules that are incorrect if the stimuli presented to them are linked in a strong prior theory. Animals will not learn to associate events if the statistical association between them falls too low. And neither animals nor humans will learn to associate events that they have not encoded properly.

Work by Holyoak, Koh, and Nisbett (1987) suggests that conditioning is also dependent on the heuristics an animal applies. Chief among these is the unusualness heuristic. Imagine a rat in a Skinner box busily pressing a lever to get its dinner in the form of food pellets. The rat hears a tone of a kind it has never heard before. It pricks up its ears, but goes busily on. Then, just as the tone comes to an end, the rat receives a painful shock through the grid floor on which it is standing. As one might expect, the next time the rat hears the tone, it stops pressing the lever and looks worriedly around the box.

Why does the rat do this? Why does the tone cause it to behave in something like the way the shock itself caused it to behave? Traditional theories of learning do not tell us. We cannot say that events that are associated will become conditioned to one another, because as we have just indicated, association is not sufficient for learning (e.g., Rescorla, 1972). According to Holyoak and his colleagues, learning takes place because the unusualness heuristic is applied. The tone is noticed because it is unusual; the shock, which immediately follows it, is also unusual. The unusualness heuristic is simply a rule suggesting that contiguous unusual events are related. This analysis implies that, if the shock is not an unusual event for the animal or if it is already perfectly predicted by some event, there will be no conditioning to the tone stimulus. In both cases the shock itself is not unusual and not unanticipated. These phenomena are well established in the conditioning literature, which indicates that a motivationally relevant stimulus may be capable of generating learning only when it is still novel or when it is not well predicted (Rescorla & Wagner, 1972).

The heuristics approach suggests that one-trial learning should be frequent. Application of the unusualness heuristic is an inferential procedure and as such should produce rapid changes in behavior. Traditional, "stamping-in" learning mechanisms, in contrast, do not lead us to expect large, abrupt behavioral changes; yet these are readily demonstrated (see, e.g., Kamin, 1968). Types of heuristics other than the unusualness heuristic also play a role in learning. The notion of preparedness can be readily stated as a heuristic principle. Animals and humans use familiar types of association as a guide to assessing potential correlates of any stimulus whose occurrence they wish to predict. Organisms will attend to stimuli of a sort that generally predict the type of stimuli in question. Once found, they will be presumed to cause, or at least to signal, the interesting event. Such an interpretation makes it clear that higher-level processes such as analogy are often involved in conditioning.

As psychologists of a cognitive persuasion come to deal with the old-fashioned phenomena of the behaviorist, it seems certain that they will acquire a new respect for the rat! It will seem less like a trial-and-error plodder and more like a scientifically minded human, armed with heuristics, categories, and analogies.

Covariation detection in humans

If a study of the heuristics of animal learning will ultimately make rats look smarter than they seem, a comparable analysis of human learning will probably have the effect of making humans seem less intelligent than they might like. A fair amount of evidence already suggests that at least some kinds of covariation detection tasks are very difficult for people.

We alluded earlier to work by Jennings and colleagues (1982), which shows that the "psychophysics" of covariation can pose serious problems for people. Those investigators asked subjects to estimate the degree of association (on a simple 100-point scale from *no association* to *perfect association*) between two columns of figures or between a column of little men and an adjacent column of their associated walking sticks. Almost none of the subjects reliably detected the associations until the correlation was in the range of .3 or .4; and not until the correlation was in the range of .6 did virtually all of the subjects see a correlation. Other work shows that people are sometimes more sensitive covariation detectors than that, but the available evidence on the psychophysics of covariation detection indicates that people are often quite poor at seeing associations.

When the task is altered so that it is no longer a purely psychophysical one and one's theories about the world can play a role, matters become worse. Chapman & Chapman (1967, 1969), in elegant studies conducted more than two decades ago, showed that people sometimes see a strong positive correlation where there is no correlation or even a negative correlation. Clinicians themselves, they observed that clinicians often saw strong associations between certain projective test "signs" (i.e., the things their clients discerned in inkblots or drew in pictures) and their clients' symptoms or personality characteristics. For example, many clinicians reported that male homosexual clients saw more genitals in Rorschach inkblots and more figures with ambiguous sexual characteristics, men dressed as women, and so on, than did heterosexuals. Similarly, many clinicians reported that paranoid clients emphasized the eyes in their drawings of the human figure or that dependent clients drew fat figures, and so on. Yet the systematic research shows that almost none of these common-sense associations is actually present. Male homosexuals are *not* more likely to see genitals, paranoid patients are *not* more likely to emphasize eyes, and so on.

The Chapmans reasoned that clinicians are subject to an illusion that we would now say is based on their *preparedness* to see certain associations. According to our theories about the world, certain concepts suggest others. Homosexuality calls to mind genitals; paranoia involves suspiciousness, which calls to mind darting or slitted eyes; and so on. To demonstrate the possibility that the clinicians in their study were subject to this illusion, the Chapmans showed that psychologically untrained undergraduates were subject to the same illusion. They showed Rorschach cards to undergraduate subjects along with a word signifying what a client had allegedly seen in the card ("genitals," "mountains," etc.) and some client characteristics ("depressed," "homosexual," etc.). The cards were carefully arranged so that there was no statistical association between "signs" and characteristics. Nevertheless, the subjects readily "discovered" the same illusory associations seen by the clinicians. They did so, moreover, under circumstances that made their task substantially easier than that confronting the clinicians: Instead of seeing the Rorschach sign at one time and being informed of the patient's characteristics at another, the subjects saw both at the same time. Moreover, they were given the cards and allowed to take all the time and perform all the calculations that they wished. Despite these advantages, even when actual negative associations were built in, the subjects still saw positive associations! The Chapmans obtained very similar results when they showed their subjects human figures that had allegedly been drawn by clients, together with alleged patient characteristics. Subjects "discovered" that suspicious clients draw funny eyes, dependent clients draw fat figures, and so on. An example of the stimulus materials for this study is given in Figure 3.2.

In a sense, the Chapmans' study demonstrates something that has been known for a long time. Social perception is often driven by *stereotypes*, that is, partially or wholly erroneous schemata that color the evidence available to us and make us see even contradictory evidence as confirmatory. The Chapmans' work, however, together with Seligman's analysis of preparedness and a consideration of parallel results in animal work, make stereotyping seem less the "devil's work" motivated by intergroup hatred than an unfortunate consequence of the way our covariation detection mechanisms work. We see the associations we are prepared to see; sometimes we also "see" them when they are not there.

The principles of preparedness and illusory correlation are also useful for understanding some of the evidence on concept formation, the topic to which we turn next.

Category and concept formation

One of the most basic of all inductive tasks is the formation of useful categories and concepts. Here we use the term *category* to refer to a mental representation of a class of instances, such as *cats*. *Concept* is a broader term that includes mental representations that do not so obviously refer to classes. Concepts can correspond to individuals (*my cat Scruffy*), properties (*furry*), as well as abstractions (*gravity*). Since the seminal work of Bruner, Goodnow, and Austin (1956), concept learning has received a great deal of attention from psychologists (see Glass & Holyoak, 1986, chap. 5, for a review). Mental representations of categories make it possible to deal with the ubiquitous variability of experience by enabling us to treat instances of the same category in the same way for certain purposes. Categories typically provide *default* expectations – assumptions about category instances that are maintained unless overridden by more specific information. For example, if a four-legged animal of a certain shape and size is classified as a *cat*, we will probably expect it to purr when petted and be surprised if it bites instead.

Concepts arise in two contrasting ways, which can be characterized as *bottom-up* versus *top-down*. Bottom-up category induction involves the detection of multiple correlated properties that make the instances of the category stand out as a natural class, distinct from other categories. A human who sees even a single giraffe, for example, could hardly fail to induce a

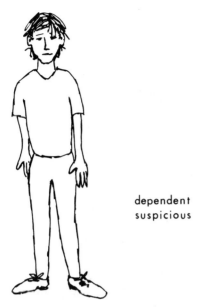

dependent
suspicious

Figure 3.2. Figure allegedly drawn by a client of the client's alleged symptoms. From Chapman and Chapman (1967).

category and classify giraffes that he or she subsequently observes as instances of it. Categories of this type correspond to what Quine (1969) termed *natural kinds*. Rosch and her colleagues (Rosch, Mervis, Gray, Johnson, & Boyes-Braem, 1976) have emphasized that natural categories emerge as a consequence of the correlational structure of the environment. Different giraffes simply look much more like one another than like anything else and hence form a natural category.

In contrast with bottom-up concept formation, the top-down variety is more directly triggered by the goals of the learner. One major type of goal is explanation. The Newtonian concept of *gravity*, for example, was generated in the process of explaining regularities in the motion of physical objects. *Gravity*, unlike *giraffe*, does not correspond to a natural cluster of properties in the world; we do not see or even feel gravity in a direct way, although we certainly feel its effects. *Gravity* is inherently an abstraction, postulated because it plays a role in an explanatory theory. Other concepts are induced because they capture aspects of situations important to goal attainment. A student of physics, for example, will acquire such concepts as *problems solvable by the first law of thermodynamics*. The instances of this goal-defined category may differ enormously in their superficial properties yet still be classified as members of the same abstract problem category (Chi, Feltovich, & Glaser, 1981).

Concepts developed by top-down mechanisms clearly illustrate the close connection between concepts and procedures that we discussed earlier. A problem concept exists simply because it helps one define appropriate procedures for solving a given class of problems. However, categories derived by bottom-up mechanisms also serve important procedural functions. As Quine (1969) emphasized, natural categories generate useful inferences. If something is known to be a giraffe, for example, we can immediately make inferences about its expected behavior and its inner biological structure (e.g., it probably has an unusually long esophagus). Concepts of all varieties are crucial components of rules for making inferences.

Bottom-up category formation

A great many proposals have been made about the mechanisms of bottom-up category formation (see Smith & Medin, 1981). One important hypothesis is that people abstract a *prototype*, or a representation of the central tendency of a category − something like an "average" or "most typical" example (Posner & Keele, 1968; Reed, 1972). The suggestion is that people abstract a prototype during learning and then classify novel instances into the category with the most similar prototype.

Knowledge of variability. Even the earliest studies indicated that people learn more than the central tendencies of categories. In the experiments of Posner and Keele, for example, subjects were sensitive to the *variability* of category instances. Although learning was slower when the training instances were relatively disparate, the subjects subsequently classifyed highly distorted, atypical patterns more accurately if they had learned from more varied examples. Later research (Fried & Holyoak, 1984; Homa & Vosburgh, 1976) provided more detailed evidence that people induce representations of the *distributions* of category instances. Fried and Holyoak presented subjects with patterns like those shown in Figure 3.3. The patterns were produced by random distortion of a standard pattern of light and dark squares on a grid. Fried and Holyoak told their subjects that they were about to view a series of geometric patterns designed by two artists, named Smith and Wilson, and that they would have to distinguish the work of Smith from that of Wilson. The two standards shown in Figure 3.3 were used to generate patterns for all subjects, but each subject saw a different random sample of distortions, and no subject saw the standard. The numbers .07 and .15 refer to the proportion of squares that were altered to make a new pattern from the standard. The .07 distortion probability defined a low-variability category, whereas the .15 distortion probability defined a high-variability category.

One experiment was designed to distinguish whether subjects classify new instances as category members on the basis of simple distance to a prototype or, instead, on the *likelihood* that the instance was generated by the cate-

STANDARDS

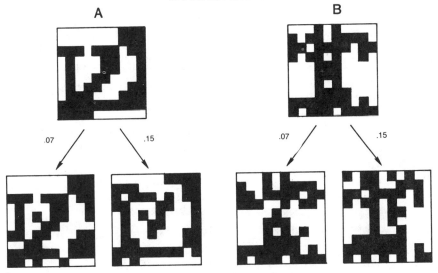

Figure 3.3. Examples of random distortions. From Fried and Holyoak (1984).

gory given its central tendency and variability. The subjects were shown patterns from one low-variability category and one high-variability category. Thus, the Smith patterns were produced by a random distortion probability centering on .07 and the Wilson patterns by a distortion probability centering on .15. In the transfer phase, the subjects were shown new works by Smith and Wilson and were required to assign each pattern to one category or the other. Some of these transfer patterns were more likely to be generated by the high-variability category, even though they were actually more similar (in terms of the number of shared squares) to the standard for the low-variability category. For these crucial items, subjects proved more likely to assign the pattern to the high-variability category, which was in fact more likely to have generated it.

The induction and use of variability information in classification are in accord with sound statistical principles for making inferences. A statistician would not wish to classify objects into categories given knowledge only of central tendencies if the properties of the alternative categories overlapped. Rather, the statistician would require some estimate of the dispersion of the dimensions defining each category and would base classification decisions on information about both central tendencies and dispersion.

Of course, people do not explicitly calculate statistics in order to perform everyday categorizations. How, then, is information about category distributions encoded and used? One possibility, emphasized by Medin and Schaffer (1978), is that people remember individual instances and classify novel instances on the basis of their similarity to remembered training instances. This is a simple version of an analogy heuristic, to be discussed below in more general terms. However, as we argue later, analogy is typically used to form more general rules, so that subsequent cases will be classified directly by rules rather than by continued use of instance representations.

Rule-based account of category formation. Anderson, Kline, and Beasley (1979) developed a rule-based computer simulation model of human categorization that is capable of accounting for the acquisition of distributional information. The program forms rules based on properties that predict category membership (e.g., "If something is small, black and furry, then it is a cat"). New rules are created using generalization and specialization mechanisms and are tagged with a measure of their "strength" − a number indicating the degree to which the rule has made accurate classifications in the past. The strength of a rule is indicative of the degree to which the properties mentioned in its condition in fact predict the category specified by the action part of the rule. A category is represented not by one "optimal" rule or by rules appropriate only for describing the prototype. Rather, a category corresponds to a set of rules with various strengths, representing the relationship between properties (singly and in combination) and category membership. These rules reflect the distribution of properties over the alternative categories. Although no explicit prototype is induced, the prototype is classified easily because it matches high-strength rules based on the properties of "typical" instances. However, if the training instances were variable, rules relating less typical properties to category membership (e.g., "If something is calico-colored, then it is a cat") will also have had the opportunity to develop moderate strength. Hence, greater variability of instances during training will lead to the induction of rules useful for classifying less typical instances.

One limitation of the model proposed by Anderson et al. is that it depends on the learner being explicitly told the category to which the training instances belong. In contrast, when categories are sufficiently distinctive, people are able to learn to classify instances quite accurately even if they never receive such information (Fried & Holyoak, 1984). How are categories induced from simple observation of instances that form natural clusters?

Learning rule clusters by focused sampling. One way to identify a category without the guidance of an external "teacher" is to learn rules that interrelate a cluster of correlated properties. Indeed, given our basic assumption that categories are represented by clusters of rules, our framework suggests that an inductive system should be particularly adapted to finding *groups* of regularities. Once one regularity has been identified, the formation of related regularities should be facilitated, since the components of the existing rule will provide promising candidates for the formation of related rules.

How can a system take advantage of clustered regularities to deal with the complexity characteristic of category learning? Billman (1983) proposed a learning mechanism that facilitates the acquisition of rules based on interrelated properties. She suggested that, in a complex learning environment in which not all properties of inputs can be encoded, learners will use whatever is predictive to guide subsequent encoding. Learners, faced with the need to encode selectively only a subset of the properties of the environment, tend to encode those that are already involved in useful regularities. Billman called this *focused sampling*, since a learner's sample of possible observations of the environment will be biased by his or her focus on those properties that have already proved useful.

The focused-sampling hypothesis makes an important prediction regarding the acquisition of groups of interrelated rules. Suppose the environment is such that when Property 1 has value a (i.e., $P\,1 = V\,a$), then Property 2 has value b. This regularity can be described by the following rule:

Rule 1: If $(P\,1 = V\,a)$, then $(P\,2 = V\,b)$.

Suppose we now compare two conditions, one in which the regularity expressed by Rule 1 is the only one that involves Properties 1 and 2 and another in which these properties are involved in additional regularities involving Property 3, such as those expressed by Rules 2 and 3:

Rule 2: If $(P\,1 = V\,a)$, then $(P\,3 = V\,c)$.
Rule 3: If $(P\,2 = V\,b)$, then $(P\,3 = V\,c)$.

The focused-sampling hypothesis predicts that Rule 1 will be learned more readily in the latter condition, in which it forms part of a group of regularities, than when it is an isolated regularity. In the grouped condition, it is possible that Rules 2 and/or 3 (or their converses) will be formed and strengthened because of their successful predictions. If the probability of using properties to form new rules increases when they are already a part of other successful rules, such focused sampling will increase the probability of forming and testing Rule 1 in the grouped condition relative to the condition in which it is an isolated regularity.

Billman tested this prediction in experiments involving the induction of syntactic categories in an artificial language. A child learning language must acquire rules representing the hierarchical structure of word classes (e.g., proper noun, noun, noun phrase) and rules representing grammatical sequences (e.g., to generate a noun phrase, one can generate a determiner followed by an adjective followed by a noun). Adults typically provide the child with sample utterances that occasionally contain errors, and they do not clearly inform the child as to which utterances are grammatical. The sheer complexity of language, coupled with the paucity of external guidance for the learner, have motivated heavily nativist accounts of the acquisition of syntax. In contrast, the approach taken by Billman and a few others (Anderson, 1983; Maratsos & Chalkley, 1980) has been to examine the effects of regularities in the data provided to the learner.

Billman tested the prediction about the ease of learning grouped regularities in a series of experiments in which subjects attempted to learn an artificial language ("Neptunese"). Subjects were not given any instruction in the language, which had properties quite unlike those of English. Rather, they were simply told to learn Neptunese by watching "spaceship maneuvers" displayed on a computer-controlled video monitor. The animated display was accompanied by a four-word "sentence" describing the depicted event (e.g., a spaceship of a particular shape striking another while a third remained passively positioned nearby; see Figure 3.4).

Billman constructed several versions of the artificial language, which differed in the degree of grouping of certain properties. The regularities of interest involved the organization of nouns into three classes, roughly analogous to a noun declension in a natural language. The system was based on three properties: (a) the shape of objects referred to by nouns, (b) the vowel in the noun's stem, and (c) the vowel in the noun's ending. In the *grouped* condition, all three of these properties were mutually predictive (e.g., a particular type of shape, such as an elongated "spaceship," would be associated with a particular stem vowel in the corresponding noun). Subjects in three *isolated* conditions were exposed to variations of the language in which only one of the three possible regularities was present. After the learning session, subjects in all conditions received a battery of tests to determine whether they had learned particular aspects of the language. It would not have been sufficient simply to have had the subjects judge whether sentence— picture pairs were correct, since of course there would have been more possible cues in the grouped condition than in the isolated conditions (i.e., in the former case the detection of a violation of any one of the three regularities would have been sufficient to reveal an error). To provide an appropriate test, Billman presented her subjects with displays in which parts were omitted so that only one regularity was available. For example, the picture might be omitted so that the property of object shape was not provided, and only the relationship between the stem and ending vowels could be assessed. Billman found that her subjects were significantly more capable of learning the individual regularities related to noun categories if they formed part of a group. This basic result was obtained both when each relationship between two properties was entirely regular and when exceptions were introduced. Thus, multiple, interrelated associations are learned more readily than single associations both when associations are deterministic and invariant and when they are merely probabilistic.

STIMULI

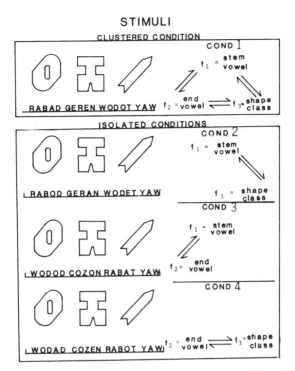

Figure 3.4. Examples of stimuli used in the clustered and isolated conditions. From Billman (1983).

The greater ease of learning a rule that forms part of a group is particularly noteworthy because there were, of course, more rules to be learned in the grouped condition. Consequently, one might have supposed that any particular rule would have received less attention than if it had been the only regularity. Billman's results, in contrast, clearly support the assumption that human mechanisms of induction facilitate the acquisition of such interrelated groups. Sometimes it is easier to learn many things at once than to learn a single isolated regularity. We should expect focused sampling to result from the use of elements found to be predictively useful in the past as building blocks for new rules. Once one rule has been formed, related rules will be easier to form because much of the encoding work has already been done.

It should be noted that Billman's results help to make sense of what otherwise would appear to be a contradiction between our description of covariation detection in the previous section and our description of category learning in this section. Learning a category amounts to learning a network of associations, whereas covariation detection as we have defined it means learning to associate only a pair of elements. It turns out that the former is probably much easier than the latter.

Top-down concept formation

Much less research has been done on top-down than on bottom-up mechanisms of concept formation (but see Flannagan, Fried, & Holyoak, 1986;
Murphy & Medin, 1985). Top-down concept formation is especially important in the induction of scientific concepts. How are scientists able to arrive
at such concepts as *black hole, electron,* and *continental drift?*

Heuristic search for constancies. There seem to be a number (perhaps a relatively small number) of heuristics that guide the induction of scientific concepts. One set of heuristics, illustrated in a series of computer simulation
models developed in the BACON project (Langley, Bradshaw, & Simon,
1983), is based on the general strategy of searching for *constant values* that
relate numerical variables. For example, Kepler's third law states that, for
each planet, the square of the period of revolution around the sun is directly
proportional to the cube of the mean radius of the planet's orbit. BACON is
given a set of data concerning the periods and locations of several planets
and seeks to find a mathematical expression to account for these data. It
notices which variables given to it are correlated and uses heuristics for trans-
forming variables to arrive at the law that d^3 / p^2 is a constant. BACON
can also induce concepts by defining *intrinsic variables* − properties of objects associated with constant values of quantities. For example, the intrinsic
variable *resistance* is postulated on the basis of measurements of current
flowing through different types of wires.

Conceptual combination. An important top-down mechanism for forming
new concepts is the combination of existing concepts in novel ways. This
process is evident in mundane aspects of language comprehension, as in
understanding adjective−noun pairs like *striped apple* and *pet fish* (Osherson & Smith, 1981; Smith & Osherson, 1984). Note that, even in such simple cases, the meaning of the combined concept is not simply the "sum"
of the meanings of the parent concepts. For example, as Osherson and Smith
pointed out, a guppy is a rather atypical pet or fish, yet it seems to be a
typical instance of *pet fish*. A new set of default expectations is associated
with the derived concept.

   Thagard (1984; also Holland et al., 1986) has described several heuristics
for resolving the conflicting expectations that may be generated when concepts are combined. One major heuristic depends on knowledge of variability: If the parent concepts conflict with respect to some property, keep the
value of the property that is less variable for its parent. Thus, fish vary with
respect to "being kept by humans" (although typically they are not), whereas pets are much less variable in this regard (and typically are indeed kept
by humans). Accordingly, we understand that a *pet fish* will typically be kept
by humans, the property value inherited from *pet*.

In the case of scientific concepts, more complex forms of conceptual combination are guided by the goal of establishing an explanation of observed phenomena. A fine example of conceptual combination in science is Darwin's notion of natural selection as the mechanism of the evolution of species. As described by Darden (1983), Darwin's idea had two sources: his knowledge of human breeders' artificial selection of domesticated plants and animals, and Malthus's view that competition for food and other resources caused by increasing population results in a struggle for survival. Starting with a concept of selection that included a rule specifying humans as the selection agent, Darwin substituted natural selection based on competition for resources. This goal-directed conceptual combination led to Darwin's new concept of natural selection driving the evolution of new species.

We shall have more to say about top-down concept formation when we discuss additional inductive mechanisms.

Generalization and specialization

As we have emphasized, concepts do not exist in isolation, but rather form hierarchies of defaults and exceptions. In order to develop such hierarchies it is necessary to form concepts and rules more general and more specific than those currently in the system. The chief inductive mechanisms for accomplishing this task are generalization and specialization.

The term *generalization* is used in several ways, both in psychology and in artifical intelligence (see Dietterich & Michalski, 1983). Here we focus on two kinds of generalization that are particularly important in rule-based systems. The first is *condition-simplifying* generalization, in which one makes an existing rule more general by dropping part of its condition. Specialization, as we describe it here, is essentially the reverse − forming a new rule by adding constraints to the condition of an existing rule. The second form of generalization is *instance-based*, in which a new rule is produced to predict properties found in observed instances of a known category. We first consider the generalization and specialization of existing rules and then instance-based generalization.

Generalization and specialization of existing rules

Condition-simplifying generalization. The most elementary form of condition-simplifying generalization is simply the elimination of part of a rule's condition. We can make the rule "If something has wings and is brown, then it can fly" more general by dropping the clause "is brown," producing the rule "If something has wings, then it can fly." In order to constrain generalization so as not to delete crucial parts of a rule's condition, we can proceed by taking the *intersection* of the conditions of two rules (Hayes-Roth & Mc-

Dermott, 1978). In taking the intersection, requirements not held in common are treated as details to be ignored. The resulting condition is satisfied by any situation that would have satisfied *any* of the conditions intersected. As a simple example, consider the intersection of the two rules "If something is large-winged, brown and feathered, then it can fly," and "If something is small-winged, brightly colored, and feathered, then it can fly." The result is, "If something is feathered, then it can fly."

Specialization. Once some reasonably strong rules have developed in the system by generalization or other means, other techniques can be used to refine the emerging default hierarchy. The need for useful rules to model the environment propels the system to generalize, but the rules may later produce erroneous predictions. It would be wasteful simply to abandon the old rules, however, since the accumulated knowledge can be transformed, and protected, by specialization.

When a strong rule is identified as the source of an error, an overgeneralization may have been detected. The rule's condition is satisfied by the situation, but the result of the rule's action is not satisfactory. For example, the condition of the rule "If something is an animal with wings, then it can fly" may be satisfied by *penguin*, yielding an erroneous expectation. This is exactly the situation in which we want to generate an exception rule by specialization.

In the above example, we want to generate such rules as "If something is a penguin, then it cannot fly," or "If something is a fat, small-winged, swimming animal, then it cannot fly." (The latter is a rule that itself admits further exceptions.) Such rules have a more specific condition than the parent, and a different action (in Anderson's, 1983, terms, *action discriminations*). In addition, it may be useful to generate rules such as "If something is an animal with wings, and not fat, small-winged, and a swimmer, then it can fly," which specify the same action as did the parent but add new restrictions to the condition (in Anderson's terms, *condition discriminations*). The net effect of specialization is the induction of a more refined default hierarchy of rules. The ACT* model of learning (Anderson, 1983) makes use of condition-simplifying generalization in combination with specialization to account for inductive learning in complex domains, such as the acquisition of English syntax.

Specialization illustrates the importance of the unusualness heuristic, described earlier. Note that, in the formation of a new rule to predict the conditions for flightlessness in birds, the unusual properties of penguins, such as their shape and small wing size − properties not associated with typical birds − are likely to be selected. The heuristic of focusing on unusual properties has been invoked in work on topics ranging from animal conditioning (Holland et al., 1986, chap. 5), to human judgments of causation (Einhorn & Hogarth, 1986), to machine learning (Salzberg, 1985).

Instance-based generalization

A second kind of generalization proceeds not from rules but from instances. The classic example is the inference that all swans are white based on a few instances of objects that are swans and white. Philosophers since Aristotle have been greatly concerned with this kind of generalization, and it has been the focus of much recent work in artificial intelligence (e.g., Mitchell, 1982; Winston, 1975).

Evaluating possible generalizations. A major question to be asked about instance-based generalization is, How can we determine whether we have enough instances of a generalization to warrant its acceptance? Mill (1843/ 1974, p. 314) noticed that the required number of instances is not constant. He asked, "Why is a single instance, in some cases, sufficient for a complete induction, while in others myriads of concurring instances, without a single exception known or presumed, go such a very little way towards establishing a universal proposition?"

On the basis of psychological research on generalization among people, which we describe below, it appears that three major types of information are useful for evaluating the acceptability of a generalization that all A's are B (or, in a probabilistic case, that many A's are B). The first is simply the number of instances of A that have been found to be B. The second involves checking for possible counterexamples — things that are A but not B (Holyoak & Glass, 1975). The third is more complex, because it concerns the background knowledge an organism has about the statistical properties of the populations it is concerned to generalize. If the A's and B's are known to be highly invariant and seldom subject to random fluctuation, then generalization from few instances will be legitimate. Conversely, if A's and B's are subject to high variability or randomness, then generalization should take place only if there are many confirming instances.

Variability assessment and propensity to generalize. For a statistician, variability considerations are clearly relevant to the evaluation of possible generalizations, just as they are to categorization decisions. Given that empirical studies have established that people are able to learn degree of variability quite accurately, we can proceed to consider evidence that such variability information is in fact used in generalizing. A number of studies on the statistical aspects of generalization were conducted by Nisbett et al. (1983). One of these studies, described below, shows the influence of assumptions about variability. The subjects were given information about several novel kinds of objects and then asked to make generalizations about the objects:

Imagine that you are an explorer who has landed on a little known island in the Southeastern Pacific. You encounter several new animals, people, and objects. You observe the properties of your "samples" and you need to make guesses about how common these properties would be in other animals, people or objects of the same type.

Suppose you encounter a new bird, the shreeble. It is blue in color. What percent of all shreebles on the island do you expect to be blue?

Why did you guess this percent?

The subjects were also told that the shreeble was found to nest in a eucalyptus tree and were asked what percentage of all shreebles they expected to nest in eucalyptus trees.

The subjects were then told to imagine that they encountered a member of the "Barratos" tribe. He was brown and obese. The subjects were asked what percentage of all male Barratos they expected to be brown and what percentage they expected to be obese. Finally, the subjects were told that they had encountered a sample of a rare element called "floridium." It was found to conduct electricity and to burn with a green flame when stretched out to a filament and heated to a very high temperature. The subjects were asked what percentage of all floridium they expected to conduct electricity and to burn with a green flame. There were two other experimental conditions. In one, the subjects were told that 3 samples of each object were encountered. In the other, the subjects were told that 20 samples of each object were encountered.

The reasons the subjects gave for proposing their estimates were coded according to their content. There were three basic types of response: (a) references to homogeneity of the kind of object with respect to the kind of property; (b) references to the heterogeneity or variability of the kind of object with respect to the kind of property, attributed to the existence of subkinds having different properties (e.g., male vs. female) or to some causal mechanism producing different properties (e.g., genetic mistakes) or to purely statistical variability ("Where birds nest is sometimes a matter of chance"); and (c) other sorts of responses, most of which were mere tautologies or other nonanswers.

The results were clear-cut. Figure 3.5 presents subjects' estimates of the percentage of objects of each kind that they would expect to have the attribute found in the sample. The subjects expected that essentially all floridium would have the properties of conductivity and of burning with a green flame. They also expected that essentially all Barratos would be brown. These expectations held regardless of the number of cases in the sample. In contrast, the subjects did not expect all shreebles to be blue or to nest in eucalyptus trees, even if 20 shreebles were observed. Subjects expected that an even smaller percentage of Barratos would be obese, and their beliefs about the percentage of obese Barratos were highly dependent on the number of cases in the sample.

The subjects' beliefs about the variability of the objects in question with

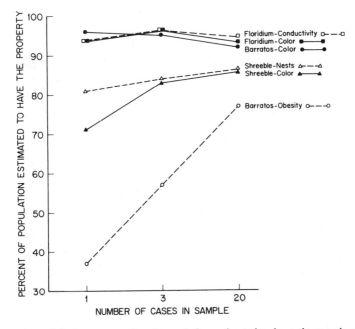

Figure 3.5. Percentage of each population estimated to have the sample property as a function of number of cases in the sample. From Nisbett, Krantz, Jepson and Kunda (1983).

respect to the property in question clearly determined this pattern of responses. The subjects reported believing that the properties of elements are invariant across samples and that isolated tribes people are homogenous with respect to color. They believed that bird types are only sometimes homogenous with respect to color and nesting location; and they believed that even isolated human groups are heterogeneous with respect to body weight. *Within* each point of the graph, individual differences in estimates of percentages were dependent on individual differences in beliefs about variability. Subjects who estimated higher percentages thought that the kind of object was not highly variable with respect to the kind of property.

For this simple type of generalization, then, people are capable of tempering the strength of their conclusions about kinds of objects according to the degree of homogeneity they expect. At one extreme, a fairly strong generalization may be formed on the basis of a single case, if homogeneity is presumed. At the other extreme, when great heterogeneity is presumed, even a fairly large number of cases will not result in a strong generalization.

It should also be clear, however, that people do not always generalize in a way that a statistician would endorse. Sometimes people do not temper their generalizations on the basis of the variability of the objects in question, and sometimes people are insensitive even to the number of instances. People's statistical failings are often seen in high relief in the context of generalizations about social objects (Nisbett et al., 1983; Nisbett and Ross, 1980). People sometimes make confident generalizations about highly variable social objects on the basis of very little evidence. For example, after a brief interview with a person, some people may feel that they have enough information to predict confidently how the person will behave in a wide variety of situations (Kunda & Nisbett, 1986). Yet the unstructured interview gives them very little basis for predicting behavior of any kind, whether school performance or job performance or even future congeniality.

People's violations of statistical requirements when they generalize about social objects seem to be understable in terms of the encoding constraint. Social variables are difficult to encode unambiquously, and sometimes it is difficult even to know what units one ought to use. Whereas the color of an object or the obesity of a person is clearly a codable variable, friendliness, honesty, or leadership qualities are much more difficult to code, and the choice of units with which to code such variables is even more problematic. Since coding and unitization pose a problem, variability estimates are difficult, if not impossible to make. Because variability estimates are essential for the use of statistical rules such as the law of large numbers, people's generalizations about social objects are often erroneous and overconfident.

Analogy

Both bottom-up category formation and instance-based generalization depend in part on comparison among multiple examples. This comparison can be very simple, as when one compares the colors of two swans. *Analogy*, in its more sophisticated forms, involves more complex comparisons involving multiple similar relations among objects that also have salient differences. Analogy and metaphor (which Miller, 1979, analyzes in terms of analogy) are often viewed as important sources of creative ideas, enabling one to apply knowledge acquired in one domain (the *source*) to another domain (the *target*). In this section, we examine the role of analogy in induction.

Solving analogy problems

One type of analogy problem is often encountered in intelligence tests. This is the "proportional" analogy, which has the general form $A : B : : C : D$, where the task is typically to select the most appropriate D term from a set of alternatives (see Figure 3.6). Such problems, along with such related tasks as sequence extrapolation (Kotovsky & Simon, 1973; Restle, 1970; Simon & Kotovsky, 1963) and Raven's Progressive Matrices Test (Hunt, 1973), have received considerable attention from psychologists. Indeed, tasks of the in-

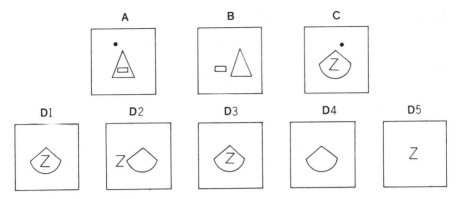

Figure 3.6. Geometric analogies examined by Evans (1968).

telligence test variety have been the major focus of psychological research on induction as the topic has been traditionally construed.

An early model of analogy problem solving was developed by Evans (1968). The model was developed as a project in artificial intelligence; however, certain general aspects of the analysis have been carried over into psychological models (Sternberg, 1977), and some predictions have been supported by studies of humans working on the problems Evans's computer program could solve (Mulholland, Pellegrino, & Glaser, 1980). Evans worked with geometric analogies of the sort depicted in Figure 3.6. The computer is given descriptions of the diagrams, which specify the locations of such features as straight lines, curved lines, and closed figures. Using general geometric knowledge, the computer elaborates this knowledge by deriving relations between components of the diagrams, such as "above," "inside of," and "left out."

The computer then matches the components of the A diagram with components of B, using a measure of similarity to determine which components should match. In the problem in Figure 3.6, the large triangle and small rectangle in A match the corresponding components of B, and the dot in A fails to find any match. The next step is to generate rules that might transform A into B. The potential rules are based on such operations as addition, deletion, and changes in location. Thus, A can be transformed into B if the rectangle is moved out of the triangle and placed to the left of it and the dot is deleted. These rules may be tentative, because in some cases the set of matches between A and B will be incomplete or ambiguous.

The components of C are then matched with the components of each of the D alternatives in a similar fashion. The candidate rules for taking A into B are used to constrain the search for rules that could take C into the D alternatives. The basic idea is to find generalized versions of the candidate rules for the source domain (A to B) that can also apply in the target do-main (C to D). The answer to the analogy problem is found by selecting the D alternative for which the possible rules are maximally similar to those proposed for the source. Thus, in our example problem, the best answer is D2. Note that we can transform C into D2 by deleting the dot (the location of which is different in C than in A) and moving a Z (rather than a rectan-gle) out of a three-sided curved form (rather than a triangle). The basis of the analogy can be captured by generalized rules such as "Delete the dot" and "Move the small figure out of the large three-sided figure." The close link between analogy and generalization highlighted in Evans's model has been emphasized in later work on the use of analogy in problem solving, to be discussed below.

Analogical problem solving

Although work on solving analogy problems provided an initial basis for understanding analogy as an inductive mechanism, the paradigm fails to ad-dress several important aspects of the everyday use of analogy in such tasks as solving problems and developing explanations. One important part of using an analogy is retrieving a useful source analog from memory. Some aspects of the target situation must provide retrieval cues to remind the problem solver of an analog (Schank, 1982). In contrast, in an analogy prob-lem, the source $A : B$ is simply given. Also, a person is asked to solve the analogy problem simply for its own sake, rather than in the service of some other goal, such as finding the solution to a different problem.

Analogies between remote problems

Gick and Holyoak (1980, 1983) investigated the use of somewhat remote analogies in solving relatively ill defined problems. The problem they stud-ied most extensively was the "radiation problem" made famous by the Ge-stalt psychologist Karl Duncker (1945):

Suppose you are a doctor faced with a patient who has a malignant tumor in his stomach. It is impossible to operate on the patient, but unless the tumor is destroyed the patient will die. There is a kind of ray that at a sufficiently high intensity can destroy the tumor. Unfortunately, at this intensity the healthy tissue that the rays pass through on the way to the tumor will also be destroyed. At lower intensities the rays are harmless to healthy tissue, but will not affect the tumor either. How can the rays be used to destroy the tumor without injuring the healthy tissue?

People often run out of ideas when they try to solve this problem. They simply do not have rules for developing a solution directly and hence find themselves at an impasse. This is just the kind of situation in which an anal-ogy could be used to generate rules that suggest actions. To test this possi-bility, Gick and Holyoak (1980) attempted to demonstrate that variations in the solution to an available source analog can lead subjects to generate qualitatively different solutions to the target. The experimenters provided their subjects with a potential source analog in the form of a story about the predicament of a general who wished to capture a fortress located in the center of a country. Many roads radiated outward from the fortress, but these were mined so that, although small groups could pass over them safely, any large group would detonate the mines. Yet the general had to get all of his large army to the fortress in order to launch a successful attack. The general's situation was thus essentially parallel to that of the doctor in the radiation problem.

Different versions of the story described different solutions to the military problem. For example, in one version the general discovered an unguarded road to the fortress and sent the entire army along it; in another version the general divided his men into small groups and dispatched them simultaneously down several roads to converge on the fortress. All of the subjects were then asked to suggest solutions to the radiation problem, using the military story as an aid. Those who read the former version were inclined to suggest sending the rays down an "open passage," such as the esophagus, so as to reach the tumor while avoiding contact with healthy tissue. Subjects who read the story in which the general divided his army into small groups were inclined to suggest a "convergence" solution — directing weak rays at the tumor from different directions. Across many comparable experiments, Gick and Holyoak found that about 75% of tested college students generated the convergence solution after receiving the corresponding military story and a hint to apply it. In contrast, only about 10% of students generated this solution in the absence of a source analog, even though most subjects agreed that the solution was an effective one once it was described to them.

Gick and Holyoak also found that subjects' ability to perceive the analogy fell far short of their ability to make use of it once it was pointed out. If they were not prompted to apply the analogy, only about 30% of the subjects generated the convergence solution to the radiation problem immediately after having read the multiple-approach-routes story. This result indicates that the initial reminding process required to access a source analog may often fail to identify a good source analog that is superficially dissimilar to the target. Later research demonstrated that increased similarity can lead to much higher rates of spontaneous analogical transfer in problem solving (Holyoak & Koh, 1987). The factors that influence analogical transfer have been the focus of much theoretical discussion in both psychology and artificial intelligence (Carbonell, 1983, 1986; Gentner, 1983; Holyoak, 1984).

Inducing a problem category

The abstract structure common to the two analogs — the idea of several converging weak forces serving the function of a single large force — can become the basis for inducing a representation of the general *type* of problem for which convergence solutions are possible. The induction of a problem category may be a side effect of using an analogy to solve a problem (Winston, 1980). Gick and Holyoak (1983) found that the induction of a problem category plays a major role in successful transfer across remote problem domains. Two groups of subjects read two convergence stories (e.g., the military story described earlier and a fire-fighting story in which converging sources of fire retardant extinguished a large blaze). Other groups read a single convergence story and a disanalogous story. All subjects summarized each story and described the points of similarity between the paired stories. The latter task was intended to trigger a mapping between the two stories, which would have the incidental effect of leading to the induction of an explicit representation of the shared schematic structure. All subjects then attempted to solve the ray problem, both before and after receiving a hint to consider the stories. Gick and Holyoak found that the subjects in the two-analog groups were significantly more likely to produce the convergence solution, both before and after receiving the hint, than were subjects in the one-analog groups. Gick and Holyoak interpreted these and other more detailed results as indicating that the induction of an explicit schema facilitates transfer. As Gick and Holyoak (1983) argued, there are important theoretical reasons to expect an abstract problem category to yield greater interdomain transfer than would a single concrete source analog. A problem category will carry rules for classifying novel instances, so that subsequent examples of the problem type can be categorized and solved by means of prestored general rules rather than by the execution of the less direct analogy mechanism.

Analogy in science

In scientific domains, analogy provides an additional top-down mechanism for concept formation. Scientific theorists working in a problematic new domain often look to areas they already understand as a source of transportable concepts and problem-solving techniques. An excellent illustration is the wave theory of light. Those who developed this theory often relied on analogies between light and sound, the latter of which they already understood in terms of wave propagation. They adopted variations of rules and concepts from the theory of sound that enabled them to solve problems in the domain of light. The theory of sound is based on the notion that sound consists of waves, from which one can predict that sound will propagate and reflect; the mapping to light generated the hypothesis that light also consists of waves, leading to the prediction that light will propagate and reflect much like sound.

Similarly, the analogy between natural selection and the artificial selection performed by breeders was important for the development and justification of Darwin's theory of evolution. Darwin argued that, just as breeders modify populations by selecting for traits produced by natural variations, so nature produces new species by selection arising from the struggle for survival. Rules and concepts about the practice of breeding were thus carried over to a new domain. As we saw earlier, Darwin used conceptual combination in conjunction with analogy to develop his natural selection theory. Analogy typically operates in combination with the other induction mechanisms we have discussed.

Improving inductive inference

As we have frequently pointed out in this chapter, people habitually make errors in the process of inductive reasoning. Are these errors the inevitable result of the trade-offs incurred by the use of imperfect heuristics under conditions in which severe constraints are usually present?

Probably they are not. At any rate, it is possible to reduce the errors that people make in at least two major ways. First, people can be helped to encode events, especially social events, in ways that make it easier for them to apply useful heuristics, especially statistical heuristics. For example, Nisbett et al. (1983) presented subjects with a problem about a high school senior who had to choose between two colleges that were similar in terms of prestige, distance from his home, and cost. He had several friends at A, who uniformly liked their school, and several friends at B, most of whom were dissatisfied on various social and intellectual grounds. He visited both schools for a day, and his own feelings, based on conversations with several people, including a few professors, and his observations of some classes, were different from those of his friends. He was impressed with B and was put off by the things he saw at A. Which school should he choose? The overwhelming majority of college student subjects said that the student should choose the school *he* liked, rather than the one his friends liked.

Other subjects were given the same problem but were helped to encode the problem as one of sampling from a population. They were told that, the night before he went to each school, the student drew up a list of all the people, classes, and places he wanted to visit. Because there were many more items on his list than he could hope to see in only a day, he randomly picked a group of people and places to concentrate on. The subjects who read his version were much more inclined than the subjects who read the first version to say that the student should go to the school his friends liked. This list manipulation helped the subjects to see that the number of students, professors, and classes was immense, whereas the number of people and places that could be visited in a single day was very small and hence the events of that day could easily have been atypical. Thus, people can improve their inductive reasoning by encoding events in such a way that statistical heuristics can be applied to the process.

Perhaps an even more powerful way to improve inductive reasoning is to improve people's statistical heuristics. Work by Fong, Krantz, and Nisbett (1986) shows that statistical training can have a profound effect on the way people reason about everyday events. They gave the following problem to college students who had or had not taken a statistics course, to graduate students who had taken one or more statistics courses, and to PhDs who had had many graduate-level statistics courses. A manufacturer's representative whose job took her to many cities was also a gourmet. Whenever she ate an excellent meal in a restaurant she returned to the restaurant as often as possible. However, she was usually disappointed, because subsequent meals were rarely as good as the first. The subjects were asked to explain why they thought this was the case. Their answers were coded as to whether they contained any recognition of the statistical aspects of the problem. Some answers were purely deterministic − for example, "Maybe the chefs change a lot" or "Maybe her expectations are too high." Other answers reflected some appreciation of the random element of dining out: "Maybe it was just by chance that she got such a good meal the first time." Still other answers recognized not merely the chance aspects but modeled the problem in sampling terms: "There are more restaurants where you could get an excellent meal occasionally than there are restaurants that consistently serve excellent meals, so the odds are she won't get an excellent meal twice in a row at the same place."

Other subjects were given a different version of the same problem. The protagonist works in Japan but does not speak the language and chooses her meals by pointing a pencil randomly at an item. It was reasoned that, like the list manipulation in the college choice problem above, the random choice manipulation would help subjects to code the restaurant problem as a statistical one involving samples from a population.

The effects of education and of the random cue manipulation can be seen in Figure 3.7. Graph A presents the frequency of statistical answers as a function of education. It can be seen that subjects with no statistical training virtually never gave a statistical answer to the problem lacking the cue and that more training was associated with a greater frequency of statistical answers. In the case of the problem containing a randomness cue, statistical answers were much more common and, again, statistical training increased the frequency. The quality of statistical answers, presented in Graph B of Figure 3.7, exhibited a somewhat different pattern. It improved with training for both problems, but the randomness cue did not improve quality. Apparently, proper encoding only helps to trigger the use of statistical rules; it cannot produce better answers than can be derived from the rules that a person possesses.

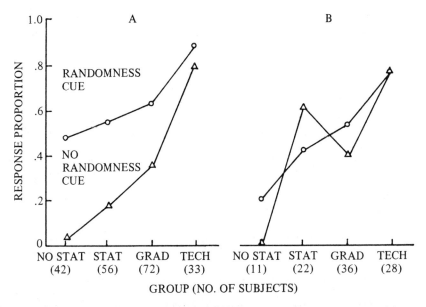

Figure 3.7. Frequency of statistical answers (A) and quality of statistical answers (B) to the restaurant problem as a function of presence versus absence of probabilistic cue and level of statistical training. (No stat = college students with no statistics course; stat = college students with one or more statistics courses; grad = graduate students in psychology, most of whom had had two or more courses in statistics and methodology; tech = technical staff at a research laboratory.)

Other work by Fong and his colleagues has shown that even brief training sessions in the abstract nature of the law of large numbers improves people's statistical reasoning about a very broad range of everyday events. This work suggests not only that people's rules can be improved, but that people can apply very abstract rules to concrete events as long as they can encode the events in ways that enable them to apply the rules.

Comparable work has been done by Cheng and her colleagues (1986) on the effects of teaching regulation schemata. The found that even brief training sessions on the abstract nature of the obligation rule helped people to solve a variety of concrete everyday problems. (In contrast, even an entire semester of training in formal logic did not improve reasoning on such problems. This finding raises questions about the extent to which people actually rely on formal logic in solving problems, because all of the problems Cheng et al. gave could be readily solved by the application of elementary formal rules.) Lehman, Lempert, and Nisbett (1987) found that training in such fields as medicine and the law, which emphasize reasoning concerning obligations, improved reasoning about problems to which the obligation schema could be applied. This work again suggests that people's reasoning can be improved, even by abstract training techniques, as long as the rule system is similar to those that people possess in at least a rudimentary, intuitive way. A task for the future is to find which rules can be taught, and how, to produce the greatest improvement in reasoning.

References

Anderson, J. R. (1983). *The architecture of cognition*. Cambridge, MA: Harvard University Press.
Anderson, J. R., Kline, P. J., & Beasley, C. M. (1979). A general learning theory and its application to schema abstraction. In G. H. Bower (Ed.), *The psychology of learning and motivation*, (Vol. 13). New York: Academic Press.
Billman, D. (1983). *Inductive learning of syntactic categories*. Unpublished doctoral dissertation, University of Michigan, Ann Arbor.
Braine, M. D. S. (1978). On the relation between the natural logic of reasoning and standard logic. *Psychological Review, 85*, 1–21.
Brown, R. (1973). *A first language*. Cambridge, MA: Harvard University Press.
Bruner, J. S., Goodnow, J. J., & Austin, G. A. (1956). *A study of thinking*. New York: Wiley.
Carbonell, J. (1983). Learning by analogy: Formulating and generalizing plans from past experience. In R. Michalski, J. Carbonell, & T. Mitchell (Eds.), *Machine learning: An artificial intelligence approach*. Palo Alto, CA: Tioga Press.
   (1986). Derivational analogy: A theory of reconstructive problem solving and expertise acquisition. In R. Michalski, J. Carbonell, & T. Mitchell (Eds.), *Machine learning: An artificial intelligence approach* (Vol 2). Los Altos, Calif.: Kaufmann.
Chapman, L. J., & Chapman, J. P. (1967). Genesis of popular but erroneous diagnostic observations. *Journal of Abnormal Psychology, 72*, 193–204.
   (1969). Illusory correlation as an obstacle to the use of valid psychodiagnostic signs. *Journal of Abnormal Psychology, 74*, 271–80.
Cheng, P. W., & Holyoak, K. J. (1985). Pragmatic reasoning schemas. *Cognitive Psychology, 17*, 391–416.
Cheng, P. W., Holyoak, K. J., Nisbett, R. E., & Oliver, L. M. (1986). Pragmatic versus syntactic approaches to training deductive reasoning. *Cognitive Psychology, 18*, 293–328.
Chi, M., Feltovich, P., & Glaser, R. (1981). Categorization and representation of physics problems by experts and novices. *Cognitive Science, 5*, 121–52.
Darden, L. (1983). Artificial intelligence and philosophy of science: Reasoning by analogy in theory construction. In P. Asquith & T. Nickles (Eds.), *PSA 1982* (Vol. 2). East Lansing, MI: Philosophy of Science Association.
Dietterich, T., & Michalski, R. (1983). A comparative review of selected methods for learning from examples. In R. Michalski, J. Carbonell, & T. Mitchell (Eds.), *Machine learning: An artificial intelligence approach*. Palo Alto, CA: Tioga Press.
Duncker, K. (1945). On problem solving. *Psychological Monographs, 58* (No. 270).
Einhorn, H. J., & Hogarth, R. M. (1981). Behavioral decision theory: Processes of judgment and choice. *Annual Review of Psychology, 32*, 53–88.
Einhorn, H. J., & Hogarth, R. M. (1986). Judging probable cause. *Psychological Bulletin, 99*, 3–19.
Evans, T. G. (1968). A program for the solution of a class of geometric-analogy intelligence test questions. In M. Minsky (Ed.), *Semantic information processing*. Cambridge, MA: MIT Press.
Fahlman, S. (1979). *NETL: A system for representing and using real-world knowledge*. Cambridge, MA: MIT Press.
Flannagan, M. J., Fried, L. S., & Holyoak, K. J. (1986). Distributional expectations and the induction of category structure. *Journal of Experimental Psychology: Learning, Memory and Cognition, 12*, 241–56.

Fong, G. T., Krantz, D. H., & Nisbett, R. E. (1986). The effects of statistical training on thinking about everyday problems. *Cognitive Psychology, 18*, 253–92.

Fried, L. S., & Holyoak, K. J. (1984). Induction of category distributions: A framework for classification learning. *Journal of Experimental Psychology: Learning, Memory, and Cognition, 10*, 234–57.

Garcia, J., McGowan, B. K., Ervin, F., & Koelling, R. (1968). Cues: Their relative effectiveness as reinforcers. *Science, 160*, 794–5.

Gentner, D. (1983). Structure-mapping: A theoretical framework for analogy. *Cognitive Science, 7*, 155–70.

Gick, M. L., & Holyoak, K. J. (1980). Analogical problem solving. *Cognitive Psychology, 12*, 306–55.

(1983). Schema induction and analogical transfer. *Cognitive Psychology, 15*, 1–38.

Glass, A. L., & Holyoak, K. J. (1986). *Cognition* (2nd ed.). New York: Random House.

Hayes-Roth, R., & McDermott, J. (1978). An interference matching technique for inducing abstractions. *Communications of the ACM, 21*, 401–10.

Holland, J. H., Holyoak, K. J., Nisbett, R. E., & Thagard, P. R. (1986). *Induction: Processes of inference, learning, and discovery.* Cambridge, MA: MIT Press.

Holyoak, K. J. (1984). Analogical thinking and human intelligence. In R. J. Sternberg (Ed.), *Advances in the psychology of human intelligence* (Vol. 2). Hillsdale, NJ: Erlbaum.

Holyoak, K. J., & Glass, A. L. (1975). The role of contradictions and counterexamples in the rejection of false sentences. *Journal of Verbal Learning and Verbal Behavior, 14*, 215–39.

Holyoak, K. J., & Koh, K. (1987). Surface and structural similarity in analogical transfer. *Memory & Cognition, 15*, 332–340.

Holyoak, K. J., Koh, K., & Nisbett, R. E. (1987). Conditioning and learning within rule-based default hierarchies. In *Proceedings of the Ninth Annual Conference of the Cognitive Science Society.*

Homa, D., & Vosburgh, R. (1976). Category breadth and the abstraction of prototypical information. *Journal of Experimental Psychology: Human Learning and Memory, 2*, 322–30.

Hunt, E. (1973). Quote the raven? Nevermore! In L. W. Gregg (Ed.), *Knowledge and cognition.* Hillsdale, NJ: Erlbaum.

Jennings, D., Amabile, T. M., & Ross, L. (1982). Informal covariation assessment: Data-based vs. theory-based judgments. In A. Tversky, D. Kahneman, & P. Slovic (Eds.), *Judgment under uncertainty: Heuristics and biases.* Cambridge University Press.

Johnson-Laird, P. N. (1975). Models of deduction. In R. J. Falmagne (Ed.), *Reasoning: Representation and process.* New York: Wiley.

(1983). *Mental models.* Cambridge, MA: Harvard University Press.

Kahneman, D., Slovic, P., & Tversky, A. (1982). *Judgment under uncertainty: Heuristics and biases.* Cambridge University Press.

Kamin, L. J. (1968). "Attention-like" processes in classical conditioning. In M. R. Jones (Ed), *Miami Symposium on the Prediction of Behavior: Aversive Stimulation.* University of Miami Press.

Kelley, H. H. (1972). Causal schemata and the attribution process. In E. E. Jones, D. E. Kanouse, H. H. Kelley, R. E. Nisbett, S. Valins, & B. Weiner (Eds.), *Attribution: Perceiving the causes of behavior.* Morristown, NJ: General Learning Press.

(1973). The process of causal attribution. *American Psychologist, 28*, 107–28.

Kotovsky, K., & Simon, H. A. (1973). Empirical tests of a theory of human acquisition of concepts for sequential events. *Cognitive Psychology, 4*, 399–424.

Kunda, Z., & Nisbett, R. E. (1986). The psychometrics of everyday life. *Cognitive Psychology, 18*, 195–224.

Langley, P., Bradshaw, G., & Simon, H., (1983). Rediscovering chemistry with the BACON system. In R. Michalski, J. Carbonell, & T. Mitchell (Eds.), *Machine Learning: An artificial intelligence approach.* Palo Alto, CA: Tioga Press.

Lehman, D., Lempert, R., & Nisbett, R. E. (1987). *The effects of graduate education on reasoning: Formal discipline and thinking about everyday-life events.* Unpublished manuscript, University of British Columbia.

Maratsos, M., & Chalkley, A. (1980). The internal language of children's syntax: The ontogenesis and representation of syntactic categories. In K. E. Nelson (Ed.), *Children's language* (Vol. 2). New York: Gardner Press.

McArthur, L. Z., & Post, D. (1977). Figural emphasis and person perception. *Journal of Experimental Social Psychology, 13,* 520–35.

Medin, D. L., & Schaffer, M. M. (1978). Context theory of classification learning. *Psychological Review, 85,* 207–38.

Mill, J. S. (1974). *A system of logic ratiocinative and inductive.* University of Toronto Press. (Original work published 1843.)

Miller, G. A. (1979). Images and models, similes and metaphors. In A. Ortony (Ed.), *Metaphor and thought.* Cambridge, MA: Cambridge Press.

Mitchell, T. M. (1982). Generalization as search. *Artificial Intelligence, 18,* 203–26.

Mulholland, T. M., Pellegrino, J. W., & Glaser, R. (1980). Components of geometric analogy solution. *Cognitive Psychology, 12,* 252–84.

Murphy, G. L., & Medin, D. L. (1985). The role of theories in conceptual coherence. *Psychological Review, 92,* 289–316.

Newell, A. (1973). Production systems: Models of control structures. In W. G. Chase (Ed.), *Visual information processing.* New York: Academic Press.

Newell, A., & Simon, H. A. (1972). *Human problem solving.* Englewood Cliffs, NJ: Prentice-Hall.

Nisbett, R. E., Krantz, D. H., Jepson, D., & Kunda, Z. (1983). The use of statistical heuristics in everyday inductive reasoning. *Psychological Review, 90,* 339–63.

Nisbett, R. E., & Ross, L. (1980). *Human inference: Strategies and shortcomings of social judgment.* Englewood Cliffs, NJ: Prentice-Hall.

Osherson, D. N., & Smith, E. E. (1981). On the adequacy of prototype theory as a theory of concepts. *Cognition, 9,* 35–58.

Peirce, C. S. (1931–58). *Collected papers,* 8 Vols. Edited by C. Hartshorne, P. Weiss, & A. Burks. Cambridge, MA: Harvard University Press.

Posner, M. I., & Keele, S. W. (1968). On the genesis of abstract ideas. *Journal of Experimental Psychology, 77,* 353–63.

Quine, W. V. O. (1969). *Ontological relativity and other essays.* New York: Columbia University Press.

Reed, S. K. (1972). Pattern recognition and categorization. *Cognitive Psychology, 3,* 383–407.

Rescorla, R. A. (1972). Informational variables in Pavlovian conditioning. In G. H. Bower (Ed.), *The psychology of learning and motivation.* New York: Academic Press.

Rescorla, R. A., & Wagner, A. R. (1972). A theory of Pavlovian conditioning: Variations in the effectiveness of reinforcement and nonreinforcement. In A. H. Black & W. F. Prokasy (Eds.), *Classical conditioning: Vol. 2. Current theory and research.* New York: Appleton-Century-Crofts.

Restle, F. (1970). Theory of serial pattern learning: Structural trees. *Psychological Review, 69,* 329–43.

Riley, M. S., Greeno, J. G., & Heller, J. I. (1983). Development of children's problem-solving ability in arithmetic. In H. P. Ginsberg (Ed.), *The development of mathematical thinking.* New York: Academic Press.

Rosch, E. (1978). Principles of categorization. In E. Rosch & B. B. Lloyd (Eds.), *Cognition and categorization.* Hillsdale, NJ: Erlbaum.

Rosch, E., Mervis, C. B., Gray, W., Johnson, D., & Boyes-Braem, P. (1976). Basic objects in natural categories. *Cognitive Psychology, 7,* 573–605.

Salzberg, S. (1985). Heuristics for inductive learning. In *Proceedings of the Ninth Joint Conference on Artificial Intelligence.* Los Altos, CA: Kaufmann.

Schank, R. C. (1982). *Dynamic memory.* Cambridge University Press.

Seligman, M. E. P. (1970). On the generality of the laws of learning. *Psychological Review, 77,* 406–18.

Siegler, R. S. (1983). How knowledge influences learning. *American Scientist, 71,* 631–8.

Simon, H. A., & Kotovsky, K. (1963). Human acquisition of concepts for sequential patterns. *Psychological Review, 70,* 534−46.

Smith, E. E., & Medin, D. (1981). *Categories and concepts.* Cambridge, MA: Harvard University Press.

Smith, E. E., & Osherson, D. (1984). Conceptual combination with prototype concepts. *Cognitive Science, 8,* 337−61.

Sternberg, R. J. (1977). Component processes in analogical reasoning. *Psychological Review, 84,* 353−78.

Taylor, S. E., & Fiske, S. T. (1978). Salience, attention and attribution: Top of the head phenomena. In L. Berkowitz (Eds.), *Advances in experimental social psychology* (Vol. 11). New York: Academic Press.

Thagard, P. (1984). Conceptual combination and scientific discovery. In P. Asquith & P. Kitcher (Eds.), *PSA 1984* (Vol. 1). East Lansing, MI: Philosophy of Science Association.

Wason, P. C. (1966). Reasoning. In B. M. Foss (Ed.), *New horizons in psychology.* Harmondsworth: Penguin Books.

(1983). Realism and rationality in the selection task. In J. St. B. T. Evans (Ed.), *Thinking and reasoning: Psychological approaches.* London: Routledge & Kegan Paul.

Winston, P. H. (1975). Learning structural descriptions from examples. In P. H. Winston (Ed.), *The psychology of computer vision.* New York: McGraw-Hill.

(1978). Learning by creating transfer frames. *Artificial Intelligence, 10,* 147−72.

(1980). Learning and reasoning by analogy. *Communications of the ACM, 23,* 689−703.

4   Thinking about causality

Miriam W. Schustack

An understanding of causality is central to our ability to deal successfully with the complex world in which we live. We have to be able to figure out cause-and-effect relationships in both directions – analyzing what causes the desirable and undesirable events we experience and analyzing the consequences of each of our actions – so that we can sustain or reproduce the desirable outcomes and terminate or avoid the undesirable ones. From the infant's progress in making sense of the overwhelming, incomprehensible, confusing, disorganized profusion of events in his or her environment to the efforts of the research biologist to understand how the AIDS virus impairs the human immune system, the comprehension of causal relationships plays a pivotal role in our lives. We are strongly focused on seeking causal explanations and tend to impose causal interpretations on events that occur close together in space and time, regardless of their underlying relationship (e.g., Michotte, 1963).

One of the important early milestones in intellectual development is that point at which the infant begins to recognize cause-and-effect relationships. According to Piaget, this ability is acquired in its most rudimentary form late in infancy; it is only after considerable experience with the world (most of the first year of life) that a baby can comprehend that actions have consequences. In the beginning, this understanding is essentially limited to the most direct sorts of physical causality: Banging on a pot with a spoon causes noise, or pushing a toy off the high-chair tray causes it to fall to the ground.

The perfecting of causal reasoning is not an accomplishment of childhood, however. Despite their impressive powers to make sophisticated causal inferences with limited and often confusing evidence, even intelligent and educated adults tend to deviate from accurate causal reasoning in many kinds of tasks. This chapter focuses on how people carry out the complex job of inferring causality in a variety of contexts and how aspects of this performance lead to both the strengths and the weaknesses observed in causal reasoning.

Philosophical background

Before we discuss the psychology of human causal reasoning, it will be helpful to look briefly at the concept of causality itself. Philosophers have been grappling for centuries with the definition of *cause* and with methods for

92

determining whether (or to what extent) a given outcome is caused by some action or event.

One approach to the definition of causality is to describe it in terms of necessary and sufficient conditions. A necessary condition for some outcome is a condition that must always be present for the outcome to be present, that is, a condition whose absence will prevent that outcome. For example, the presence of oxygen is a necessary condition for combustion. If there is no oxygen, there is no combustion. If there is combustion, we know there must be oxygen. Of course, combustion does not always occur given the presence of oxygen – oxygen is not a sufficient condition for combustion. A sufficient condition is one whose presence guarantees that the outcome will occur, that is, a condition that can never be present in the absence of the outcome. For example, going without food and water for a month is a sufficient condition for a person's death. If the outcome did not occur (and the person is still alive), we know that the person did not go without food and water for a month. Of course, a person can die in many other ways – the occurrence of the outcome does not allow us to conclude that a particular sufficient cause of that outcome is present. No particular sufficient cause is necessary for the occurrence of the outcome, and necessary causes are not sufficient for the occurrence of the outcome. A third class of conditions consists of those that are both necessary and sufficient for the outcome. Some philosophical treatments of causality (e.g., Skyrms, 1966) take this distinction to be essential to any discussion of causation, requiring any proposal of methods of determining causality to specify the kind of causal condition (necessary, sufficient, or both necessary and sufficient) that is involved.

Other philosophers take a more pragmatic approach, which seems much closer to our everyday, informal, natural-language sense of the meaning of *cause*. According to this view, a cause is a condition whose presence makes a critical difference to the occurrence of an outcome: an "incident or action which, in the presence of those conditions that usually prevail, made the difference between the occurrence or nonoccurrence of the event" (Copi, 1978). This definition seems to capture more of the psychological sense of *cause*. If you asked someone what had caused a recent explosion at the fireworks warehouse, you would probably accept an answer like "The night watchman dropped a lit cigarette," as an adequate explanation of the cause, even though that would not strictly be either a necessary or a sufficient condition. And you might be quite unsatisfied with answers like "There was oxygen in the air inside the warehouse" (which would be a necessary condition) or "Many of the fireworks ignited within a short period of time" (which would be a sufficient condition). The definition of *cause* given above, with its inclusion of the notion that "the conditions that usually prevail" are not in themselves good candidates for the cause, captures some of the essense of why these answers differ in their acceptability as causal explanations. A more formal version of this notion, acknowledging the complexity of necessity and sufficiency relations in real-world causation, is attempted by Mackie (1965).

Several methods for inferring causality have been proposed in the philosophical literature. They are relevant to the psychological study of causal reasoning because they provide some normative models (prescriptions for ideal performance) against which human performance can be judged. Unlike the situation in many other domains of logic, there is no single accepted set of procedures for the valid determination of causality. David Hume (1739/1888) proposed a set of "rules by which to judge of causes and effects," basically a set of rules for diagnosing the existence of a causal relationship. According to Hume, in order to know what leads to what, one needs an "experimental method of reasoning."

Hume's notion was developed by John Stuart Mill (1843) into a set of "methods of experimental inquiry," often called "Mill's canons." These methods can be generally characterized as a set of procedures by which it is possible to determine a necessary or a sufficient cause of some outcome, given complete information about the presence and absence of all (previously identified) potential causes and the presence and absence of the outcome in each of many observed situations. Given a complete listing of the circumstances in each observed situation, the methods make it possible to compute the necessary or the sufficient cause by a process of elimination. For example, by means of one of Mill's methods, the "Direct Method of Agreement," we can isolate a necessary cause of some outcome by listing situations in which the possible causes that are present and those that are absent are varied and the outcome is observed to occur (or to fail to occur). Any of the possible causes that are absent in any situation in which the outcome occurs are eliminated from consideration, since they cannot be necessary causes. This process is continued until only a single possible cause, which is always present when the outcome is present, is isolated; the unique condition that "agrees" with the outcome is the cause. The logic underlying Mill's approach has much in common with the standard scientific method of controlled experimentation, the goal of which is to find the cause responsible for some observable outcome.

Normative models and human performance

Three main problems arise in applying this type of approach to people's normal causal reasoning: It neglects the critical processes of generating or identifying candidate causes (causal hypotheses), it ignores the usual incompleteness of the set of observed or observable situations in the real world, and it ignores the limitations of human cognitive abilities. Each of these problems is discussed in this section.

First, the success of these methods requires that the set of potentially causal conditions be well defined, relatively small, and known to the reasoner and that the actual (true) cause be included in the set. The methods in themselves provide no guidance for this critical and difficult process of hypothesis generation. If we analyze naturalistic causal reasoning within this framework, we see that many of its observed shortcomings arise at precisely this point, when people fail to include the true cause in the set of potential causes. In the same vein, what is striking about many major scientific discoveries is that the true cause came to be hypothesized — that someone managed to conceive of a causal role for some agent or entity that was previously unknown or thought to be irrelevant. The subsequent demonstration of the causal role of that hypothesized cause is often not as impressive an achievement. For example, once it had been hypothesized that a particular type of mosquito was responsible for transmitting yellow fever, proving its role was not very difficult. Formulating the hypothesis was the hard part of the task: Even after centuries of experience with the disease, no one apparently even considered the mosquito vector before Walter Reed. Unless the actual cause is included in the set of candidate causes, even the most assiduous application of causal reasoning procedures will not lead to the correct conclusion.

Conversely, one of the strengths of human causal reasoning (relative to mechanical approaches) is our ability to focus on potential causes for which we can construct some plausible underlying connection to the outcome. Including what will turn out to be the actual cause in the set of potential causes is required for success in causal analysis. In identifying the set of possible causes, we utilize much of our knowledge about the kinds of conditions that can reasonably be expected to cause particular kinds of outcomes. In making these decisions, we use heuristics that usually serve us well but can also mislead us. It is also at this stage that we use our knowledge of the world to exclude the normal, routine, usual, ever-present aspects of the observed situations from the infinite set of possible conditions that might be the cause. This allows us to pare down the set of potential causes and focus on the ones that are likely to differentiate the situations in which the outcome occurs from those in which it fails to occur. If we did not have this ability, every causal analysis that we attempted would be likely to include ever-present potential causes like the presence of gravity on earth, the vertebrate status of humankind, and the universality of the incest taboo, regardless of the relevance of these factors to the outcome of interest. Any of these potential causes might be good candidate causal hypotheses in a very limited set of situations. For example, if the question is why astronauts sometimes do and sometimes do not float around inside a spacecraft, the presence of gravity on earth is an important causal hypothesis that differentiates the occurrence of the outcome from its absence. In the majority of causal situations to be analyzed, however, considering the presence of gravity as a potential cause would be an unnecessary burden. The process of identifying potential causes of some outcome of interest is very complex in itself and is not well addressed in the normative approach.

The second major problem in applying these normative approaches to everyday causal reasoning is that we are not always blessed with nature's perfect experiment – we may not have information about every potential cause in every observed situation. Either we may be given incomplete information, or we may fail to identify some potential cause until after the opportunity to observe it in many of the situations is gone. In addition, the set of observed situations may not include enough variation in the set of conditions that are present and absent. (This is not a problem if the reasoner can design and carry out a controlled experiment, but it is a serious problem if the reasoner has information only about the set of situations that happened to occur and cannot construct sets of conditions to determine whether they will or will not produce the outcome.)

The third major problem is that these normative approaches make demands on memory and processing capacity that are unrealistic for everyday reasoning problems. They would require the reasoner to observe and remember many attributes of each of many observed situations and then carry out complex combinatorial procedures to isolate the cause. Without some kind of external aids (at least pencil and paper), a person could use these formal methods only with the simplest of causal problems. Given the limitations of human information processing, people have only "bounded rationality" (Simon, 1957) and cannot be expected to make perfectly rational attributions of causality (Fischhoff, 1976).

In the discussion that follows we look at some of the ways in which human reasoning deviates from these normative approaches, often failing to be as "rational" as the prescriptions, but often managing to be more sensible than the normative models can capture.

Detecting contingency between two variables

Correlation and causality

If some condition is the cause of some outcome, the condition and the outcome will, over multiple situations, tend to covary. The outcome will tend to occur when the cause is present (and vice versa) and will tend not to occur when the cause is absent (and vice versa). The ability to detect such covariation accurately is crucial to people's success at causal analysis.

We can measure the degree of correlation (covariation) between two variables (e.g., between a cause and an outcome) as a ratio of their common variability to their individual variability. When we speak of a "perfect correlation," we refer to a situation in which any change in one variable is always accompanied by a proportionate change in the other variable. In such a case, all the variation within each variable is also common variability between the variables, so the ratio of the common variance (of the two variables) to the individual variances (of each variable) is equal to 1, which is the maximum possible correlation. (Actually, depending on the form of the relationship and the way the variables are measured, perfectly correlated variables have correlation coefficients of either 1 or -1, which reflect equivalent degrees of covariation.) For example, the height of a stack of pennies is perfectly correlated with its weight. Any change in height (by the addition or subtraction of pennies) is accompanied by a perfectly proportional change in weight: If the height of a stack is reduced by one-tenth, its weight will be reduced by one-tenth as well.

At the other extreme is zero correlation, in which there is no tendency toward proportional change − for example, the shoe sizes of a group of people and the house numbers in their addresses. A change in the composition of the group such that there are more people with big feet has no predictable effect on the distribution of house numbers, and knowledge of someone's house number is no help in predicting his or her shoe size. In this case there is no common variation between the two variables, so the ratio of common to individual variance is 0, the minimum possible degree of correlation. (Remember that all negative values reflect the same degree of correlation as their corresponding positive values.)

We can compute the degree of correlation between any pair of variables that can be jointly observed, whether the variables are numerical ones that reflect measurable quantities (e.g., pounds, number of children, or parts per million) or dichotomous variables that can be described only in terms of presence/absence or categories (e.g., alive vs. dead, flammable vs. nonflammable, success vs. failure, male vs. female). Things that are closely causally related will show correlations that are commensurate with the strength of the relationship − a cause that is both necessary and sufficient for some outcome will be perfectly correlated with that outcome. But although the presence of a causal relationship will produce a nonzero correlation (barring problems of measurement and nonlinearity), the presence of a nonzero correlation does not allow us to draw conclusions about causality. For example, there is a substantial correlation between people's body weight and their age. Babies and small children usually weight much less than adults, but a gain in weight does not make one any older. There is also a correlation between household income and the number of televisions in a household. Buying an additional television is not likely to improve one's financial situation, but if one's income should double, one is likely to buy more television sets. A third example is the correlation in the overall American population between pregnancy and the wearing of high-heeled shoes: This should not be taken as evidence of the contraceptive benefits of flat shoes, but only as a consequence of both pregnancy and high heels being much more prevalent among women than among men.

What the examples demonstrate is a cardinal rule of interpreting correlation: Correlation does not imply causality. Two entities (some variables A and B) can be correlated because A causes B, because B causes A, or because there is some unmentioned other variable that, as it changes, produces or contributes to the changes in both A and B. As mentioned earlier, however, causality will manifest itself in correlation. Thus, correlation can be an important diagnostic tool in the assessment of causality, but it is easily misinterpreted.

Evaluating simple contingency

Being able to detect the relationship between some condition and an outcome accurately is critical both to noticing that some condition (potential cause) is correlated with an outcome of interest and to evaluating whether some suspected cause is actually responsible for the outcome. Whether or not we already have an idea of what the cause is, we must analyze the covariation (correlation) between the states or events to infer a causal relationship.

Most research on the way people perform this task has focused on the relatively simple situation in which the two events, that is, the possible cause and the outcome, are explicitly identified; in which each has only two possible states, present and absent (i.e., where they are dichotomous variables rather than ones measured on a continuum); in which subjects are not likely to have any prior beliefs about the relationship between the possible cause and the outcome; and in which no other potentially causal variables are involved. The task of the subjects in these studies is simply to evaluate the degree of relationship between the causal variable and the outcome variable, given information about several situations. For each situation, subjects are told (or they observe for themselves) whether the cause is present or absent and whether the outcome is present or absent. For example, they might be asked to evaluate the relationship between a symptom and a disease, given information for each of a number of patients about whether that particular symptom was present and whether the patient turned out to have the disease. One way to summarize such information is to construct a contingency table, such as those shown in Table 4.1. Contingency Table 4.1a shows the labeling of the cells and Tables 4.1b and c provide sample data. The contingency table format shows the frequency of occurrence of each possible combination of presence and absence of cause and outcome. For example, for each situation in which the cause is present and the outcome occurs, the count in cell a of Table 4.1a is incremented by 1.

The true relationship between the purported cause and the outcome is measured by the extent to which the outcome is more likely to occur in the presence of the cause than in its absence. Measuring this relationship requires information from all four of the cells of the contingency table. More formally put, the presence of a relationship will lead to a conditional probability of the occurrence of the outcome in the presence of the cause that differs from the conditional probability in the absence of the cause. That is,

Table 4.1. *Sample contingency tables*

| | Cause | | |
Outcome	Present	Absent	Total
(a) Present	a	b	a + b
Absent	c	d	c + d
Total	a + c	b + d	—

| | Cause | | |
Outcome	Present	Absent	Total
(b) Present	50	25	75
Absent	25	50	75
Total	75	75	—

| | Cause | | |
Outcome	Present	Absent	Total
(c) Present	10	2	12
Absent	5	1	6
Total	15	3	—

if the purported cause C is really producing outcome O, the probability of the outcome in the presence of the cause $(p(O)|C)$ will be greater than the probability of the outcome in the absence of the cause $(p(O)|\sim C)$. The numerical examples in Table 4.1 show two different situations. In Table 4.1b, the outcome occurs 67% of the time when the cause is present (the outcome occurs in 50 of the 75 situations when the cause is present) but only 33% of the time when the cause is absent (25 of 75). Thus, in this case, the presence of the purported cause is associated with a substantial increase in the probability of occurrence of the outcome. In Table 4.1c, the outcome occurs 67% of the time in the presence of the cause (10 out of 15 situations) and 67% of the time in the absence of the cause (2 out of 3 situations). Here, the presence of the purported cause has no influence on the likelihood of the outcome, neither increasing nor decreasing its probability of occurrence. Even though the most prevalent kind of observed situation in Table 4.1c is in cell a, where the outcome and the cause co-occur, the cause does not in fact have any influence on the probability that the outcome will occur.

Under most circumstances, however, people do not make judgments in accordance with this optimal approach, which calls for using the difference in conditional probabilities to infer a relationship. The strategies that people do appear to use, however, vary somewhat across the experiments that have been done with this paradigm (Beyth-Marom, 1982). One important influence on the level of sophistication of the strategies people spontaneously use is the manner in which information is presented. When it is presented case by case (e.g., when subjects are informed about the symptom and disease status of one patient at a time), the task seems most difficult and subjects exhibit the crudest performance. The greater the degree of summarization in the data presented, the more appropriate (accurate) is the approach. Subjects show the best performance when the data are presented in the form of a contingency table. With tabular presentation, less demand is made on memory in general, the salience of the different kinds of relationships is equated (all cells are equally accessible), and selective recall of the cases presented has less potential influence.

The simplest strategy subjects tend to use is simply to look at the prevalence of instances in which the cause and the outcome are jointly present (cell *a*). As Table 4.1c shows, this can be a very misleading analysis. This crude strategy characterizes the performance of early adolescents (Inhelder & Piaget, 1958) and, in some tasks, even of adults (e.g., Smedslund, 1963). A slightly more sophisticated strategy (e.g., Einhorn & Hogarth, 1978) involves taking two cells into account, looking at all situations in which the cause is present, and subtracting those cases in which the outcome fails to occur (cell *c*) from those in which the outcome does occur (cell *a*). A different strategy that also involves the use of only two of the cells of the contingency table takes into account the fact that a causal relationship can be confirmed by the joint absence of the cause and the outcome: Some situations seem to evoke a strategy in which subjects are sensitive to not only the joint presence of cause and effect (cell *a*), but also consider their joint absence (cell *d*) (Ward & Jenkins, 1965). Note that the first and third of these strategies (cell *a* alone and cell *a* with cell *d*) focus exclusively on the cases that confirm the causal hypothesis and ignore the cases that disconfirm it. An even more sophisticated strategy (but one that will not guarantee accurate judgment) takes all four cells into account but does not analyze conditional probabilities. Using this strategy, subjects count the confirming cases (summing the frequencies of cells *a* and *d*) and count the disconfirming cases (summing cells *b* and *c*) and compare the two sums. The greater the amount of confirmation relative to disconfirmation, the greater is the judged relationship between the variables (e.g., Shaklee & Tucker, 1980). This "difference-of-diagonals" strategy does not always lead to an accurate evaluation of the causal relationship; its accuracy depends on the equivalence of the row and column marginal frequencies. In situations such as the one in Table 4.1c, the sum of the confirmatory diagonal is greater than that of the disconfirmatory diagonal, even though there is no true covariation. This strategy is, however, closer to the optimal strategy in that it takes all the cells into account. Inhelder and Piaget (1958) claim that this approach is characteristic of the older adolescent.

In addition to being influenced by the format in which cases are presented, subjects' strategies are also sensitive to the nature of the variables being queried. When these variables take the form of simple presence/absence (e.g., symptom present vs. not present) versus having two values (high/low or dark/light), there is a greater tendency to underutilize the disconfirming information. Subjects are more likely to use the difference-of-diagonals or conditional-probability strategies when the variables have two values that are more symmetric. The presence/absence variables seem to lead to a selective focus on presence, whereas more symmetric values seem to lead to a more balanced consideration of all the cells (Beyth-Marom, 1982). It can be argued, however, that the bulk of causal analysis that people actually perform on dichotomous variables involves presence/absence more often than two symmetric values.

Illusory correlation: the influence of prior beliefs

All of the contingency-evaluating strategies described above were found in studies in which people were asked to evaluate relationships between previously unknown variables or between variables that were not fully described (e.g., symptom X and disease Y). By and large, subjects had no prior familiarity with the variables and no prior beliefs about the nature of their relationship. By way of contrast, we can also look at situations (like many in the real world) in which subjects do have preexisting beliefs about the relatedness of the variables and see how such beliefs influence their analysis of data. One very prevalent finding is that when people have a prior belief about the causal relatedness of two variables, they perceive the two variables co-occurring in sets of observations in which there is no objective correlation (or even in sets with a negative objective correlation, in which the occurrence of one variable actually predicts the absence of the other). If subjects actually see a set of observations of the joint values of two variables and the subjects have strong prior beliefs about the relationship between those variables, they tend to perceive the degree of correlation they anticipated rather than the degree that is present. This phenomenon is termed *illusory correlation* (e.g., Chapman & Chapman, 1969). In the Chapmans' original experiments, subjects were presented with a set of pictures that had supposedly been drawn by mental patients. Each picture was a drawing of a person and was accompanied by a clinical diagnosis of the fictitious patient who had drawn it. Subjects were asked to estimate the frequency with which certain features of the drawings co-occurred with certain diagnoses. When a feature was combined with a diagnosis that fit the subjects' expectations of what such a patient's drawing would look like, the subjects reported high frequencies regardless of the actual frequencies. For example, subjects erroneously reports that there was a very high frequency of pictures with peculiar eyes drawn by paranoid patients. This distortion of perception led the subjects to see correlations that were not present (but were expected) and to miss the ones that were present (but were not expected). Just as in the case of an optical illusion, subjects perceive something that is not there and do not see what is there.

This influence of prior beliefs on perceived relationships has important consequences for causal reasoning. One implication is that, in reviewing the evidence about the relatedness of some pair of variables, we tend to see the data we have as confirmation of our causal hypotheses regardless of what the data actually show. Once we have a hypothesis that A causes B, we tend to conclude that it is correct (that in fact A does cause B) even if A does not tend to cause B or, worse still, even if A tends to cause B not to occur. Making an effort to gather and review data relevant to our hypothesis is not a guarantee that we will make a rational (accurate) evaluation of that hypothesis once we have the data.

Illusory correlation can be seen as an instance of *confirmation bias*, a pervasive tendency of human reasoners to perceive data erroneously as confirmatory of their hypotheses, to seek out data selectively that are confirmatory of their hypotheses, and to undervalue evidence that is contrary to their hypotheses. (Some of this tendency is captured in the popular humorous phrase "My mind is made up; don't confuse me with the facts.") Other instances of this bias will be discussed in the sections below.

Prior causal beliefs influence people's estimates of the relationship of two variables in a set of data in a number of ways. In any data set, the degree of correlation between A and B is identical to the degree of correlation between B and A. The accuracy of prediction of B from A is equivalent to the accuracy of prediction of A from B (unless A and B have markedly different distributions). However, people incorrectly perceive the symmetric relationship of correlation as an asymmetric one, dependent on the direction of causality. For example, Tversky and Kahneman (1980) asked subjects about the relative accuracy of predictions of a father's height from his son's height versus a son's height from his father's height. The correct response is that they are equally predictable, but more than 40% of the subjects made the error of saying that the father's height predicted the son's more accurately than the son's height predicted the father's. In these and similar problems, there is a real or perceived causal link in one direction and not in the other: A father's height influences the height of his son via the father's genetic contribution to his son, but since the father's height is already fixed before the son even exists, the son cannot be seen as influencing his father's height. Notice that there is a true asymmetry of causality; bias arises from reasoners' extension of the causal asymmetry to an asymmetry of correlation.

Inferring causality from correlation

On the side of the coin opposite illusory correlation (where judgments of correlation are influenced by causal and associative relationships) is the inference of causality from the presence of correlation. The strength of a cor-relation tells us only the degree to which the presence or extent of one variable predicts the presence or extent of another, and vice versa. As men-tioned earlier, underlying this relation can be causality in either direction or causality arising from some other, unobserved variable. Thus, even if the degree of correlation is accurately perceived, a difficult cognitive task in itself, people can still make erroneous (or at best unsupported) inferences about the underlying causal relation.

Many factors influence what causal relation is perceived by an observer from a set of covarying events or entities. We are influenced by the time at which events or conditions hold, relative to one another. If *A* precedes *B* in each observed instance, we are more likely to conclude that *A* causes *B* than vice versa. Normative models (including those of Mill and Hume) provide limited support for this influence of temporal precedence on inferred causal-ity. According to the normative approaches, temporal priority of a condi-tion is necessary but not sufficient for attributing causal status. If *A* is the cause of *B*, then condition *A* cannot follow condition *B* in time − but simply preceding *B* is not sufficient proof of the causal role of *A*. In everyday rea-soning, however, people often overextend the significance of temporal or-dering. It is a very prevalent logical fallacy to infer causality on the basis of order of occurrence. The human tendency to do this (and the logical unac-ceptability of doing so) has been known for hundreds of years, and genera-tions of students have been warned against reasoning on the basis of *post hoc ergo propter hoc* (after that, therefore, because of that).

There are many situations in which we want to draw conclusions about causal relations, but the only data available are correlational. Correctly in-terpreting the causal implications of such data requires our having knowl-edge about how the data were gathered and analyzed. One common domain in which the interpretation of correlational data is required is epidemiology. Most epidemiological studies of the relationship between diseases and be-haviors are correlational, although we really want information about causal relationships. For example, virtually every study of smoking and lung cancer has shown that there is a tremendous correlation between them. The correla-tion captures the difference in the prevalence (conditional probability) of the disease if one is a member of the nonsmoking group versus a member of the smoking group. These studies do not themselves prove that smoking causes lung cancer − it is always possible that there is some other unmeasured variable on which the smoking and nonsmoking groups differ that is the true cause of lung cancer. No matter how carefully researchers rule out other potentially causal factors that may be correlated with smoking (e.g., age, sex, occupation, and alcohol consumption) and use temporal precedence to rule out a causal effect in the other direction (in which people with lung cancer are more likely to take up smoking than people without lung cancer), correlation alone can never prove the existence of a direct causal effect. The studies can, of course, provide overwhelmingly strong evidence − so strong that no one but the tobacco industry would question the riskiness of smoking. The only way to achieve logical certainty of the direct causal relationship would be to perform a (clearly unethical) experiment: Assign children randomly at birth to smoking and nonsmoking groups, and force members of the smoking group to smoke at least a pack of cigarettes each day and prevent members of the nonsmoking group from ever smoking a cigarette. Since we obviously cannot perform such experiments and are limited to interpreting correlational data, we are obligated to exercise great skepticism and great care in drawing causal conclusions.

Causal reasoning with more than one possible cause

In the preceding sections we reviewed findings on the ways in which people evaluate the contingency between two variables when those variables are the only ones to be considered. People's performance in more complex situations reveals some of the same characteristics seen in the simpler situations and some characteristics that are unique to the multiple-variable situation.

In a series of experiments involving multiple possible causes, subjects evaluating the causal strength of a hypothesized cause showed biases similar to those discussed above (Schustack & Sternberg, 1981). The subjects were presented with a list of situations relevant to the same outcome, as well as information about the presence and absence of many potentially causal variables in each situation. In some of the experiments, the causes and outcomes were represented abstractly, as letters of the alphabet; in others, they were real-world events that were plausibly related as cause and effect, such as a sewage spill causing a disease epidemic or a corporate embezzlement scandal lowering stock value. The results were the same with both abstract and concrete materials. The evidence relating the outcome to the single target cause (the one that the subjects were asked to evaluate) can be analyzed in terms of a simple contingency table as shown in Table 4.1a (although this, of course, leaves out the influence of the other potentially causal variables). This contingency-table analysis showed that the subjects were strongly biased toward overreliance on the cases in which cause and effect were jointly present (cell a). These instances were given disproportionate weight in the subjects' numerical evaluation of the strength of a relationship. The subjects were somewhat sensitive to the disconfirming evidence from both cells b and c (which show violations of the necessity and the sufficiency of the cause, respectively). They also showed a small influence of confirmation of the relationship by the joint absence of cause and effect (cell d).

Causal discounting and minimum causation

The same study (Schustack & Sternberg, 1981) also provided substantial evidence of the way in which subjects used information about other potentially causal variables in evaluating the target cause. Even though the subjects had no reason to believe that the targeted causes were particularly strongly related to the outcome (relative to the other potential causes mentioned in a problem) they behaved as though they were. Simply by virtue of having been singled out for evaluation, these target causes were seen as moderately related to the outcome. Moreover, this focus on the evidence relevant to the target cause led to a greatly diminished use of information about the other potentially relevant variables. Even the presence of alternative variables that had a much stronger causal relationship to the outcome had only a small effect on the causal strength attributed to the target cause. A similar procedure was used in another group of studies, in which the subjects were explicity asked to evaluate the causal strength of a combination of potentially causal variables. Under these conditions (Downing, Sternberg, & Ross, 1985), the subjects failed to consider any of the potential causes other than those explicitly being evaluated. The small influence of the strength of alternative hypotheses in the earlier study was diminished to no influence when subjects had to evaluate a more complex cause that included multiple variables.

One common observation in multicausal tasks is that people do not follow the optimal strategy of discounting − of taking alternative causes into account and reducing the judged causal strength of one cause on the basis of the strength of alternative causes (Kelley, 1972). Instead of discounting, people seem to follow a principle of minimum causation (Shaklee, 1977). Subjects seem to interpret the known presence of one possible cause as sufficiently explaining the outcome, and they greatly decrease their estimate of the importance of other causes, even when these other causes are unrelated (i.e., when they are completely independent, with no appearance of mutual exclusivity). Even in realistic situations in which there could actually be multiple causation (i.e., when a given outcome could actually be the result of multiple causal factors acting simultaneously), subjects behave as though they are seeking a unique cause. The subjects in one study were presented with hypothetical situations in which there were multiple possible causes and were asked to choose what additional information they would find helpful in making their judgments (Shaklee & Fischhoff, 1982). The initial presentation of the problem included evidence favoring one of the possible causes, and the subjects were more likely to seek further information about that implicated cause than to seek any information about the other potential causes. They were more interested in acquiring further information that could verify that the implicated cause was the true cause than they were in finding out whether one of the other causes might be a better candidate. They seemed to be following a "satisficing" strategy, trying to find a cause that was "good enough" rather than following optimizing strategies of either trying to find the best cause or trying to clarify the relative contribution of each cause.

Scientific reasoning

In the following discussion of tasks requiring scientific reasoning, which can be defined as the explicit specification of a causal relationship and its chain of supporting evidence, it will sometimes be useful to break the task down into components and to look at each of them separately. In our analysis, the task can be seen as having three parts: (a) the generation of one or more hypotheses from preexisting knowledge and/or from the observation of relevant situations, (b) the selection of appropriate tests of the hypotheses (either the construction of experiments to be performed or the search for naturally occurring situations that are relevant), and (c) the interpretation of the outcome of those tests. These steps may be performed once or many times in the course of causal reasoning about some outcome; they may occur within a very brief time (seconds or minutes) or over a longer time span (hours, days, even years).

Normative approaches to scientific reasoning (e.g., Platt, 1964; Popper, 1959) require that we test hypotheses not by attempting to confirm them, but by trying to falsify them (to prove them false). It is insufficient to generate tests where the outcome would occur if the hypothesis were correct: We are required to construct experiments that could prove our hypothesis wrong rather than to focus on repeated testing to show that it is right. We are urged to consider alternative hypotheses when our current ones are supported by the data, rather than only to consider alternatives when we are forced to abandon our current ideas. These normative ideas should be kept in mind as the data on actual performance are discussed below.

Developmental background

The initial development of scientific reasoning in individuals occurs during adolescence (in the stage that Piaget terms *formal operations*). It is only with the attainment of formal operations that people begin to think in terms of generating hypotheses and devising ways to test them. What is required for this kind of reasoning is an ability to think in terms of "what if," that is, to follow out the logic of a hypothesis to some expected outcome that can be tested. This requires the reasoner to think hypothetically, as follows: "I've seen that when both factors A and B are present, this outcome occurs. If factor A, and not factor B, were the cause of this outcome, then if I could construct a situation in which A was present and B was absent, the outcome would occur there. And, if I could construct some other situation in which B was present and A was absent, the outcome would not occur there."

Younger (or less intellectually developed) people, when faced with the same problems, are able to guess what causes the outcome, but they are unable to perform the hypothetical reasoning about what would occur in other (as yet unobserved) situations if the hypothesis were true or about how to construct or seek out situations that would appropriately test the hypothesis. Note that adolescents (and adults and even scientists) are not always successful in carrying out these tasks – what differentiates this kind of causal thinking from more primitive and concrete approaches is that an attempt is made to use hypothetical reasoning, even though there may be errors in executing that hypothetical reasoning.

In his original work in this area, Piaget explored the growth of scientific thinking by observing individual children solving problems involving logical relations of causality and having the children answer questions as they worked (Inhelder & Piaget, 1958). One problem required the children to ascertain what factors determine the degree of flexibility of a rod. The children were presented with a set of rods of uniform length made of different materials and having different shapes and sizes (in cross section). These rods could be clamped horizontally at any point along their length onto the edge of a shallow pan of water (allowing the functional lengths of the rods to differ), and dolls of different weights could be placed on the end of any rod to test its flexibility. The children's experimentation with these materials was observed, and they were asked what factors determined whether the rod would bend down to the water when a doll was placed on it.

For optimal solution, this task requires the systematic generation of hypotheses about relevant factors and systematic tests of these hypotheses. The youngest children did not generate hypotheses, much less test them – they often seemed not even to understand the task. They simply enjoyed putting the dolls on the rods and seeing if the rods touched the water. For example, when the experimenter showed a five-year-old child that a heavy weight on a long thin rod made the rod touch the water and asked the child why this occurred, the child replied, "Because it has to."

Slightly older children observe some of the relevant relationships from instances presented to them or from instances that they themselves create unsystematically, and guess that these might be important, but they cannot construct systematic experiments that will test them. These children do experiment, but in a rather haphazard fashion. The most common deficiency in their gathering of data is that they focus on a variable of interest (the one that they hypothesize to be the cause of differential flexibility) but fail to take the other potentially causal variables into account (neither keeping them constant nor varying them systematically). For example, such a child might want to compare a thick rod with a thin one as a test of the hypothesis that thin rods are more flexible than thick rods. But rather than carefully construct an experiment to isolate the influence of the hypothesized cause, she uses whatever situations happen to be available. She might compare a short thin rod and a long thick one, or rods of different materials, or dolls of different weights (or any combination of these).

It is only at the highest level of Piaget's developmental hierarchy (the stage of formal operations) that hypothesis testing (experimenting) is carried out with the necessary systematicity, leading to a high rate of success in isolating the correct causal variables. However, successful performance at this level is not attained by every person (even with continued schooling, not all students reach this stage), nor is success at one problem or type of task completely predictive of success at others.

Note that the set of experiments required for correct identification of the causal variable or variables will depend on what the subjects already know about the nature of the causal problem. When subjects are told that there is a single variable or element that is alone responsible for the outcome (i.e., when there is a single necessary and sufficient condition), there is no need to gather data relevant to interactions among variables. In the more common case, in which the variables may potentially inhibit the outcome as well as cause it and the influences of the variables on the outcome may interact, a larger and more complex set of experiments is required.

Adult performance

In domains like the ones Piaget investigated, where all the possibly relevant factors are fairly obvious and rather few in number, adults (or at least the college students that form the bulk of the adult subject population) tend to be systematic and careful experimenters. They usually succeed at the "formal operations" tasks, isolating the relevant variables efficiently. We might take this as a very positive reflection on adult reasoning in scientific tasks. However, if we consider a broader set of tasks, we can observe the limitations of performance.

One important group of studies (Mynatt, Doherty, & Tweney, 1977, 1978) involved a situation in which the set of possibly causal factors was not as obvious as in Piaget's tasks. In a more complex environment such as this, generating the class of potential hypotheses is in itself a difficult task, which may account for the decline in performance seen in such situations. Whether subjects were constructing their own experiments or were testing their hypotheses by performing "experiments" chosen from a set that had already been constructed, there was a consistent trend toward choosing potentially confirming tests over potentially disconfirming ones. Subjects also tended to ignore the existence of alternative hypotheses that were consistent with the outcome of the "experiments" when those experiments confirmed current hypotheses. As an extreme example of confirmation bias, there was some evidence that subjects became so committed to their hypotheses that they would not reject or revise them even in the face of direct disconfirmation: About one-fifth of the "experiments" that disconfirmed the current hypothesis were followed by another test of the identical hypothesis.

Many of the limitations discussed here are not specific to the scientific-reasoning context – they are general characteristics of human reasoning. For example, the focus on seeking confirming rather than disconfirming (falsificatory) data is seen in the classical concept-formation experiments in which subjects have to determine what rule determines category membership, given information about whether particular exemplars are or are not members of the category. Although the concept-formation paradigm presented in this section has been criticized as being unrepresentative of the way people form concepts in the real world (e.g., Smith & Medin, 1981), the data are nonetheless very relevant to issues of hypothesis generation, hypothesis testing, and hypothesis revision. This paradigm can be related to the causal framework if we view the task as one of deciding what features cause items to be considered members of a category.

The prototypical experiment in this paradigm (e.g., Bruner, Goodnow, & Austin, 1956) involves stimuli that vary in color, shape, and size. In an easy task, the rule determining category membership would include one or two of these features. For example, the rule might be "All red figures are members of the category," or "All large circles are members of the category." Even with these very simple stimuli, however, the rules to be discovered can be quite complex: "all figures that are red or circles, but not both" or "all figures that have more than three sides." Usually, the subjects see the stimuli one at a time and are told after they view each figure whether the figure is a member of the category. Sometimes the subjects initially guess whether each item is a category member. Sometimes the subjects are shown the exemplars in an order determined by the experimenter, and sometimes they themselves select which exemplar to "test" next. In some experiments, the subject has to state aloud his or her current hypothesis about the rule on every trial, whereas in others the subject states a hypothesis only once, when he or she is satisfied that the hypothesis is correct.

Each of these procedures (and their combinations) can be seen to be analogous to different causal reasoning situations. For example, being given the choice of which exemplar to check next is similar to the situation in experimental science in which the reasoner constructs the experiment that will test the current hypothesis. The alternative case, having to make do with whatever situation happens to occur next, corresponds more closely to reasoning in nonexperimental domains. Although each procedure can provide slightly different information about subjects' performance, there are some clear generalizations that hold true for the paradigm.

Subjects are overwhelmingly subject to confirmatory bias. This shows up in many aspects of their behavior. First, when they have a hypothesis, they select figures for testing that would be members of the category if the current hypothesis were correct and neglect figures that would not be members. (If they think the rule is "red squares," for example, they will test only figures that are red squares.) This bias in acquiring evidence relevant to the hypothesis prevents subjects from finding out that a more general rule is true (say, "all squares"), because they never attempt to falsify their hypothesized rule. Second, subjects do not make good use of information that disconfirms (falsifies) their hypotheses. Rather than use the attributes of a disconfirming instance to modify a current hypothesis, subjects often respond to disconfirmation as though it provided no useful information other than that the current hypothesis is wrong (i.e., as though the only alternative were to abandon the current hypothesis completely and start over). Third, to the extent that subjects use information from prior trials to formulate new hypotheses when current ones are disconfirmed and abandoned, they preferentially consider information from the positive exemplars that have been seen. Their new hypothesized rules are likely to be possibly correct descriptions of the set of previously seen positive exemplars, but to be incorrect if the entire set of previously seen figures (both exemplars and nonexemplars) is considered.

In a much simpler but elegant experiment, Wason (1960) demonstrated many of the same limitations on people's hypothesis generation, testing, and revision. The subjects were presented with a sequence of three numbers (say, 2 : 4 : 6), their task being to discover the rule by which the experimenter had generated the sequence. They were not allowed to ask direct questions about the rule, but could generate sequences of their own to present to the experimenter, who would indicate whether the new sequence could be generated by the rule. Almost every subject began by testing sequences like 4 : 8 : 12, 6 : 8 : 10, 20 : 40 : 60, and 3 : 6 : 9. They were asked to stop testing as soon as they believed they had the correct rule and then to state the rule. Four-fifths of the subjects stated the wrong rule. The most common pattern subjects followed was to propose many tests that confirmed their hypothesized rule. When they had proposed enough sequences that the experimenter said could be generated by the rule, they were sure they knew the rule. In almost all cases, the incorrect rules that subjects announced were much more restrictive than the correct rule (which was simply that the sequence ascended). No amount of testing of sequences conforming to a more restrictive rule (such as $X : 2X : 3X$ or $X : X + 2 : X + 4$) would ever lead to the discovery of the more general correct rule. Simply accumulating evidence that confirms a current hypothesis is inadequate − successful testing of a hypothesis requires both attempting to falsify that hypothesis and considering alternative hypotheses in the face of confirmation of the current hypothesis. Of course (as Wason points out), in real life there is no experimenter to tell us when we have the wrong rule. The findings of this study (and others) are that people increase their degree of belief in their hypotheses as more and more confirmatory evidence is generated. To the extent that this characterizes behavior outside the experimental setting (and there is much evidence that is does), all of us probably hold many erroneous beliefs for which we can adduce much evidence − convincing ourselves and others of generalizations that are, at best, overly narrow.

Scientific reasoning by scientists

Most of us would like to believe that the shortcomings and biases that characterize the causal reasoning of ordinary people untrained in logic and scientific method are overcome by the trained scientist on whose findings so many important decisions rest. We (as individuals and as a society) rely on scientists to tell us about causal relationships in domains where they are experts. For example, they tell us about the safety of substances in our environment, how to reduce our risk of acquiring various diseases, what psychotherapeutic treatments work most effectively, how various economic changes would influence different groups of people in our society, and how early experience affects children's development.

It would be comforting to believe that these scientific findings, which influence so many lives and involve so much money, are based on the most careful and logical of reasoning processes. Attempts to assess the "scientific reasoning" of scientists have shown, however, that scientists are subject to many of the same biases and limitations as the person on the street or the subject in the psychology laboratory (e.g., Chalmers, 1976; Mitroff, 1974). The limited amount of research that has been carried out suggests that working scientists tend to seek confirmation of their hypotheses rather than follow the normative scientific goal of falsification and consideration of alternative hypotheses (as advocated by, e.g., Platt, 1964, and Popper, 1959). Although experimental scientists who use common statistical tests are forced by the structure of those tests (analysis of variance, t-tests, etc.) to falsify rather than confirm their hypotheses, this can be done as a formality, not necessarily forcing scientists to make any real attempt to falsify their hypotheses.

The confirmation bias in working scientists operates in many ways. There is evidence that these scientists design experiments that attempt to confirm rather than falsify their current hypothesis. If the experiment does not "work" (i.e., if it produces results that do not strongly support the hypothesis), they often try it again and again with slight variations until it produces evidence supporting their initial hypothesis. They change instruments, laboratory assistants, subject sampling, minor aspects of the procedure – change whatever can be changed without abandoning the hypothesis, until the experiment finally "works." Logically, of course, the eventual production of the desired result may be artifactual (i.e., due to extraneous factors unrelated to the hypothesis of interest), just as the scientist believes the "failures" are artifactual. The parallel tendency seems to hold true for studies in nonexperimental domains (e.g., certain areas of astronomy or geology). Researchers seek out naturally occurring situations supportive of their hypotheses and make excuses for the observed data that are not in accordance with their hypotheses. With either type of approach, experimental or observational, the possibility that the hypothesis is wrong is usually far down on the list of potential reasons for "failure."

In some domains, experimenters' expectations about the outcome (i.e., their conviction that their hypothesis is correct) can actually influence the outcome (Rosenthal, 1966). This *experimenter expectancy effect* biases the outcome in favor of the experimenter's hypothesis. If two experimenters have opposite beliefs about what will happen in a given experiment, they are likely to get somewhat different results even if they follow what seem to be the same procedures. This influence can be seen as a consequence of the experimenter's desire to confirm (not to falsify) his or her hypothesis. The expectancy effect is not limited to experiments in which the behavior of a human subject is being judged or rated by an experimenter who is interacting with the subject. In such experiments, we could easily imagine that the experimenter gives subtle and unintentional cues to the subject or that the experimenter misperceives the subject's performance in accordance with his or her beliefs about how the subject should behave. But even the performance of rats being trained in a Skinner box tends to vary with the experimenter's expectancy (Rosenthal & Lawson, 1964).

The most extreme example of this confirmatory bias in the production or gathering of data is the (fortunately rare) practice of concocting supporting data when no amount of tuning of the experiments or observational procedures seems to "fix" them. It is painfully clear from such unethical behavior that the scientist can differ from our stereotypical notion of an objective, detached judge of evidence. Even working within the standards of the scientific community, scientists are committed to their hypotheses, often to an extent that interferes with the advancement of scientific knowledge. (Perhaps it is not to the credit of the scientific community that sincere attempts at falsification are made most frequently when the hypothesis being tested is that of some rival group or individual.)

Social reasoning

One of the major areas of everyday life in which causal reasoning is important is the attribution of causal responsibility in social and interpersonal domains. Although many of the characteristics of general causal reasoning apply to this domain as well, it has some special characteristics.

A frequent reasoning task in this domain is to determine why someone reacted as she did (or behaved as he did) in response to some event or person or state of affairs. For example, someone might want to know why she did poorly in a course, why his roommate threw a screaming fit when the trash can overflowed, or why her mother is afraid of her new dog. What all of these cases have in common is that causal responsibility for the event can be analyzed in terms of three classes of variables: attributes or dispositions of the person involved (e.g., self, roommate, mother), attributes of the stimulus (e.g., the course, the overflowing trash can, the dog), or attributes of the situation in which the behavior occurred.

One normative approach to this task of social attribution was proposed by Kelley (1967, 1972). Kelley's idea was that causal analysis should consist of an examination of the statistical variation in the three potential variables along the lines of a three-way analysis of variance. The reasoner should assemble information about many instances of each of the potentially causal variables and observe which variable covaries with the outcome. For example, in analyzing the cause of her mother's fear of the new dog, the ideal social reasoner would look at each of the variables. She would note whether her mother is afraid of many other things in addition to the new dog (attributing the fear of the new dog to the mother's fearful nature). She would ascertain whether many other people are afraid of this new dog (if they are, she would attribute the mother's fear to characteristics of the stimulus, in this case, to the ferociousness of the dog). She would also determine whether certain characteristics of the situation in which she observed her mother's fear of the dog tended to produce a fear response, such as the dog jumping out of the darkness as she watched a horror movie on television (if the situation evoked the response, she would attribute the behavior to the situation). This analysis-of-variance approach is both analytic and predictive. If the mother of our ideal social reasoner is afraid of many things, she will probably be afraid of the new dog. If the new dog scares many people, it will probably scare the mother. If the situation itself produces fright, other people would probably react fearfully to other stimuli in the same situation.

What differentiates this kind of social reasoning from causal reasoning in general is that the potentially causal variables can be so neatly classified. Research in this framework on people's actual attributions of causality shows that the optimal statistical approach is not rigorously followed in many cases but that the framework itself is a powerful analytic tool for examining the way causal attribution occurs. One interesting finding is that people see the data differently when it is their own behavior that is to be explained. For example, people tend to attribute their own failures to the external factors of stimulus and situation (e.g., the course was difficult, the teacher was unfair, the umpire was biased), whereas they attribute corresponding failures by others to the internal factors of attributes and dispositions of the person (e.g., the student is unintelligent, she did not work hard in the course, he is a poor ballplayer).

Conclusions

The overall picture of human causal reasoning shows us to be knowledgeable and sophisticated users of many complex strategies. Although we do not behave optimally in many situations, our causal analyses often enable us to focus on the correct causal account. If we are aware of the nature of our shortcomings (e.g., memory limitations, confirmation bias, and tendency to ignore alternative hypotheses), we can make an effort to avoid these pitfalls and thereby improve our performance.

References

Beyth-Marom, R. (1982). Perception of correlation reexamined. *Memory & Cognition, 10,* 511–19.

Bruner, J. S., Goodow, J. J., & Austin, G. A. (1956). *A study of thinking.* New York: Wiley.

Chalmers, A. F. (1976). *What is this thing called science? An assessment of the nature and status of science and its methods.* St. Lucia, Queensland: University of Queensland Press.

Chapman, L. J., & Chapman, J. P. (1969). Illusory correlation as an obstacle to the use of valid psychodiagnostic signs. *Journal of Abnormal Psychology, 74,* 271–80.

Copi, I. M. (1978). *Introduction to logic* (5th ed.). New York: Macmillan.

Downing, C. J., Sternberg, R. J., & Ross, B. H. (1985). Multicausal inference: Evaluation of evidence in causally complex situations. *Journal of Experimental Psychology: General, 114,* 239–63.

Einhorn, H. J., & Hogarth, R. M. (1978). Confidence in judgment: Persistence of the illusion of validity. *Psychological Review, 85,* 395–416.

Fischhoff, B. (1976). Attribution theory and judgment under uncertainty. In J. H. Harvey, W. J. Ickes, & R. F. Kidd (Eds.), *New directions in attribution research* (Vol. 1, pp. 421–52). Hillsdale, NJ: Erlbaum.

Hume, D. (1888). *Treatise of human nature.* New York: Oxford University Press. (Original work published 1739.)

Inhelder, B., & Piaget, J. (1958). *The growth of logical thinking from childhood to adolescence.* New York: Basic.

Kelley, H. H. (1967). Attribution theory in social psychology. In D. Levine (Ed.), *Nebraska Symposium on Motivation* (Vol. 15, pp. 192–238). Lincoln: University of Nebraska Press. (1972). *Attribution in social interaction.* Morristown, NJ: General Learning Press.

Mackie, J. L. (1965). Causes and conditions. *American Philosophical Quarterly, 2,* 245–64.

Michotte, A. (1963). *The perception of causality.* New York: Basic.

Mill, J. S. (1843). *A system of logic, ratiocinative and inductive.* London: Parker.

Mitroff, I. I. (1974). *The subjective side of science.* Amsterdam: Elsevier.

Mynatt, C. R., Doherty, M. E., & Tweney, R. D. (1977). Confirmation bias in a simulated research environment: An experimental study of scientific inference. *Quarterly Journal of Experimental Psychology, 29,* 89–95. (1978). Consequences of confirmation and disconfirmation in a simulated research environment. *Quarterly Journal of Experimental Psychology, 30,* 395–406.

Platt, J. R. (1964). Strong inference. *Science, 146,* 347–53.

Popper, K. R. (1959). *The logic of scientific discovery.* London: Hutchinson.

Rosenthal, R. (1966). *Experimenter effects in behavioral research.* New York: Appleton-Century-Crofts.

Rosenthal, R., & Lawson, R. (1964). A longitudinal study of the effects of experimenter bias on the operant learning of laboratory rats. *Journal of Psychiatric Research, 2,* 61–72.

Schustack, M. W., & Sternberg, R. J. (1981). Evaluation of evidence in causal inference. *Journal of Experimental Psychology: General, 110,* 101–20.

Shaklee, H. (1977). Limited minds and multiple causes: Discounting in multicausal attributions (doctoral dissertation, University of Oregon, 1977). *Dissertation Abstracts International, 37,* 4764.

Shaklee, H., & Fischhoff, B. (1982). Strategies of information search in causal analysis. *Memory & Cognition, 10,* 520–30.

Shaklee, H., & Tucker, D. (1980). A rule analysis of judgments of covariation between events. *Memory & Cognition, 8,* 459–67.

Simon, H. A. (1957). *Models of man.* New York: Wiley.

Skyrms, B. (1966). *Choice and chance: An introduction to inductive logic.* Belmont, CA: Dickenson.

Smedslund, J. (1963). The concept of correlation in adults. *Scandinavian Journal of Psychology, 4,* 165–73.

Smith, E. E., & Medin, D. L. (1981). *Categories and concepts.* Cambridge, MA: Harvard University Press.

Tversky, A., & Kahneman, D. (1980). Causal schemas in judgements under uncertainty. In M. Fishbein (Ed.), *Progress in social psychology* (Vol. 1, pp. 49–72). Hillsdale, NJ: Erlbaum.

Ward, W., & Jenkins, H. (1965). The display of information and the judgment of contingency. *Canadian Journal of Psychology, 19,* 231–41.

Wason, P.C. (1960). On the failure to eliminate hypotheses in a conceptual task. *Quarterly Journal of Experimental Psychology, 12,* 129–40.

5   Deduction

Lance J. Rips

Imagine that sometime in the future a team of psychologists is sent to another galaxy to report on the mental abilities of a newly discovered, intelligent life form. The team makes observations, conducts tests, and finally compiles its findings. When we read the report they publish in the *Journal of Extraterrestrial Psychology*, we probably are not very surprised to learn that the perceptual systems of these creatures are different from our own. Nor are we astonished that these creatures have a memory capacity that exceeds ours. But suppose we are also told that the creatures reject simple, familiar inference principles in favor of equally simple, but to our minds obviously incorrect principles.

To us earthlings, an intuitively straightforward inference principle is the one logicians call *modus ponens*. According to this principle, from the statement *IF so-and-so is true, THEN such-and-such is true* and the statement *So-and-so is true*, we are entitled to conclude that *Such-and-such is true.*[1] For example, from the information *If Calvin deposits 50 cents, Calvin will get a Coke* and *Calvin deposits 50 cents*, it follows that *Calvin will get a Coke*. We can write this in the form shown in (1), where the sentences above the line are called *premises* and the sentence below the line the *conclusions*:

(1) If Calvin deposits 50 cents, Calvin will get a Coke.　　⎫　　PREMISES
　　　Calvin deposits 50 cents.　　　　　　　　　　　　　　　⎬
　　　―――――――――――――――――――――――――　　⎭
　　　Calvin will get a Coke　　　　　　　　　　　　　　　　　CONCLUSION

Now suppose the creatures in our sci-fi example have exactly the same inference skills that we do, with one important exception. They reject all modus ponens arguments like (1) and adopt instead a contrary principle that we might call *modus shmonens*: From *IF so-and-so is true, THEN such-and-such is true* and *So-and-so is true*, they conclude that *Such-and-such is NOT true*. For instance, they would say that the conclusion of (1) does not follow from its premises, but the conclusion of (2) does follow:

(2) If Calvin deposits 50 cents, Calvin will get a Coke.
　　　Calvin deposits 50 cents.
　　　―――――――――――――――――――――――――
　　　Calvin will not get a Coke.

I am grateful to Fred Conrad, Judy Florian, Reid Hastie, Julie Johnson, Russ Revlin, Ed Smith, and Bob Sternberg for their comments on an earlier version of this chapter. Work on the chapter was supported by NIMH Grant MH39633.

The existence of creatures who systematically deny modus ponens and accept modus shmonens would be extremely surprising − much more surprising than the existence of creatures who differ from us in basic perceptual or memory abilities. In a situation like this one, we would probably be more apt to blame the translation of whatever language the creatures speak than to accept the idea that they sincerely believe in modus shmonens (Davidson, 1970; Dennett, 1980; Quine, 1970, chap. 6). Indeed, our reluctance to attribute exotic inferences even to exotic creatures is an interesting property of our *own* thought processes. Modus ponens and other inference principles like it are so well integrated with the rest of our thinking − so central to our notion of intelligence and rationality − that contrary principles seem out of the question. Deep-rooted modes of thought like these are important objects of psychological investigation, since they may well turn out to play a crucial role in the organization of people's beliefs and conjectures.[2]

This chapter emphasizes deductive reasoning as a basis for thinking. That is, it explores the idea, which we call the *deduction system hypothesis*, that principles like modus ponens underlie many other forms of higher cognition. The approach views deduction as analogous to a general-purpose programming system: Just as we can use a computer language like *Basic* or *Pascal* to keep track of our finances or to solve scientific or engineering problems, we can use deductive reasoning to accomplish a variety of mental activities.[3] In particular, we shall see how deduction enables us to answer questions from information stored in memory, to plan actions in order to obtain goals, and to solve certain kinds of puzzles.

The deduction system hypothesis is not the only way, nor even the most popular way, of understanding the role of deduction in human thinking. Other theories view deduction as a more peripheral part of cognition, analogous to the role played by special-purpose mental skills such as the ability to tell time on a standard clock. Handy as it sometimes is, telling time is not a central cognitive function since it is not critical to other mental skills or actions. According to the theories in question, deduction is also a specialized task that is useful mainly in solving logic puzzles or proving theorems in mathematics. Some psychologists have also claimed that people have few if any cognitive abilities that are peculiar to deduction, unless of course they happen to acquire them through formal training in logic. Faced with a problem that calls for deduction, untutored people use varied strategies that do not guarantee the correct solution but that may yield enough right answers to serve practical ends. We call this type of view the *deduction heuristics hypothesis* to contrast it with the deduction system hypothesis just proposed.

The heuristics view gains initial support from psychological experiments suggesting that people are prone to making mistakes in reasoning, mistakes that appear when people's judgments are compared with the answers that logic dictates. For example, although it is extremely rare to find someone who disagrees with (1) and agrees with (2), it is not at all uncommon to find people who agree with (3). Yet the conclusion of (3) does not follow logically from its premises, at least according to some ways of interpreting these three sentences. Arguments of this form are sometimes branded "fallacies of affirming the consequent" in textbooks on elementary logic.

(3)   If Calvin deposits 50 cents, Calvin will get a Coke.
      Calvin gets a Coke.
      _____

      Calvin deposited 50 cents.

This leaves us with a dilemma. Argument (1) looks so obvious that it is hard to imagine anyone mistaking it. It is therefore tempting to assume that (1) must be part of our core cognitive abilities, in accord with the deduction system hypothesis. At the same time, Argument (3), which is incorrect from a certain logical point of view, is judged acceptable by many college students. If deduction really is an important component of thought, why are people apparently so error prone in cases like (3)? This tension between the obviousness of some arguments and the obscurity of others raises fundamental questions within the psychology of deduction.

Before delving into such issues, however, we must find out more about what cognitive scientists have in mind when they talk about deductive reasoning. In the first section of this chapter we explore the properties of deductive arguments and the differences between deduction and other modes of reasoning. The second section describes a possible deduction system and shows how the system can be used to carry out cognitive tasks. The final section looks at some of the psychological evidence that could help decide between the system and the heuristics hypotheses.

The nature of deduction

Clearly, not all of the arguments that we care about are deductively correct arguments like (1), in which the conclusion is a logically certain result of the premises. We are often forced to come to a conclusion in situations where the evidence we have is insufficient to rule out alternatives. The best we can do in these cases is to accept the conclusion that is most probable on the basis of the facts we have at hand. If we have to decide, for instance, which suspect put the poisoned chocolate in Mr. Southport's candy box, we might come to accept the following argument:

(4)   Twenty witnesses testify that Max put a chocolate in the box.
      Lab tests revealed cyanide in the chocolate found in the box.
      _____

      Max put a poisoned chocolate in the candy box.

Although things look bad for Max, the case is not logically unimpeachable – the lab may have made an error, or the witnesses may be conspiring against him. The same uncertainty surrounds conventional decisions about how much to pay for a used car, whether our symptoms warrant a visit to the doctor, or when to leave for the airport in order to catch a 2 p.m. flight. It is traditional to distinguish between *inductively* correct arguments like (4) and deductively correct arguments like (1), and clarifying this distinction should help us see what is unique about deduction.

Before going on, it may be helpful to clarify some terms that we have already come across and that will continue to be important in what follows. I shall use the term *argument* in a technical sense to mean a series of sentences, the last of which is the conclusion and the rest of which are the premises. Examples (1)−(4) are arguments. The term *inference* will mean a particular type of mental process through which conviction in one set of beliefs comes to affect conviction in another. *Reasoning* and *inference* will be used interchangeably. We may want to place further restrictions on what should qualify as a genuine inference, but the present point is simply that an inference is a psychological activity whereas an argument (in our technical sense) is not. Sometimes it will be useful to think of an inference as aligned with an argument: A person forms a set of beliefs corresponding to the premises, passes through an intermediate set of mental states, and finally comes to believe in the conclusion. But as we shall see, the relationship between an inference and an argument may be more complex. For example, a person might begin with a conclusion, working backward to ascertain whether there are other beliefs that support it.

Deduction versus induction

One way to define a deductively correct argument is to say that its conclusion is true in any state of affairs in which its premises are true. In a state of affairs in which Calvin deposits 50 cents and in which if he deposits 50 cents he will get a Coke, it will certainly be true that Calvin gets a Coke; so Argument (1) is deductively correct. We call arguments that meet this standard of correctness *deductively valid*, and they are the main subject of this chapter.

It is important to remember that the validity of an argument depends on the *relation* between the premises' truth and that of the conclusion: In a valid argument the conclusion is true in every state of affairs in which the premises are true. This means, first, that an argument can still be valid even though its premises or its conclusion happen to be false in some state of affairs, including our actual state. For example, Calvin's not depositing 50 cents would make the second premise in (1) false in our current state of affairs, but the argument remains valid. What is important is that, whenever the premises are true, the conclusion is true as well. Second, it is not enough for validity that both the premises and the conclusion happen to be true in the present state of affairs. Although it is true both that Jane Austen wrote *Emma* and that Charlotte Brontë wrote *Shirley*, the following is not a valid argument: Jane Austen wrote *Emma*; therefore, Charlotte Brontë wrote

Shirley. This is because there are possible states of affairs in which Austen wrote *Emma*, but Brontë did not get around to writing *Shirley*.

Aside from (1), none of the examples discussed so far lives up to this validity standard. For example, it is possible, though unlikely, that Max is innocent even when both the premises in (4) are true, and this means that Argument (4) is not deductively valid. However, this is not to say that all deductively invalid arguments are worthless. The premises of (4) are certainly good reasons for believing that Max planted the poisoned chocolate. To distinguish cases like these, we might call an argument *inductively strong* if, as in (4), it is not deductively valid but the truth of the premises nevertheless makes it likely that the conclusion is true (Skyrms, 1966). The strength of inductive arguments is an important topic in its own right, one that is taken up in other chapters in this volume. However, two points about it are worth mentioning here, because they bring out the relationship between induction and deduction. First, inductive strength is a matter of degree, depending as it does on how much support the premises lend to the conclusion. If only a single witness testified to Max's guilt, the resulting argument would still be reasonable, but it would be considerably weaker than (4). By contrast, deductive validity is an all-or-none matter according to our account. Second, some arguments are neither deductively valid nor inductively strong. Argument (2) provides such an example, since when its premises are true the conclusion not only *can* be false but is certain to be false.

Thus, of the argument examples, (1) is deductively valid, (4) is inductively strong (but not deductively valid), and (2) is worthless in having neither deductive validity nor inductive strength. Argument (3) poses some tricky problems that we shall confront later in the section on empirical issues.

Validity and provability as tests of deductive correctness

The notion of validity that we just discussed provides one way to check whether an argument is deductively correct, but in order to apply this standard, we must determine the relation between the premises' and the conclusion's truth in every possible state of affairs. Luckily, there is a second method of determining deductive correctness that does not depend on truth relations among sentences. With this method, we attempt to *prove* that the argument is correct using techniques familiar from proofs in mathematics.

There are several ways of formalizing proof procedures for deductive arguments, but one simple procedure is as follows. We start with a (usually small) set of rules that tell us when sentences of one form follow immediately from sentences of another. To determine whether a particular argument is deductively correct, we apply one of these rules to the premises of the argument and see what sentence follows from them. If the conclusion of the argument is identical to this newly derived sentence, we have succeeded in proving the argument correct. If not, we continue by again applying a rule, this time to the larger set of sentences formed by the original premises and the derived item. We continue in this way. The argument is deductively correct if there is some sequence of rules that will produce the conclusion. At this stage, the entire set of sentences that we have derived is the *proof* of the argument, and the argument itself is said to be *provable*. Of course, if the argument is deductively incorrect, we will never succeed in deriving the conclusion. Either we will reach a point at which we will no longer be able to derive new sentences or we will continue indefinitely adding new sentences to our set.

To understand what a simple proof is like, let us suppose our system includes the following rule:

R1 (modus ponens): From a sentence of the form *IF p THEN q* and another of the form *p*, the sentence *q* follows.

Here, *p* and *q* stand for arbitrary sentences. This rule suffices to show that Argument (1) is deductively correct, since the conclusion can be derived in one application of R1 to the premises. The premise *If Calvin deposits 50 cents, then Calvin gets a Coke* exactly matches the *IF p THEN q* form in the rule, with *p* equal to *Calvin deposits 50 cents* and *q* equal to *Calvin gets a Coke*. Similarly, the second premise is *Calvin deposits 50 cents*, which is the sentence we have just set equal to *p*. *Calvin gets a Coke* therefore follows from R1; and since this is the conclusion of (1), the argument is provable.

One-step arguments like (1) are not much fun, so let's try something slightly meatier. Suppose we want to show that the following argument is provable:

(5)   If Calvin deposits 50 cents, Calvin will get a Coke.
      If Calvin gets a Coke, Calvin will buy a burger.
      Calvin deposits 50 cents.
      _____

      Calvin will buy a burger.

A proof of this argument might be the following (where the comments on the right explain how the corresponding sentence was derived):

(6)   a. If Calvin deposits 50 cents,   [First premise of (5).]
         Calvin will get a Coke.
      b. Calvin deposits 50 cents.   [Third premise of (5).]
      c. Calvin will get a Coke.   [Follows from R1 applied
                                             to a and b.]
      d. If Calvin gets a Coke,   [Second premise of (5).]
         Calvin will buy a burger.
      e. Calvin will buy a burger.   [Follows from R1 applied
                                             to c and d.]

Line e in the proof is the conclusion of (5), and so (5) is provable. Here we have used R1 twice in order to derive this result.

The arguments that we can prove will depend on the rules that we include in our system. Rule R1 helps us capture arguments based on *conditional* sentences (ones of the IF . . . THEN form), but we will probably want to add rules for other sentence types. For example, proof systems in formal logic have been devised for arguments based on sentence connectives (words like AND, OR, NOT, as well as IF . . . THEN), quantifiers (phrases like FOR ALL or FOR SOME), terms dealing with knowledge (e.g., KNOW and BELIEVE), temporal terms (e.g., BEFORE and AFTER), terms of moral obligation (e.g., OUGHT and CAN), terms of possibility (e.g., POSSIBLE and NECESSARY), and others. Some of the systems that logicians have proposed are simply extensions of others, since all of the arguments that are provable in the smaller systems remain provable in the larger ones. For example, most books on elementary logic (e.g., Thomason, 1970) show how to extend a system for sentence connectives (called *classical propositional* or *sentence logic*) to a system that includes quantifiers (called *classical predicate logic*). Other logical systems, however, are incompatible; they disagree about what is provable with the very same logical terms (Haack, 1974). Since human deduction is often judged by comparison with formal logic, we must be specific in such cases about which logic we are dealing with. In this chapter, correctness in "standard logic" will refer to classical logic, which is the system that logicians have most deeply explored. However, this does not rule out the possibility that other systems of logic are more faithful to psychology and to natural language.

Validity and provability are two separate ways of marking correct deductive arguments, but we would hope that these criteria would agree. That is, it would be convenient if all arguments that are valid were also provable and if all arguments that are provable were also valid. In standard systems this agreement does indeed exist, and in these systems it doesn't matter which criterion we use, as long as all we want to know is whether a given argument is correct. However, there are two reasons for keeping both validity and provability in mind. One is that there are some domains in which not all valid arguments are provable (such domains are said to be *incomplete*). Another is that there is debate within psychology about whether human deduction more closely resembles proving arguments or testing them for validity (for contrasting views on this issue, see Johnson-Laird, 1983; Rips, 1986).

The deduction user's manual

Checking arguments for deductive correctness is sometimes useful − for example, in understanding mathematics. However, deduction can be of more general use as a way of carrying out basic cognitive tasks such as answering questions or planning actions. The role of deduction in these tasks gives us a clue to why inference principles like modus ponens seem so deep-seated in thinking, for if these principles underlie even simple question answering and planning, then we should not be surprised to find ourselves committed to them. To understand why this is true, however, we have to be more explicit about the mechanisms that are responsible for deduction. Until now, we have focused on arguments − sequences of sentences − possessing abstract properties such as provability or validity; but we must shift to a more concrete perspective if we want to examine the actual process of drawing inferences. A number of insights about this process have come from research in artificial intelligence, in which investigators have produced programs that draw deductive inferences in order to solve problems (for more on deduction in this field, see Charniak & McDermott, 1985; Nilsson, 1980.)

We start by outlining a simple deduction system that is capable of directing cognitive tasks. The point of doing this is to develop some idea of the parts of such a system, rather than to account for any particular body of psychological data. We will discuss psychological plausibility later in the chapter; for now we will merely try to get a view of the terrain. Then in the rest of this section we will look at an example of the way our sample deduction system can solve a problem on the basis of information in memory. Although the example is small in scale, it should illustrate how deduction could prove helpful in larger applications.

Principles of operation

Let's suppose that our system includes a temporary storage area, or *working memory*, that has limited capacity but that allows fast access to information saved there. In addition, the system obeys a set of deductive operating principles (somewhat similar to Rule R1 in the previous section) that apply to *propositions* stored in working memory. These propositions are essentially mental sentences, internal representations, with a special format that we discuss below. Propositions reach working memory from the senses or from long-term storage; and once in working memory, they are controlled by the operating principles, which have the power of deleting old propositions or adding new ones.

The most important fact about working memory, for our purposes, is that it normally contains two different kinds of propositions, which we will refer to as *assertions* and *goals*. Assertions are memory propositions that are currently accepted; they are beliefs that we hold, if only temporarily, in order to see where they lead us. Goals are propositions that we would like to prove true on the basis of the assertions. We can think of them as questions to be answered during the course of deduction, and for that reason, we will follow the convention of placing a question mark after them. To return to our earlier example, suppose we accept the propositions *If Calvin deposits 50 cents, then Calvin will get a Coke* and *Calvin deposits 50 cents*. We can then ask, *Calvin will get a Coke?*; that is, our goal will be to show that *Calvin will get a Coke* follows from the assertions. Once we find that it does follow, this goal will be fulfilled and will itself become an assertion.

In general terms the deduction system works like this: When a question is posed to the system in the form of a goal, the system principles will transform working memory (by adding new propositions) in an attempt to connect the goal to relevant assertions. If this attempt is successful, the goal will be fulfilled and the question answered. The pattern of connections that the system establishes will in essence form a proof somewhat similar to the ones described in the preceding section. If the attempt is unsuccessful, the system will have to admit that it does not know the answer to the original question.[4] Obviously, the key to this process is the nature of the principles themselves; so to understand the system, we will have to take a closer look at them.

Forward and backward principles. Corresponding to our two types of propositions are two general types of principles the system obeys. The first sort, *forward* principles, deal entirely with assertions. The other type, *backward* principles, are associated with goals. Forward principles inspect the propositions in working memory, and if they find assertions of a specified form, add new assertions. As an example, we have the following forward principle, which is similar to the modus ponens rule that we considered earlier:

Principle 1 (forward modus ponens): Whenever working memory contains an assertion of the form *IF p THEN q* and also contains the assertion *p*, then the assertion *q* will be added to working memory if it is not already there.

Naturally, this means that if working memory contains both *If Calvin deposits 50 cents, then Calvin will get a Coke* and *Calvin deposits 50 cents* as assertions, then *Calvin will get a Coke* will become an assertion as well.

Backward principles oversee working-memory goals, adding new subgoals when appropriate. The point of these principles is the common-sense idea that if we want to achieve some complicated goal we can break the problem into simpler parts. For instance, if we are interested in winning a chess game (the main goal), we might concentrate on developing a positional advantage or capturing an important piece (a subgoal), on the assumption that the subgoal will eventually lead to the fulfillment of the main goal. Likewise, if we wish to prove some proposition (the main goal), we might go about it by working backward, checking whether there are other propositions (subgoals) that would lead to the first. In terms of our well-worn example, if our goal is to show that *Calvin will get a Coke?* and we already have the assertion *If Calvin deposits 50 cents, then Calvin will get a Coke*, then it may be worthwhile trying to show that *Calvin deposits 50 cents?* since if we can prove it, the main goal follows immediately. This suggests the following backward principle:

Principle 2 (backward modus ponens): Whenever working memory contains a goal of the form *q?* and an assertion of the form *IF p THEN q*, then the subgoal *p?* will be added to working memory.

Principle 2 is just the backward version of Principle 1, since both express the same logical relationship. We will also find it convenient if our deduction system incorporates another backward principle for dealing with goals containing the word AND:

Principle 3 (backward AND introduction): Whenever working memory contains a goal of the form p_1 *AND* p_2*?* then the subgoals p_1*?* and p_2*?* will be added to working memory.

This is simply to say that if we want to show p_1 *AND* p_2*?* we should try to show p_1*?* and p_2*?* separately. For example, we can answer yes to *Skidmore is in New York and Swarthmore is in Pennsylvania?* if we can answer yes both to *Skidmore is in New York?* and to *Swarthmore is in Pennsylvania?*

Variables and instantiation. The principles just formulated are sufficient to help us deal with questions whose answers are either yes or no − for example, *Did Madonna write "The Logical Structure of the World"?* or *Is the Sears Tower the tallest building?* However, we also want the deduction system to deal with questions whose answers are particular individuals, such as *Who wrote "The Logical Structure of the World"?* or *What is the tallest building?* As usual, we want to be able to put these questions to the system as goals and to answer them on the basis of assertions. Thus, our working-memory propositions must have ways of naming things (e.g., Madonna or "The Logical Structure of the World" or the Sears Tower) and ways of describing the things named (e.g., Is-the-writer-of and Is-the-tallest-building).

For these purposes, we build our assertions and goals from *atomic propositions* consisting of a simple descriptor, or *predicate*, and one or more names, or *arguments*. For example, the proposition that Madonna wrote "The Logical Structure of the World" will be expressed as *Wrote(Madonna, "The Logical Structure of the World")* and the proposition that the Sears Tower is the tallest building will be *Tallest-building(Sears Tower)*. This separation between predicates and arguments allows us to ask questions about individuals, since we can indicate our uncertainty about which name correctly fills in a proposition. To ask who wrote "The Logical Structure of the World," we can use the goal *(WHICH x) Wrote(x, "The Logical Structure of the World")?*; that is, which thing (or things) is such that it wrote "The Logical Structure. . ."? Similarly, *(WHICH x) Tallest-building(x)?* asks which thing is such that it is the tallest building.

The x's in these propositions are *variables*, and they play much the same role in our system as variables in mathematics and programming. If we solve for x in an equation like $x = 3y + 2$, we want the value of x that makes the equation true (for a given value of y). In the same way, our system is supposed to "solve" goal questions like *(WHICH x) Tallest-building(x)?* for the value of x (the building) that makes the proposition true, thereby answering the question.

Variables have another benefit, since they enable us to state general relationships among predicates. Suppose, for instance, that we want to express the fact that a polygon with three sides is a triangle. It clearly is not possible to list the names of all three-sided polygons and label each of them a triangle. What we can do, however, is state that any x that happens to be a polygon and have three sides is a triangle. In symbols this becomes *(FOR ALL x) IF Polygon(x) AND Three-sided(x) THEN Triangle(x)*, where the phrase *(FOR ALL x)* is called a *universal quantifier*. This means that if we happen to have the assertion that a specific figure *ABC* is both a polygon and three-sided [i.e., *Polygon(ABC) AND Three-sided(ABC)*], we can immediately assert that *ABC* is a triangle [*Triangle(ABC)*]. In fact, this is just a more general case of Principle 1, adapted to our new predicate–argument notation.

Table 5.1 contains a reformulation of the principles that allows the system to use them with variables. The central idea in handling variables is that the system should try to match *(WHICH x)*-type goals with assertions that have names in place of the variable. For example, the goal *(WHICH x) Tallest-building(x)?* will be fulfilled by the assertion *Tallest-building(Sears Tower)*. When this happens, the variable is said to be *instantiated* by the name, and hence the name provides the answer to our goal question. Of course, if the goal has no variables, it will be fulfilled only by an assertion that matches it exactly. Thus, the goal *Tallest-building(Sears Tower)?* (i.e., *Is the Sears Tower the tallest building?*) will be fulfilled by the assertion *Tallest-building(Sears Tower)* (i.e., *The Sears Tower is the tallest building*). This rule about goal fulfillment appears as Principle 0 in Table 5.1.

The rest of the principles in the table are analogs of the ones described above. There are yet more general ways to formulate these rules that buy greater inference power (see the artificial intelligence references cited earlier); however, the Table 5.1 principles get us surprisingly far, as we can see by considering the example in the next subsection.

Deduction for planning

We are in a cave of twisting passages (Figure 5.1). Beginning at the entrance, we must find our way to the room containing the treasure, taking care not to run into the dragon. We will assume that the only information

Table 5.1. *Deduction system principles*

Principle 0 (matching)
a. A goal *(WHICH x_1, . . ., x_k) $P(x_1$, . . ., x_k,)?* is fulfilled by an assertion $P(m_1$, . . ., m_k).
b. A goal *P?* is fulfilled by assertion *P*.
c. A goal is fulfilled whenever all of its subgoals are fulfilled.

Principle 1 (forward modus ponens)
a. Whenever *(FOR ALL x) IF P(x) THEN Q(x)* is an assertion and *P(m)* is an assertion, then *Q(m)* will become an assertion.
b. Whenever *IF P THEN Q* is an assertion and *P* is an assertion, *Q* will become an assertion.

Principle 2 (backward modus ponens)
a. Whenever *(FOR ALL x_1, . . ., x_i, . . ., x_k) IF P(x_1 . . ., x_i, . . ., x_k) THEN Q(x_1, . . ., x_i)* is an assertion and *Q(m_1, . . ., m_i)?* is a goal, *(WHICH x_{i+1}, . . ., x_k) P(m_i, . . ., m_i,x_{i+1}, . . ., x_k)?* will become a subgoal.
b. Whenever *IF P THEN Q* is an assertion and *Q?* is a goal, then *P?* will become a subgoal.

Principle 3 (backward AND introduction)
a. Whenever *(WHICH x) P_1(x) AND P_2(x) AND . . . AND P_k(x)?* is a goal, then *(WHICH x) P_1(x)?* will become a subgoal. If the subgoal is fulfilled with *x* instantiated to *m* then *P_2(m)?* will become a subgoal. . . If this subgoal is fulfilled, *P_k(m)?* will become a subgoal.
b. Whenever *P_1 AND P_2 AND . . . AND P_k* is a goal, then *P_1?* will become a subgoal. If this subgoal is fulfilled, then *P_2?* will become a subgoal. . . If this subgoal is fulfilled, *P_k?* will become a subgoal.

Note: In these principles, *m* denotes a name (e.g., "Grand Canyon" or "Veronica Lake") and *x* denotes a variable. The letters *P* and *Q* stand for arbitrary propositions, *P(x)* and *Q(x)* are expressions containing the variable *x*; similarly, *P(x_1, . . ., x_k)* and *Q(x_1, . . ., x_k)* are expressions containing the variables x_1, . . ., x_k. All goals end in question marks.

about the cave that we have at the beginning is local information concerning which rooms are directly connected to others. The problem is to string this information together in order to find a complete route to the treasure. To plan our course through the maze, we will need some assertions to represent the local features of the layout. To do this we might use the predicate *Passage(x, y)* to mean that there is a direct passageway connecting Room *x* to Room *y*. (The passages are indicated by arrows in Figure 5.1 and can be traversed in only one direction in this maze, as shown by the direction of the arrows.) Thus, the important features of the cave can be captured by the assertions in (7):

(7)   a. Passage (Entrance, A)
      b. Passage(A, B)
      c. Passage(Entrance, B)
      d. Passage(A, Dragon)
      e. Passage(B, C)
      f. Passage(C, Dragon)
      g. Passage(C, Treasure)

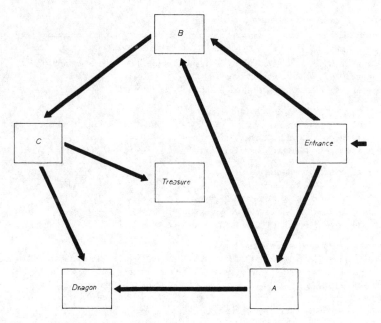

Figure 5.1. A map of a hypothetical cave with arrows indicating the direction of one-way passages from room to room.

In addition, we will need some way to represent which rooms are safe to traverse, which we might do with the predicate *Safe*:

(8) a. Safe(Entrance)
     b. Safe(A)
     c. Safe(B)
     d. Safe(C)
     e. Safe(Treasure)

That is, all of the rooms can be entered, except the one containing the dragon.[5]

Finally, in order to plan our route, we need some general assertions about getting from one place to another. Let the predicate *Route(x, y)* mean that one can find a series of safe moves from Room x to Room y. Clearly, if there is a single passageway from x to y and y is safe, then we have a route from x to y. In other cases, however, we will have to go through a series of intermediate rooms to get to our destination. We might express this by saying that there is a route between x and y if there is a passage from x to some (safe) intermediate room z and a route from z to y. This breaks the problem down into a series of simpler problems. These two pieces of knowledge can be stated in the following assertions:

(9) (FOR ALL x, y)   IF Passage(x, y)
                         AND Safe(y)
                         AND Report(y)
                         THEN Route(x, y)
(10) (FOR ALL x, y, z) IF Passage(x, z)
                         AND Safe(z)
                         AND Route(z, y)
                         AND Report(z)
                         THEN Route(x, y)

The *Report* predicate in (9) and (10) is a special expression that causes the system to report something – for example, by announcing it aloud or recording it in memory for later mention. *Report(z)* will announce whatever instantiates its variable. For instance, if the *z* in *Report(z)* is instantiated to *treasure*, then the system will report "treasure." This will come in handy, since we can use the *Report* predicate to announce the sequence of rooms along a correct route if we are successful in finding one. We shall see how this works later.

We shall assume for simplicity that the assertions in (7)–(10) are all in working memory at the start of the problem. In a more realistic system, we might want to place stricter bounds on the number of propositions that working memory can contain. In that case, we would need additional procedures (somewhat similar to *Report*) that would move information between working memory and long-term memory in order to overcome this capacity limit. But we shall ignore this complication for present purposes.

Now in order to find the path to the treasure, we should consider the goal

(11) Route(Entrance, Treasure)?

That is, is there a route from the entrance to the treasure? In order to answer this question, the system principles examine the contents of working memory to determine whether the information there suffices to fulfill the goal. Of course, the easiest way to fulfill it would be to use Principle 0 of Table 5.1 to find an assertion of the form *Route(Entrance, Treasure)*. This match would correspond to a "yes" response, meaning that we already knew about this route. But the fact is that working memory contains no straightforward assertions about routes, so we have to try a more indirect strategy.

A key to the right strategy is that the *THEN* parts of both (9) and (10) contain the *Route* predicate. Principle 2 applies in this situation, allowing us to reduce the main goal in (11) to subgoals. For example, Principle 2 can be applied to (9) and (11), yielding the subgoal *Passage(Entrance, Treasure) AND Safe(Treasure) AND Report(Treasure)?* Unfortunately, this is no help since there is obviously no direct passageway from the entrance to the treasure. (Remember that a passage is a single link in the map of Figure 5.1.)

We still have the option, however, of using the same Principle 2 in connection with (10), our only other way of establishing a route. That is, we can try to show that there is a route between the entrance and the treasure by finding a passage between the entrance and an intervening room z and then finding a route between z and the treasure. We can depict the state of things in working memory by means of the following diagram, in which we show the main goal at the top connected to Assertion (10) and to the new subgoal (E denotes Entrance, T Treasure):

Route (E, T)?

(WHICH z) Passage (E, z)
    AND Safe (z)
    AND Route (z, T)
    AND Report (z)?

(FOR ALL x, y, z) IF Passage (x, z)
    AND Safe (z)
    AND Route (z, y)
    AND Report (z)
    THEN Route (x, y)

The sense of this is that if we can fulfill the subgoal at the left, the assertion at the right will allow us to fulfill the main goal. Of course, working memory also contains the other propositions mentioned above; but to keep the diagrams simple, we include only information that is contributing to the solution.

The next step is to try to fulfill the subgoal: to find a safe intermediate room from which we will get to the treasure. This subgoal is composed of parts connected by *AND*s, which suggests that Principle 3 ought to help at this stage. This principle tries to fulfill the subgoal by fulfilling its parts one at a time; thus, it first attempts to find out *(WHICH z) Passage(Entrance, z)?* That is, which rooms are connected to the entrance? Here we have a choice, since there is a passage from the entrance to either Room A or Room B; but let's suppose that we decide to start with A [i.e., we use Principle 0 to fulfill this last subgoal by matching it to *Passage(Entrance, A)* in (7). We can also easily establish that *Safe(A)?* since this is just one of the assertions in (8). (Principle 3 allows us to plug in A here, since A instantiated variable z when the principle was first applied.) The result is the following working-memory structure:

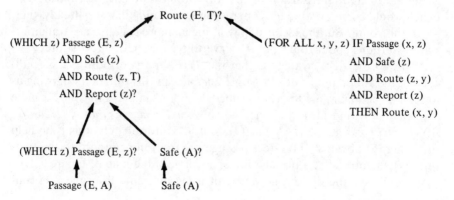

However, we are still not finished with the *WHICH* subgoal at the upper left of the diagram, since there are two remaining parts that we must fulfill. Next in line is *Route(A, Treasure)?* The form of this subgoal is exactly the same as that of the original goal (11), except that we are now one step closer to the treasure. The same possibilities are available for fulfilling this subgoal as were available for fulfilling the original goal, namely, using Principle 2 with either (9) or (10). Inspection shows that (9) will be just as fruitless as it was before and that (10) will result in a new, possibly helpful subgoal, which is shown at the bottom of the next diagram — slow but sure progress.[6]

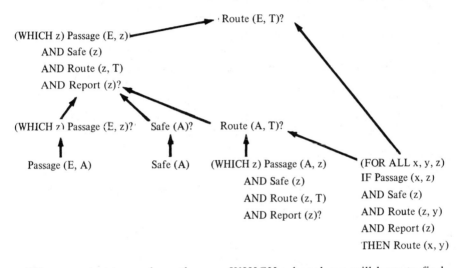

When we start to work on the new *WHICH* subgoal, we will have to find something satisfying *(WHICH z) Passage(A, z)?* from the list in (7). *Passage(A, Dragon)* might work, if it were not for the fact that we would then have to show that *Safe(Dragon)?* which plainly is not possible. So our only hope is to try *Passage(A, B)*.

At this point, we have plotted our route from the entrance to A to B. The step from B to C proceeds in exactly the same way, as illustrated in Figure 5.2, which contains the complete solution. There is only a single passage leading from B, so in effect this move is forced. At C we will be faced with fulfilling the goal *Route(C, Treasure)?* and here at last Assertion (9) will come into play. Principle 2 and Assertion (9) tell us that all we need to do is to satisfy the subgoal *Passage(C, Treasure) AND Safe(Treasure) AND Report (Treasure)?* and these three parts are easily carried out.

Notice that the word *"treasure"* will be the first thing to be reported. This is because in tackling the complex *WHICH* subgoals, we never got to *Report* anything: In trying to fulfill the *Route* predicates in these goals, we went one further level into the problem, as illustrated in Figure 5.2. Now that we have found our way to the end, we must return to those remaining *Reports*. The result will be our successful route reported in reverse order: Treasure, C, B,

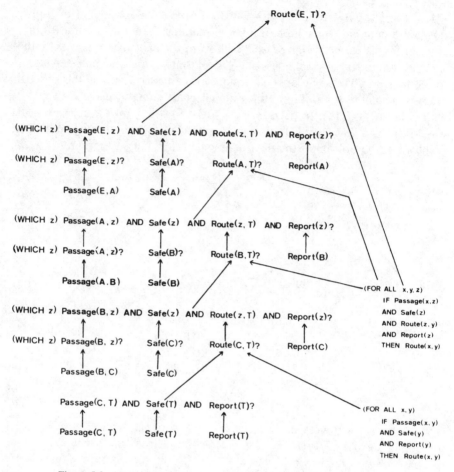

Figure 5.2. A working-memory proof that there is a route from the entrance (E) to the treasure (T); A, B, C correspond to the rooms in Figure 5.1.

A. This is not the most direct route, of course, but it is a perfectly correct one.

Summary

The advantage of a system like this one is that it is quite general. It will work correctly with assertions and goals concerning any subject matter, as long as we can express them in a form compatible with the principles of Table 5.1. (As already mentioned, it is possible to formulate the principles in ways that allow even greater flexibility in the propositions' structure.) Moreover, predicates like *Report* in the last example give the system power to control other parts of its environment − for example, retrieving information from long-term or sensory memories, focusing attention, and carrying out motor plans. This generality and power are attributes we would hope for in a core cognitive system. Artificial intelligence research has also revealed ways to make the deduction process more efficient, either by improving the inference principles (e.g., Chang & Lee, 1973), adding higher-level control mechanisms (Doyle, 1980; Genesereth, 1983; Weyhrauch, 1980), or providing heuristics for special domains (Gelernter, 1959). Although other artificial intelligence investigators (e.g., Hewitt, 1985; Minsky, 1985) argue that deduction has inherent limitations, it is at least worth contemplating the possibility that deduction forms a basis for human thinking.[7] In the rest of this chapter we look at some psychological evidence that bears on this proposal.

Empirical issues

We started this chapter with the intuition that certain deduction principles are central components of thinking, and it was this intuition that led us to consider a possible cognitive system in which deduction does indeed hold center stage. This intuition is important, but of course we eventually have to confront the question of how well this system fits relevant experimental findings.

This is not an easy question; and in trying to answer it, we must be clear about what is at stake. In the first place, although the principles in Table 5.1 seem to be plausible candidates for the beginnings of such a system, it would not be surprising if they were formulated somewhat differently or were supplemented by other rules in a correct psychological theory. As we mentioned earlier, formal logic can accommodate rules for quantifiers and connectives other than FOR ALL, AND, and IF . . . THEN, and we might want to expand our stock of principles in a similar way. What seems crucial is that there be some collection of principles that conform to the following specifications: that they respond to specifically logical properties of working-memory propositions; they direct cognition by adding, deleting, or modifying propositions; they allow forward and backward reasoning; they provide for variables and their instantiation; and they are consistent. The only new point is the last one, and it means that, if working memory contains no contradictory propositions [e.g., *Dates(Charlotte Brontë, Norman Mailer)* and *NOT Dates(Charlotte Brontë, Norman Mailer)*], the principles will not produce any.

Second, we must know what sort of psychological evidence is relevant to our deduction system. In one sense, of course, any evidence is potentially relevant. Since we are conceiving of deduction as a general-purpose mechanism for governing other complex cognitive tasks, the failure of the system to explain one of these tasks would be reason to suppose that the system is incorrect. Some of the debate within the artificial intelligence community has centered on this type of issue (Hayes, 1977, and Moore, 1982, take the prodeduction side of this debate, and Hewitt, 1985, and Minsky, 1985, the antideduction side). Within psychology, however, there is the possibility of a more direct test from a large body of experiments devoted specifically to deductive reasoning. Research in this area began around the turn of the century (see Woodworth, 1938, chap. 30) and has continued to the present, though somewhat on the periphery of experimental and social psychology. At first glance, this evidence would seem especially pertinent for evaluating the psychological status of the deduction system, and we consider it in this section. (Evans, 1982, and Wason & Johnson-Laird, 1972, provide book-length reviews of this area.)

The typical experiment in the psychology of deduction is very simple. As the subject, you receive a booklet containing a number of problems. Usually, each problem consists of a group of premises and a conclusion, as in our earlier examples (1)−(3). The experimenter tells you that your job is to decide whether the conclusion "follows logically" from the premises (or whether the conclusion "must be true when the premises are true"). You check a box marked "follows" or one marked "doesn't follow" to indicate your answer and then go on to the next problem. The basic dependent variable is the percentage of subjects who believe that the conclusion follows. The plain fabric of this experimental situation can be embroidered. For example, you may be asked to think aloud as you work the problem. Or the experimenter may record the amount of time it takes you to reach your decision. Or the experimenter may give you just the premises and ask you to write down a conclusion that follows logically from them. The main idea is that the experimenter wants to determine how variations in the nature of the problems affect the subjects' judgments about deductive correctness.

Reasoning experiments like these have special relevance to our contemplated deduction system because they explicitly call for a deductive judgment. Although question answering and other tasks also engage this system (according to the scheme of the preceding section), reasoning experiments can − at least in theory − directly probe the system's logical properties. They give us a tool for diagnosing the kind of system we are dealing with. For instance, if the system is built around a principle like modus ponens (e.g., Principles 1 and 2 of Table 5.1) and if the subjects are given a problem like the Calvin example in (1), we would expect the subjects to be in very good agreement that the conclusion follows from the premises, all else being equal. But as we shall see shortly, a great deal rides on the qualification that "all things are equal." After all, the experimenter cannot simply insert propositions into the subject's working memory. We have no guarantee that subjects correctly understand the request to decide whether the conclusion "logically follows." Similarly, we cannot be sure that subjects comprehend the sentences of the problem in the way the experimenter intends. If subjects understand them in some other way, the propositions that appear in working memory are not the ones the experiment was supposed to test. These ambiguities have given rise to long-standing controversies about the proper interpretation of reasoning experiments (e.g., Cohen, 1981, and commentaries in the same issue of *Behavioral and Brain Sciences*). Nevertheless, these experiments may still be the best tools we have for finding out whether a psychological deduction system is plausible.

Since the mid-1970s several researchers have proposed cognitive models of deductive reasoning that are in good agreement with the deduction system hypothesis (Braine, 1978; Braine, Reiser, & Rumain, 1984; Johnson-Laird, 1975; Osherson, 1974–6; Rips, 1983). According to these models, subjects have mental principles or rules similar to those of Table 5.1 that they employ in solving deduction problems. Although the details vary, the models share the idea that subjects represent the premises of a problem in propositional form and apply principles to the premises in order to prove the conclusion. If subjects obtain a (mental) proof, they respond that the conclusion follows; if no such proof is forthcoming, they respond that it doesn't follow. The proofs themselves may resemble the one in Figure 5.2. Obviously, subjects' success in finding a proof depends on whether they have the requisite principles. In addition, success will be a function of the complexity of the proof. If the conclusion follows by a short proof, subjects should be quite likely to get the right answer. More complex proofs are liable to failure because they may run up against memory or processing limitations.

Models of this type have been tested against data from experiments on a fairly wide class of problems and have in general received good empirical support (Braine et al., 1984; Osherson, 1974–6; Rips, 1983; Rips & Conrad, 1983). However, there are a number of findings in the research literature that challenge these models. One issue concerns the way people reason about sentences with explicit quantifiers such as *All* and *Some*. Certain theories about this kind of reasoning have a different flavor than the one we sampled in the previous section, and this may cast doubt on the deduction system approach. A second issue concerns the way the topic of a problem influences subjects' decisions. In many studies these decisions depend on more than logical properties. Since deduction systems are supposed to respond only to logical properties, these experiments too may give us pause about accepting the models. In the rest of this chapter, we take up these two issues in turn.

Reasoning with categorical syllogisms

Syllogisms are two-premise arguments with a fixed form for both the premises and the conclusion. The study of syllogisms comprised the subject matter of traditional logic, beginning with Aristotle's *Prior Analytics* and continuing until around the end of the nineteenth century (Kneale & Kneale, 1962). Syllogisms are no longer an important topic in logic, since by means of modern methods we can describe a vastly more general set of arguments. Nevertheless, psychologists have often chosen syllogisms as stimuli, perhaps for historical reasons or perhaps because their tidy structure lends itself to simple experimental manipulation. Recently, there has been a welcome trend away from this preoccupation with syllogisms, as psychologists have become more interested in the techniques of modern logic (e.g., Osherson, 1974–6), but we will deal with syllogisms here because they raise difficulties for the deduction system hypothesis.

The two premises and the conclusion of a categorical syllogism contain quantifiers, either the universal quantifier *All* or the existential quantifier *Some*. The same sentences can be negative or positive, producing four different sentence types: *Some . . . are . . ., All . . . are . . ., Some. . . are not . . ., and No . . . are . . .* (the last being equivalent to *All . . . are not . . .*). Thus, (12) and (13) are examples of categorical syllogisms:

(12)   All employees of Grapefruit Computing are enemies of
       Plum Systems.
       Some members of Club Avocado are employees of
       Grapefruit.
       _____
       Some members of Club Avocado are enemies of
       Plum Systems.

(13)   All employees of Grapefruit Computing are enemies of
       Plum Systems.
       Some members of Club Avocado are not employees of
       Grapefruit.
       _____
       Some members of Club Avocado are not enemies of
       Plum Systems.

All syllogisms of this sort have three terms [*employees of Grapefruit Computing, enemies of Plum*, and *members of Club Avocado* in (12) and (13)]. One of these terms must appear in the first premise and the conclusion, another in the second premise and the conclusion, and the third (or *middle* term) in both the premises. The order of the terms within the sentences can vary, however; so an argument like *All enemies of Plum are employees of Grapefruit; Some employees of Grapefruit are members of Club Avocado; Therefore, some members of Club Avocado are enemies of Plum* also qualifies as an (invalid) syllogism (Adams, 1984, provides a discussion of syllogistic form).

Results on categorical syllogisms exhibit a great range of performance from problem to problem. In one study, for example, Dickstein (1978) presented subjects with syllogistic premises and asked them to choose a conclusion from five alternatives: *All . . . are . . ., Some . . . are . . ., Some . . .*

are not . . ., No . . . are . . ., and no valid conclusion.[8] For premises similar to those in (12) and (13), most subjects chose the response corresponding to the conclusions shown in these examples; 100% chose *Some . . . are . . .* for (12) and 86% chose *Some . . . are not . . .* for (13). However, only the first of these is correct in standard logical systems: The right answer to the premises in (13) is "none of the above." [To convince yourself that (13) is invalid, consider the case in which the premises are true and in which even non-Grapefruit members of Club Avocado are enemies of Plum. This makes the conclusion false; and since the premises are true, the syllogism must be invalid.] Thus, 100% of subjects were correct on (12) but only 14% were correct on (13).

Johnson-Laird and Bara (1984, Experiment 3) obtained similar findings in a study in which they presented premises and required the subjects to produce any conclusion that necessarily followed. In that experiment 90% of the subjects responded with the correct conclusion to premises like those in (12), whereas only 10% correctly said that no valid conclusion followed from premises like those of (13). Again, the usual error on the latter problem (65% of responses) was *Some . . . are not . . .*

Theories of syllogisms. Psychologists have invoked a variety of factors to explain the results of these experiments. These factors can be divided into three classes, which we can call *shallow processing* theories, *comprehension* theories, and *analytic* theories. Although it is unlikely that any one type of theory can account for all of the data, taken together they may give a fairly complete picture of the results.

Shallow processing theories emphasize the way simple nondeductive features influence subjects' answers. In the shallow processing class, for example, are proposals that subjects are more likely to accept a syllogism as valid if they believe that its conclusion is true (e.g., Janis & Frick, 1943; Morgan & Morton, 1944). Similarly, Revlis (1975) presents evidence suggesting that subjects are biased against making the response "none of the above are valid." The most famous of these hypotheses, however, is Woodworth and Sells's (1935) proposal that subjects tend to choose existentially quantified conclusions (i.e., either *Some . . . are . . .* or *Some . . . are not . . .*) just in case either of the premises is existential and to choose a negative conclusion (either *Some . . . are not . . .* or *No . . . are . . .*) just in case either premise is negative. This proposal, called the *atmosphere hypothesis*, correctly accounts for the dominant responses to Syllogisms (12) and (13). In (12) the second premise is existentially quantified; hence, the conclusion should also be existential. However, since neither premise is negative, the conclusion will be positive. The existentially quantified, positive conclusion is *Some . . . are . . .*, which is indeed the most popular answer. In (13) the second premise is both existential and negative. Thus, according to the atmosphere hypothesis, the conclusion should also be existential and negative, producing *Some . . . are not . . .*, which is again the modal response.

According to comprehension theories, syllogism responses can be explained in terms of the way subjects understand a problem's meaning. Subjects may interpret a sentence of the type *Some X are Y* as suggesting that some *X* are *not Y* and, conversely, interpret *Some X are not Y* as suggesting that some *X are Y* (Ceraso & Provitera, 1971; Wilkins, 1928; Woodworth & Sells, 1935). In addition, several investigators have proposed that subjects understand *Some X are not Y* as implying *Some Y are not X* and understand *All X are Y* as implying *All Y are X* (Ceraso & Provitera, 1971; Chapman & Chapman, 1959; Revlis, 1975; Wilkins, 1928). This two-way interpretation of universally quantified sentences can explain why subjects are so willing to accept Syllogism (13). If *All employees of Grapefruit Computing are enemies of Plum* implies that all enemies of Plum are employees of Grapefruit, these two classes of people are identical. Hence, if some members of Club Avocado are *not* employees of Grapefruit (as asserted in the second premise), it follows that some members of Avocado are not enemies of Plum.

The final class of explanations, analytic theories, assume that subjects deal with syllogisms through some deductively correct procedure that tests whether the conclusion follows. For good reason, most current accounts are analytic (though they often combine an analytic mechanism with shallow processing or comprehension factors). Pure shallow processing explanations account for only a modest proportion of the results. For example, despite the success of the atmosphere hypothesis with Syllogisms (12) and (13), it predicts only about 50% of the responses in Dickstein's (1978) study and only 43% in the study of Johnson-Laird and Bara (1984). Even Woodworth and Sells (1935) saw the atmosphere hypothesis as an explanation of error tendencies, not as a full theory of syllogistic reasoning. Similarly, pure comprehension theories do not explain how subjects use the meaning of sentences to evaluate syllogisms. Psychologists who have championed comprehension theories have joined them with an analytic approach, often assuming that subjects reason correctly from the premises as they construe them (e.g., Henle, 1962; Revlin & Leirer, 1978).

Most analytic theories of categorical syllogisms suppose that subjects mentally represent the premises and conclusions in some sort of diagrammatic form (Erickson, 1974; Guyote & Sternberg, 1981; Johnson-Laird & Bara, 1984). As examples, Figure 5.3 shows how the premises of Syllogism (12) are depicted in the theories of Erickson and Johnson-Laird and Bara. In Erickson's view, subjects represent each premise as combinations of *Euler circles*, in which each circle denotes a class mentioned in the sentence. Overlapping areas correspond to members shared by the classes. Thus, *All employees of Grapefruit are enemies of Plum* appears in two guises: either as a circle for Grapefruit employees (dotted lines) inside a larger circle for ene-

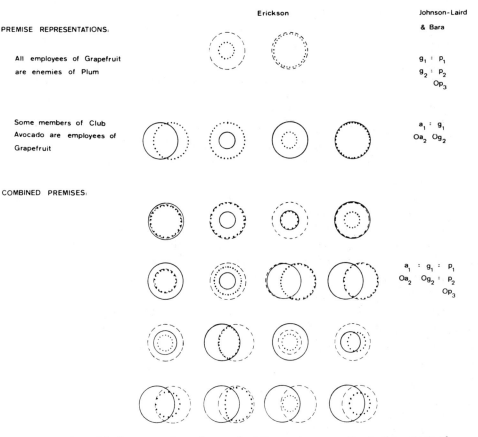

Figure 5.3. Representations of two syllogistic premises, according to the systems of Erickson (1974) and Johnson-Laird and Bara (1984). The solid circles stand for members of Club Avocado, the dashed circles for enemies of Plum Systems, and the dotted circles for employees of Grapefruit Computing.

mies of Plum (dashed lines) or as two coincident circles. The first combination portrays the one-way interpretation in which there are enemies of Plum that are not Grapefruit employees; the second gives the two-way interpretation in which Grapefruit employees and enemies of Plum are one and the same.

Johnson-Laird and Bara's representation achieves similar ends by more economical means. Here letters stand for individuals ("g" for a Grapefruit employee and "p" for a Plum enemy), an equal sign indicating that the connected people are the same. Thus, g_1 is the same person as p_1, and g_2 is p_2. A zero in front of a letter denotes a person who may or may not exist. The zero in front of p_3 (like the presence of two sets of Euler circles) means that there may or may not be enemies of Plum who do not work for Grapefruit.

To evaluate or produce a conclusion, we must combine the premise representations into a representation of the syllogism as a whole. In general there will be more than one possible combination. If a potential conclusion holds true in all of them, the conclusion deductively follows from the premises. In Erickson's theory multiple combinations occur both because each premise can usually be represented in more than one way and because each pair of premise representations can be put together in several ways. Figure 5.3 shows the 16 distinct combinations for the premises of (12). The conclusion of (12) is true in all of them; other potential but invalid conclusions (e.g., *Some members of Club Avocado are not enemies of Plum*) may be true in some but not all.

According to Johnson-Laird and Bara's account, subjects form an initial combination from the premise representations and then read from it a possible conclusion. For Syllogism (12) the combination might look like the diagram at the bottom right of Figure 5.3. Notice that equal signs connect Avocado member a_1 to Plum enemy p_1, so one candidate conclusion is *Some members of Club Avocado are enemies of Plum*. According to this approach, subjects then attempt to find alternative combinations that are consistent with the premises but that refute the first conclusion. These alternatives can be formed by changing the alignment of the letters or adding new ones. For example, by adding a new optional Avocado member, we could produce this combination:

$$
\begin{array}{lll}
a_1 = & g_1 = & p_1 \\
0a_2 & 0g_2 = & 0p_2 \\
0a_3 & & 0p_3
\end{array}
$$

But this new diagram is also consistent with the original conclusion. In fact, there are no further combinations that can refute it, and so a careful subject will choose that conclusion as the correct answer. In other syllogisms, however, new combinations will contradict the conclusion the subjects started with, and they will therefore have to revise their choice in order to make a correct response.

Analytic theories explain the difficulty of a problem in terms of the amount of processing that subjects require to arrive at a correct answer. Both Erickson's and Johnson-Laird and Bara's models attribute errors to subjects failing to consider all of the relevant combinations of the premises. The more combinations, the more difficult it is to keep track of all of them and hence the greater the likelihood of error. Both models, however, also allow for shallow processing and comprehension factors. These can affect the way subjects represent the premises or the way they derive the conclusions from the combined diagrams.

Implications for the deduction system hypothesis. In summary, people's accuracy in evaluating the validity of syllogisms varies enormously according to the type of problem. For ones like (12), subjects' judgments almost always concur with standard logical formulations. For many others there is no such agreement. None of the pure approaches just considered seems sufficient to explain this variation. Models in the shallow processing class are too simple to account for the data. Comprehension models are incomplete, presupposing some type of reasoning mechanism. Most current investigators have therefore adopted an analytic approach, supposing that people reason correctly within limits imposed by their information-processing capacity and by their understanding of the problems.

In one sense, analytic theories are in agreement with the type of deduction system outlined in the second section of this chapter. If the deduction system hypothesis is correct, we would expect subjects to be able to reason correctly in many cases, since their thinking is ultimately guided by logical rules. However, a problem in reconciling current analytic theories with deduction systems is that the diagram representations of these theories run counter to the propositional representations of Table 5.1. Of course, we could make the deduction system manipulate diagrams, just as we could make it plot a route through a maze; so the two ideas are not contradictory.

It is also possible to argue that diagram theories presuppose deduction principles in order to set up the diagrams in accord with the premises, to interpret the diagrams, and to recognize when a diagram is consistent with, or contradictory to, a conclusion (Pylyshyn, 1980; Rips, 1986). Nevertheless, it is of interest to consider whether there are deduction principles similar to those of Table 5.1 that could directly predict syllogism data. Braine and Rumain (1983) and Osherson (1976) offer suggestions along these lines, though neither of these models has been fully tested against the results of syllogism experiments. Thus, it is far from clear at this point whether deduction systems can provide a direct account of categorical syllogisms that predicts the results more accurately than the diagram theories.

At the beginning of this chapter, we distinguished the deduction system hypothesis from the deduction heuristics hypothesis. According to the heuristics view, deductive reasoning is a specialized cognitive task, suited to problems such as categorical syllogisms. The task itself may be carried out through "quick and dirty" methods that do not guarantee a correct decision. Shallow processing models are perfect examples of the heuristics approach, and the general failure of shallow processing to predict syllogism responses tends to cast doubt on its adequacy. Of course, heuristic methods may well be part of the story of why subjects commit the errors they do (see Pollard, 1982, for a defense of heuristics and biases in deductive reasoning). But the weight of evidence seems to favor the idea that people's deductive reasoning is deeper and more systematic. This situation contrasts strikingly with the state of the art in inductive reasoning, in which shallow processing is very much in favor (Tversky & Kahneman, 1974, 1983).

The issue of problem content

Subjects' answers in reasoning experiments sometimes depend on the way the problems are framed. Subjects give different answers to problems with seemingly identical logical properties if these problems have different content. These findings are a potential challenge to the deduction system hypothesis, since the actions of such a system are triggered only by the logical properties of working-memory propositions. It should not matter what these propositions are about: As long as they have the same logical form – are built up in the same way from logical connectives like IF and AND and quantifiers like FOR ALL – the system should treat them identically.

We must be careful, however, in interpreting experiments on content. Changes in the wording of a problem can influence performance for reasons that are independent of subjects' reasoning strategies. For example, in an early demonstration Wilkins (1928) presented subjects with syllogisms couched in either everyday language (e.g., *All people taking part in the play are trained actors*), meaningless letters (*All x's are y's*), or scientific or pseudoscientific terms (*All cosmanthi are phacelia*). Over all problems, the subjects were somewhat more accurate with everyday wording, even when the conclusions ran counter to common sense. Of the problems they attempted, the subjects were correct on 85% of the syllogisms with familiar wording and neutral conclusions, 80% correct for familiar wording and misleading conclusions, 76% correct for letters, and 75% correct for jargon. However, this small advantage for familiar wording does not necessarily mean that the subjects were reasoning in different ways about the four problem types. People's experience with meaningful terms may help them encode sentences and remember them, and better encoding and memory could by themselves account for the slightly higher scores.

In other experiments, however, differences in content cannot be as easily pinned on low-level cognitive factors. These studies use commonplace language throughout but vary the relations named in the problem. Content effects of this sort appear in experiments with categorical syllogisms (Revlis, 1975; Revlin & Leirer, 1978) and with related arguments based on conditional sentences (Rips & Marcus, 1977; Staudenmayer, 1975). Most of the relevant research, however, concerns a task that is somewhat different from the argument evaluations we have looked at, and it is therefore worth taking a moment to describe it.

The selection experiment. Suppose you have in front of you four index cards. On the first card is the letter E, on the second K, on the third the numeral 4, and on the last 7. The experimenter tells you that each card contains a numeral on one side and a letter on the other, although you are not allowed to look at the flip sides of the cards. The experimenter also informs you that you are to "decide which cards [you] would *need* to turn over in order to determine whether the experimenter was lying in the following statement: If a card has a vowel on one side, then it has an even number on the other side" (Wason, 1966, p. 146). (In later versions of the problem, subjects were asked to "name those cards and only those cards, which need to be turned over in order to determine whether the rule is true or false"; see Wason & Johnson-Laird, 1972).

Despite its apparent simplicity, this problem is extremely difficult. The most popular responses are that both the E and the 4 cards should be turned over (46% of responses according to Wason & Johnson-Laird, 1972) or that only the E card should be turned over (33%). Neither of these responses is correct. Certainly, the E card should be turned, since if it had an odd number on its flip side, the rule would be false. The K, however, is consistent with the rule no matter whether it is paired with an even or an odd number, so this card cannot discriminate a true from a false rule. What about the number cards? If the 4 card has a vowel on the other side, it is consistent with the rule; and if it has a consonant, it is also consistent. The 4 card is therefore irrelevant to the test. This leaves the 7 card. If its flip side contains a vowel, this card contradicts the rule, whereas if the flip side has a consonant, the card conforms to the rule. Therefore, the E and 7 cards must be turned over, but Wason and Johnson-Laird found that only 4% of their subjects made this response. In later replications, the percentage of correct responses for materials like these varied from 6 to 33% (Evans, 1982, chap. 9). Nor is the difficulty confined to undergraduates, who are the usual subjects in such experiments. Dawes (1975) reported that the correct answer was obtained by only one of five mathematical psychologists, whom he described as "highly regarded members of their field."

Of special concern to the content issue is the effect of framing the selection task with different types of rules. Early results seemed to indicate that almost any content more familiar than arbitrary letters and numbers would aid subjects in making the right choice (Wason & Johnson-Laird, 1972, chap. 14), but these findings have proved extremely difficult to replicate (Griggs & Cox, 1982; Manktelow & Evans, 1979). Although some types of everyday content do improve scores, others apparently do not. As an example, one type that *does* help involves regulations about drinking (Griggs & Cox, 1982; Wason & Green, 1984). Griggs and Cox found that 74% of subjects gave the correct answer when the rule was rephrased as "If a person is drinking beer, then the person must be over 19." The cards in this instance referred to four people sitting at a table, with their age indicated on one side of the card and the beverage they were drinking on the other side. The cards were marked "drinking beer" (analogous to the E card in the original problem), "drinking Coke" (analogous to the K card), "22 years of age" (analogous to the 4 card), and "16 years of age" (analogous to the 7 card).

By contrast to the benefits of the drinking regulation, there appears to be no advantage to be gained from rephrasing the rule as "If I eat haddock, then I drink gin" and indicating on one side of the cards "what I ate" and on the other "what I drank" at a particular meal (Manktelow & Evans, 1979). In this experiment, the cards might be marked "haddock," "macaroni," "gin," and "champagne." Only 7% of subjects correctly chose the "haddock" and "champagne" cards, a figure quite comparable to the success rate in the original letters-and-numbers experiment.

What makes content helpful in one situation and not in the other? The best current hypothesis is that content aids the decision process only if the subjects know before the experiment about the relation between the values mentioned in the IF part of the rule and the values mentioned in the THEN part (or know of a closely similar relation; Griggs, 1983). Subjects certainly know before the experiment about the required relation between age and drinking but, of course, have no idea about the arbitrary pairing of food and beverage. This hypothesis also helps to explain findings in other sorts of experiments with conditional sentences (Rips & Marcus, 1977) and can therefore claim some generality. It is not clear, however, why prior knowledge should be beneficial.

Implications for the deduction system hypothesis. The moral that we should draw from content effects depends on way these effects come about. So it might be useful to list ways in which content could guide subjects to a correct answer in problems like the selection task. Four possibilities suggest themselves:

1. Effects on low-level cognition: As we suggested earlier, subjects' performance will be better if a problem is simple to encode and to remember. In the case of the selection task, well-known relations between the parts of a rule may make the rule more memorable and hence easier to deal with. (This hypothesis is slightly different from the one mentioned earlier in connection with Wilkins's experiment. There we attributed the advantage to the memorability of individual predicates in the problem; here we are concerned with relations among predicates.)
2. Effects on comprehension: Subjects may not grasp the exact meaning of logical connectives such as IF in the selection "rule." There may be distinct varieties of IFs in natural language, and subjects may be uncertain about which of them the experimenter intends. Perhaps, then, prior knowledge can guide subjects to the correct meaning.
3. Effects on reasoning: The reasoning procedures subjects employ in dealing with familiar relationships may be different from those they use with unfamiliar relationships. This may be because they are more practiced at thinking about situations with which they have had experience. Unfamiliar settings may leave them without an obvious algorithm to fall back on.
4. Effects of associated long-term-memory information: Knowledge about the topic of a problem could bring with it associated information from long-term memory. For instance, a conditional like *If a person is drinking beer, then the person must be over 19* is related to other facts: that potential offenders are younger individuals, that to be an offender one has to drink an

alcoholic beverage, and so on. These additional facts may provide a strong clue to the right choice.

In the present state of knowledge, it is hard to tell which of these factors are responsible for subjects' performance, though some seem more likely than others. Low-level processes could certainly be involved, but the magnitude of the differences in selection experiments makes it doubtful that this factor is solely responsible. It is also important to remember that content can sometimes make subjects' performance *less* accurate. As we mentioned in connection with syllogisms, there is evidence that subjects' prior belief in a conclusion can induce them to accept an invalid argument. The effect is small but relatively consistent from experiment to experiment. For example, Wilkins (1928) noted that subjects tend to accept the following argument but correctly reject it when it is rephrased in less familiar terms:

(14)   No oranges are apples.
       No lemons are oranges.
       No lemons are apples.

If content influenced reasoning merely by streamlining information processing, this "negative" content effect would be hard to explain.

Comprehension effects might be powerful enough to account for content differences and may well be responsible for the findings of some studies of conditional and quantificational reasoning. To explain the selection task, however, proponents of this hypothesis have to maintain that the sentence *If a person is drinking beer then the person must be over 19* lends itself to a different or more definite meaning for *if–then* than *If I eat haddock, then I drink gin*. Perhaps, but it is unclear what sort of interpretation could produce the pattern of results just described. One possibility is that subjects take the sentence *If I eat haddock, then I drink gin* to mean both *IF haddock THEN gin* and *IF gin THEN haddock* (i.e., *Haddock IF AND ONLY IF gin*). This would correspond to the two-way interpretation of *All* mentioned in connection with syllogisms. But although such an interpretation is indeed appropriate in many real-world contexts (Fillenbaum, 1977; Geis & Zwicky, 1971), it should induce subjects to turn over all four cards in the selection task, since all four could potentially confirm or disconfirm the rule. Hence, it cannot by itself explain the prevalence of E and E−4 choices.

Much the same can be said about reasoning differences, for although these differences are sometimes assumed without argument, advocates of this idea owe us a concrete proposal before we can accept this hypothesis as a credible one.[9]

The last of our four factors, long-term memory information, seems to be a plausible account of many content effects. In the context of the selection task, one version of this hypothesis is that subjects do not engage in reasoning at all when given the drinking regulation; they simply choose the cards that name possible instances that could violate the rule (i.e., the 16-year-old and the beer drinker). Another version of this proposal is that subjects combine the facts explicitly mentioned in the problem with the associated long-term-memory information and use the combined knowledge to reason to the right answer. The latter version stands up better in light of other experiments that show facilitation for odd rules (*Anyone consuming Coca Cola on these premises must be at least 100 years old*; Wason & Green, 1984) and abstract rules (*If one is to take action A, one must first satisfy precondition P*; Cheng & Holyoak, 1985) that are analogous to familiar relationships but have no exact counterpart in memory. This hypothesis (in either version) is also consistent with the negative content effects mentioned earlier.

If Factors 1, 2, or 4 account for content effects, either alone or in combination, the deduction system hypothesis has little trouble accommodating the results. According to Factor 1, content makes it more likely that certain facts will be remembered; according to 2, content determines which interpretation of the sentences subjects use; according to 4, content controls the facts from long-term memory that enter into consideration. Thus, in terms of the system described earlier, these factors affect which propositions are part of working memory during the reasoning process. If content changes subjects' responses, that may be because they are using different sets of propositions. Factor 3, however, could pose a greater problem; if content alters the reasoning process itself, it could challenge the idea of a unified system that responds to the logical structure of propositions. The issue is complicated conceptually because it presupposes thorny distinctions between logical structure and nonlogical "content" and between comprehension and reasoning. It is also an area in which we need more discriminating experiments.

Conclusions

Deductive reasoning has a special status among cognitive processes, since the ability to recognize simple deductive arguments is a core property of rational thought. People who lack knowledge of ordinary concepts may seem to us woefully ignorant but not irrational. However, people who violate principles like modus ponens would be unfathomable. How could we convince them or teach them? How could we understand what they believe? From another perspective, however, it is difficult to see why this is so. Except for mathematical contexts, deduction is not in the cognitive foreground. Unless we are taking a math or logic course, or taking an intelligence test like the GRE Analytic, we do not spend much time worrying about whether arguments are deductively correct. So, on one hand, deduction appears to be a deep and necessary part of cognition, but on the other, it seems infrequently exercised.

One way to resolve this dilemma is to conceive of deduction as a system for controlling other aspects of thinking. Consider the contributions of a director to a movie: Although we may never see the director on the screen, each scene can carry his or her stamp. In the second part of this chapter, we sketched one possible design for such a cognitive deduction system. Its main features are a set of principles, which actually carry out the inferences, and a working-memory storage area, which holds propositions for input and output. This system is highly speculative and is no more than a starting point in theorizing about deduction. However, it gains some support from research in artificial intelligence (e.g., Nilsson, 1980) and in cognitive psychology (e.g., Braine et al., 1984; Osherson, 1974–6; Rips, 1983).

In the third part of the chapter, we discussed what seem the most problematic empirical questions that such a theory faces. The evidence comes from studies in which subjects judge the deductive correctness of arguments (in the case of syllogisms) or use deduction to solve a problem (in the case of the selection task). These experiments show that factors other than raw deduction enter into subjects' judgments, but the experiments do not disconfirm the basic features of the theory. Admittedly, theories like this one are difficult to test, because their very generality insulates them from direct confirmation or disconfirmation. We can obtain only limited information from the results of individual experiments, since these results can very often be "explained away" by factors that are independent of the processes of interest. Ideally, we want a snug fit to the facts with as few special alterations as possible.

In addition to explaining experimental results, we would also like the theory to be compatible with other higher cognitive processes. In this connection, we looked at some ways deduction could be useful in question answering and planning, which are not typically thought of as deductive processes. This should not be taken to mean that deduction is all there is to thinking. Certainly, inductive reasoning is crucial in many everyday situations, as we noticed early on. However, deduction is often presented in introductory textbooks as a rather esoteric process, used mainly in dealing with logic brain teasers. By contrast, the illustrations in the second section suggest that deduction may be far more pervasive in ordinary pursuits than you might have expected.

Notes

1 *Modus ponens* means "affirming mode," since we are affirming the IF part of the original sentence in order to affirm the THEN part. Modus ponens contrasts with *modus tollens* ("denying mode"), which is the argument from *IF so-and-so THEN such-and-such* and *NOT such-and-such* to *NOT so-and-so*. These terms come from traditional logic. For a discussion of a potential counterexample to modus ponens, see McGee (1985).

2 People's intuitions about mental activities assign reasoning an important place. In a recent study, subjects rated each of a series of activities according to their importance in "how our

minds work" (Rips & Conrad, 1984). The average rating for "reasoning" was 7.78 on a scale from 0 to 10, where 0 meant *not at all important* and 10 meant *couldn't be more important*. This mean rating surpassed those for all other mental acts on the list, including "solving problems" (7.57), "learning" (7.50), "remembering" (7.36), "planning" (6.14), and "imagining" (6.00).

3   In fact, the comparison between deduction and programming languages is more than an analogy. There are now general-purpose languages that use deduction to carry out their activities. The best-known language of this sort is PROLOG, which has received publicity because of its connection with the Japanese Fifth Generation Project. An excellent guide to PROLOG is Clocksin and Mellish (1981). The examples in the second section of this chapter are based in part on that reference. Kowalski (1979) contains a more general discussion of deduction as programming.

4   In some special cases, we can safely assume that failing to find a proof indicates that the question should get a negative answer. If you cannot retrieve the fact that you have shaken hands with Ronald Reagan, then it is safe to believe you haven't done so (Collins, 1978). This assumption has been called *circumscription* or the *closed-world assumption*, and formal methods have been developed for incorporating it in a deduction system (McCarthy, 1980; Reiter, 1978).

5   Of course, we could use *NOT Safe(Dragon)* rather than the list of assertions in (8). To handle propositions like this, however, we would have to add principles for NOT to those in Table 5.1. This no doubt *should* be done in a full-scale deduction theory, but to keep our illustrations simple, we have omitted these extra principles. Braine (1978) and Rips (1983) give rules for negation that would work in this context.

6   Progress in this problem is ensured by the fact that the cave in Figure 5.1 contains no loops (i.e., we cannot double back to a room we have already visited). In the more general case, we would have to keep track of the rooms we had been to in order to avoid going in circles. One way to do this would be to introduce a predicate similar to *Report* that would construct a room list, adding to it whenever we entered a new room. Notice, also, that at more than one place in our march through the maze, we choose goals in just the right order to avoid dead ends. In normal circumstances, we would not be so lucky. For this reason, a complete deduction system would have to include provisions for noticing when a subgoal could not be fulfilled and backing up to a previous goal in order to make a fresh start. For some empirical evidence on maze searching, see Hayes (1965).

7   The main alternatives to deduction systems in both artificial intelligence and cognitive psychology are production systems (e.g., Anderson, 1983) and frame systems (e.g., Brachman & Schmolze, 1985; Fikes & Kehler, 1985). However, the differences among them may be more a matter of emphasis than a substantive dispute about the character of thinking. In production systems a fundamental distinction is made between certain *if–then* propositions (production rules) and all other propositions. There are usually a large number of these production rules, and they have the capacity to inspect working memory and carry out actions (via predicates like *Report*). They are themselves governed by some type of rule applier that resolves conflicts among rules, instantiates variables, and carries out other housekeeping tasks. The rule applier, in effect, uses forward modus ponens on the production rules and the contents of working memory. Thus, it is possible to view production systems as a type of deduction system consisting of one general principle (forward modus ponens) and a large number of special *if–then* propositions that can themselves perform actions.

  Frame systems are essentially theories about how memory is organized. According to this view, knowledge is divided into frames or concepts that have internal structure and have specified relations to neighboring concepts. These systems perform some inferences automatically by virtue of the built-in relations, but these inferences are far too limited for carrying out tasks like those discussed in this chapter. Clearly, frame systems require additional procedures, but the nature of these routines has not been clearly specified. At least on first glance, they could be consistent with the deduction framework described above. That is, we can understand frame systems as hypotheses about representation and deduction systems as hypotheses about processing.

It should be clear that all three systems are very general. To some extent, each is capable of simulating the behavior of the other two. More important for our purposes, each appears to incorporate deduction at some level in order to take advantage of the logical structure of propositions, rules, or relations among concepts.

8   Dickstein used letters rather than natural language terms in his problems. Thus in one trial, subjects would have seen the following pair of premises:

All *M* are *P*.
Some *S* are *M*.

They would have been asked to choose among the following conclusions: *All S are P, Some S are P, No S are P, Some S are not P,* or none of the above. This example has the structure of (12), with *S* replacing *members of Club Avocado*, *M* replacing *employees of Grapefruit*, and *P* replacing *enemies of Plum Systems*.

9   Cheng and Holyoak (1985) have advanced a proposal that comes close to the differences-in-reasoning idea for the selection task. According to their view, performance on the drinking problem is improved if subjects call to mind abstract "reasoning schemata" associated with permissions or obligations. Other ways of stating the problem will evoke other schemata or perhaps no schema at all, yielding poorer performance. Cheng and Holyoak may well be right in stating that permission giving is the crucial ingredient in boosting subjects' scores, but it is hard to tell whether this factor causes subjects to reason differently in the relevant sense. For example, it is possible that permission contexts remind subjects of specific incidents that provide clues to the correct answer (a Factor 4 explanation, as discussed below). Alternatively, it may be that people have special logical connectives that enable them to represent conditional permission or obligation. (The field of *deontic* logic, in fact, is devoted to the study of just such operators; see, e.g., Føllesdal & Hilpinen, 1971; Lewis, 1974.) If so, it may be that the permission context influences subjects' comprehension of the problem by substituting the conditional permission connective for ordinary *if*. This is a Factor 2 explanation. (Of course, a change in the interpretation of a logical operator will force a change in reasoning: If someone misreads AND as OR in a problem, then his or her reasoning will probably be different. What is at stake here, however, is whether there can be a change in reasoning with the very same logical form.)

References

Adams, M. J. (1984). Aristotle's logic. In G. H. Bower (Ed.), *Psychology of learning and motivation* (Vol. 18, pp. 255–311). New York: Academic Press.

Anderson, J. R. (1983). *The architecture of cognition.* Cambridge, MA: Harvard University Press.

Brachman, R. J., & Schmolze, J. G. (1985). An overview of the KL-ONE knowledge representation system. *Cognitive Science, 9,* 171–216.

Braine, M. D. S. (1978). On the relation between the natural logic of reasoning and standard logic. *Psychological Review, 85,* 1–21.

Braine, M. D. S., Reiser, B. J., & Rumain, B. (1984). Some empirical justification for a theory of natural propositional logic. In G. H. Bower (Ed.), *Psychology of learning and motivation* (Vol. 18, pp. 313–71). New York: Academic Press.

Braine, M. D. S., & Rumain, B. (1983). Logical reasoning. In J. H. Flavell & E. M. Markman (Eds.), *Handbook of child psychology* (Vol. 3, pp. 263–340). New York: Wiley.

Ceraso, J., & Provitera, A. (1971). Sources of error in syllogistic reasoning. *Cognitive Psychology, 2,* 400–10.

Chang, C. L., & Lee, C. T. (1973). *Symbolic logic and mechanical theorem proving*. New York: Academic Press.

Chapman, L. J., & Chapman, J. P. (1959). Atmosphere effect re-examined. *Journal of Experimental Psychology, 58,* 220−6.

Charniak, E., & McDermott, D. (1985). *Introduction to artificial intelligence*. Reading, MA: Addison-Wesley.

Cheng, P. W., & Holyoak, K. J. (1985). Pragmatic reasoning schemas. *Cognitive Psychology, 17,* 391−416.

Clocksin, W. F., & Mellish, C. S. (1981). *Programming in PROLOG*. Berlin: Springer-Verlag.

Cohen, L. J. (1981). Can human irrationality be experimentally demonstrated? *Behavioral and Brain Sciences, 4,* 317−70.

Collins, A. (1978). *Studies of plausible reasoning: Vol. I. Human plausible reasoning* (Report no. 3810). Cambridge, MA: Bolt Beranek and Newman.

Davidson, D. (1970). Mental events. In L. Foster & J. W. Swanson (Eds.), *Experience and theory* (pp. 79−101). Amherst: University of Massachusetts Press.

Dawes, R. M. (1975). The mind, the model, and the task. In F. Restle, R. M. Shiffrin, N. J. Castellan, H. R. Lindman, & D. B. Pisoni (Eds.), *Cognitive theory* (Vol. 1, pp. 119−29). Hillsdale, NJ: Erlbaum.

Dennett, D. C. (1980). True believers: The intentional strategy and why it works. In A. F. Heath (Ed.), *Scientific explanation* (pp. 53−75). New York: Oxford University Press. (Clarendon Press).

Dickstein, L. S. (1978). The effect of figure on syllogistic reasoning. *Memory & Cognition, 6,* 76−83.

Doyle, J. (1980). *A model for deliberation, action, and introspection* (Report No. AI TR-581). Cambridge, MA: MIT, Artificial Intelligence Laboratory.

Erickson, J. R. (1974). A set analysis theory of behavior in formal syllogistic reasoning tasks. In R. L. Solso (Ed.), *Theories in cognitive psychology* (pp. 305−329). Hillsdale, NJ: Erlbaum.

Evans, J. St. B. T. (1982). *The psychology of deductive reasoning*. London: Routledge & Kegan Paul.

Fikes, R., & Kehler, T. (1985). The role of frame-based representation in reasoning. *Communications of the ACM, 28,* 904−20.

Fillenbaum, S. (1977). Mind your p's and q's: The role of content and context in some uses of *and, or,* and *if.* In G. H. Bower (Ed.), *Psychology of learning and motivation* (Vol. 11, pp. 41−100). New York: Academic Press.

Føllesdal, D., & Hilpinen, R. (1971). Deontic logic: An introduction. In R. Hilpinen (Ed.), *Deontic logic: Introductory and systematic readings* (pp. 1−35). Dordrecht: Reidel.

Geis, M. L., & Zwicky, A. M. (1971). On invited inference. *Linguistic Inquiry, 2,* 561−6.

Gelernter, H. (1959). Realization of a geometry-theorem proving machine. *Proceedings of an International Conference on Information Processing* (pp. 273−82). Paris: UNESCO.

Genesereth, M. R. (1983). An overview of metalevel architecture. *Proceedings of the National Conference on Artificial Intelligence, 3,* 119−24.

Griggs, R. A. (1983). The role of problem content in the selection task and in the THOG problem. In J. St. B. T. Evans (Ed.), *Thinking and reasoning* (pp. 16−43). London: Routledge & Kegan Paul.

Griggs, R. A., & Cox, J. R. (1982). The elusive thematic-materials effect in Wason's selection task. *British Journal of Psychology, 73,* 407−20.

Guyote, M. J., & Sternberg, R. J. (1981). A transitive-chain theory of syllogistic reasoning. *Cognitive Psychology, 13,* 461−525.

Haack, S. (1974). *Deviant logic*. Cambridge University Press.

Hayes, J. R. (1965). Problem topology and the solution process. *Journal of Verbal Learning and Verbal Behavior, 4,* 371−9.

Hayes, P. J. (1977). In defense of logic. *International Joint Conference on Artificial Intelligence, 5,* 559−65.

Henle, M. (1962). On the relation between logic and thinking. *Psychological Review, 69*, 366–78.

Hewitt, C. (1985). The challenge of open systems. *Byte, 10*, 223–42.

Janis, I. L., & Frick, F. (1943). The relationship between attitudes toward conclusions and errors in judging the logical validity of syllogisms. *Journal of Experimental Psychology, 33*, 73–77.

Johnson-Laird, P. N. (1975). Models of deduction. In R. J. Falmagne (Ed.), *Reasoning: Representation and process in children and adults* (pp. 7–54). Hillsdale, NJ: Erlbaum.

(1983). *Mental models.* Cambridge, MA: Harvard University Press.

Johnson-Laird, P. N., & Bara, B. G. (1984). Syllogistic inference. *Cognition, 16*, 1–61.

Kneale, W., & Kneale, M. (1962). *The development of logic.* New York: Oxford University Press. (Clarendon Press).

Kowalski, R. (1979). *Logic for problem solving.* Amsterdam: North Holland.

Lewis, D. (1974). Semantic analyses for dyadic deontic logic. In S. Stenlund (Ed.), *Logical theory and semantic analysis* (pp. 1–14). Dordrecht: Reidel.

Madonna (1936). *The logical structure of the world.* London: Routledge & Kegan Paul.

Manktelow, K. I., & Evans, J. St. B. T. (1979). Facilitation of reasoning by realism: Effect or non-effect? *British Journal of Psychology, 70*, 477–88.

McCarthy, J. (1980). Circumscription: A form of nonmonotonic reasoning. *Artificial Intelligence, 13*, 27–39.

McGee, V. (1985). A counterexample to modus ponens. *Journal of Philosophy, 82*, 462–71.

Minsky, M. (1985). *The society of mind.* New York: Simon and Schuster.

Moore, R. C. (1982). The role of logic in knowledge representation and commonsense reasoning. *Proceedings of the National Conference on Artificial Intelligence, 2*, 428–33.

Morgan, J. J. B., & Morton, J. T. (1944). The distortion of syllogistic reasoning produced by personal convictions. *Journal of Social Psychology, 20*, 39–59.

Nilsson, N. J. (1980). *Principles of artificial intelligence.* Palo Alto, CA: Tioga Press.

Osherson, D. N. (1974–6). *Logical abilities in children* (Vols. 2–4). Hillsdale, NJ: Erlbaum.

Pollard, P. (1982). Human reasoning: Some possible effects of availability. *Cognition, 12*, 65–96.

Pylyshyn, Z. W. (1980). Computation and cognition: Issues in the foundations of cognitive science. *Behavioral and Brain Sciences, 3*, 111–69.

Quine, W. V. (1970). *Philosophy of logic.* Englewood Cliffs, NJ: Prentice-Hall.

Reiter, R. (1978). On reasoning by default. *Theoretical Issues in Natural Language Processing, 2*, 210–18.

Revlin, R., & Leirer, V. O. (1978). The effect of personal biases on syllogistic reasoning: Rational decisions from personalized representations. In R. Revlin & R. E. Mayer (Eds.), *Human reasoning* (pp. 51–81). Washington, D. C.: Winston.

Revlis, R. (1975). Syllogistic reasoning: Logical decisions from a complex data base. In R. J. Falmagne (Ed.), *Reasoning: Representation and process in children and adults* (pp. 93–133). Hillsdale, NJ: Erlbaum.

Rips, L. J. (1983). Cognitive processes in propositional reasoning. *Psychological Review, 90*, 38–71.

(1986). Mental muddles. In M. Brand & R. M. Harnish (Eds.), *The representation of knowledge and belief* (pp. 258–86). Tucson: University of Arizona Press.

Rips, L. J., & Conrad, F. G. (1983). Individual differences in deduction. *Cognition and Brain Theory, 6*, 259–85.

(1984). *The centrality of mental acts.* Unpublished manuscript, University of Chicago.

Rips, L. J., & Marcus, S. L. (1979). Suppositions and the analysis of conditional sentences. In M. A. Just & P. A. Carpenter (Eds.), *Cognitive processes in comprehension* (pp. 185–220). Hillsdale, NJ: Erlbaum.

Skyrms, B. (1966). *Choice and chance.* Belmont, CA: Dickenson.

Staudenmayer, H. (1975). Understanding conditional reasoning with meaningful propositions.

In R. J. Falmagne (Ed.), *Reasoning: Representation and process in children and adults* (pp. 55–79). Hillsdale, NJ: Erlbaum.

Thomason, R. H. (1970). *Symbolic logic*. New York: Macmillan.

Tversky, A., & Kahneman, D. (1974). Judgment under uncertainty: Heuristics and biases. *Science, 185*, 1124–31.

(1983). Extensional versus intuitive reasoning: The conjunction fallacy in probability judgment. *Psychological Review, 90*, 293–315.

Wason, P. C. (1966). Reasoning. In B. M. Foss (Ed.), *New horizons in psychology* (pp. 135–51). Harmondsworth: Penguin Books.

Wason, P. C., & Green, D. W. (1984). Reasoning and mental representation. *Quarterly Journal of Experimental Psychology, 36A*, 597–610.

Wason, P. C., & Johnson-Laird, P. N. (1972). *Psychology of reasoning*. Cambridge, MA: Harvard University Press.

Weyhrauch, R. (1980). Prolegomena to a theory of mechanized formal reasoning. *Artificial Intelligence, 13*, 133–70.

Wilkins, M. C. (1928). The effect of changed material on ability to do formal syllogistic reasoning. *Psychological Archives, 16*, whole no. 102.

Woodworth, R. S. (1938). *Experimental psychology*. New York: Holt.

Woodworth, R. S., & Sells, S. B. (1935). An atmosphere effect in formal syllogistic reasoning. *Journal of Experimental Psychology, 18*, 451–60.

6   Judgment and decision making

Baruch Fischhoff

Some of life's decisions are easy to make. By midwinter, regular television viewers should have a fairly good idea of what program to choose at eight o'clock on Saturday night. By midsemester, introductory chemistry students know whether it is better to fudge their lab results or report what they really observed. By midterm, a president should know whether to approach Congress directly for support on a piece of legislation or to "go over its head" and appeal to the American people. What makes these decisions fairly easy to make is the relative certainty about both the facts and the values involved in them. The decision makers know what they want from each decision (e.g., an effortlessly good time, a good grade with minimal work, looking like a winner). And they know what they will get if they take each possible course of action (e.g., how enjoyable each program will be, how the teaching assistant will respond to real and fabricated results, how the news media will report different political stances).

These decision-making processes might be just as easy, but lead to different conclusions, if the people making them saw the world the same way but wanted different things from it (e.g., a viewer for whom the weekend was the time to be reminded of the burning political issues of the day, a student for whom candor was more important than grades, a president for whom impact was more important than image). Different easy decisions might also be made by individuals who had the same values but saw the facts differently (e.g., fun-loving viewers who disagreed over whether NBC's sitcom was more fun than ABC's, lazy students who disagreed over whether the teaching assistant cared more about truth than conclusions, presidents who disagreed over whether the news media really wanted to see a good show).

Decision making becomes difficult when there is uncertainty, either about what will happen or about what one wants to happen. For example, a viewer's decision would be complicated by not knowing what the networks are going to offer during "Sweeps" month (a question of facts) or by not knowing whether education or entertainment is more important (a question of values). A president's decision would be complicated by not knowing just how the Congress, the news media, or the American people would respond to different appeals or by holding conflicting values about the presidency.

My thanks to Robyn Dawes and Lita Furby for thoughtful comments on earlier drafts. Support for this work was provided by the National Science Foundation and is gratefully acknowledged.

Decisions that are easy to make are not necessarily better or worse than decisions that are hard to make. The appropiate level of difficulty depends on the particulars of the decision. Making a decision can be too easy if one fails to consider significant complicating factors (e.g., ignoring the uncertainty created by this being Sweeps month, ignoring one's confusion over the relative importance of personal enjoyment and social responsibility). Making a decision can be too difficult if one fails to recognize important simplifying facts about the world (e.g., as far as one is concerned, the networks' special efforts are just more of the same programming) or about oneself (e.g., one does not just want to have fun and feels bad about becoming too self-absorbed).

Thus, uncertainty sometimes is a fact of life in decision making and sometimes is not. When it is, it can often be *the* fact of life, for individuals must wrestle with understanding the world and understanding themselves before they can make their decisions. Not surprisingly, the importance of the way people grapple with uncertainty has not escaped the attention of psychologists − or of philosophers, economists, political scientists, sociologists, operations researchers, geographers, statisticians, or management scientists. Somewhat surprisingly, however, in today's age of specialization, researchers in these different disciplines have talked and even worked with one another. Indeed, some of the earliest experiments on decision making were conducted by joint teams of psychologists, economists, and philosophers. Although these interactions have often been fitful and strained, there has been enough continuity to create a loosely structured interdisciplinary (and international) field, usually known as *behavioral decision theory* (Edwards, 1961; Pitz & Sachs, 1984; Slovic, Fischhoff, & Lichtenstein, 1977). In addition, researchers have repeatedly been challenged to show how much they know by somehow being useful to people faced with real-life decisions, ranging from insuring against floods and earthquakes and investing in the stock market to choosing medical procedures and dealing with hazardous technologies (Beach & Beach, 1982; Bettman, 1979; Dreman, 1982; Elstein, Shulman, & Sprafka, 1978; Fischhoff, Lichtenstein, Slovic, Derby, & Keeney, 1981; Kunreuther et al., 1978; Slovic, 1969). The result of drawing on diverse disciplines and experiences is a field that is probably both richer and more chaotic than any field that would have developed had psychologists simply followed the internal dictates of their own research programs and responded to the criticisms of other psychologists.

Perhaps the best way to understand the present state of this interdisciplinary field is to examine the contributions made by some of its contributors, each with somewhat different perspectives on uncertainty and different methods for studying the way people deal with it. Although the emphasis will be on psychology's contribution to the understanding of these complex thought processes, the story cannot be told without a consideration of the sometimes restraining, sometimes liberating influence of these other fields. Considering the interaction as a whole suggests some general conclusions about the potential strengths and weaknesses of psychology as a discipline.

Subjective expected utility

The psychological study of decision making took its initial marching orders from the models of optimal decision making developed by philosophers and economists (Coombs, Dawes, & Tversky, 1970; Edwards, 1954). These models describe how individuals should go about determining the best possible course of action for themselves, given what they believe about the world and what they want from it. People who follow these rules are said to be *rational* and the decisions that they make are said to be *optimal*, in the sense of *maximizing* what these decision makers can hope to get from them (given their beliefs and desires).

Although the models take very strong positions on the process of decision making, they are mute with regard to its content. They say, given one's wants and beliefs, here are the procedures one must follow in deciding what option to choose (if one wants to be considered rational). As a result, in a particular situation (e.g., choosing television shows, preparing lab reports), two different people could make different rational choices. If they have different beliefs and desires, they are, in effect, facing different decisions. Criticizing a decision made by a rational process means doubting the appropriateness of the beliefs or desires that it reflects. Although such doubts are certainly possible, they are not the department of decision theorists. Questions about what one should want are left to ethical experts (i.e., philosophers, religious leaders, political figures); questions about what one should expect in the future are left to technical experts (i.e., those who know most about the facts of a matter).

These models are also mute regarding how pleasant the outcomes of rational decisions will be. In some cases, a rational choice means taking the best of several unattractive options (e.g., eating less than one wants vs. weighing more than one wants). In other cases, the best option may not be a certain one, so that a wise choice can be followed by a disappointing outcome (e.g, a fastened seat belt is much more likely to save your life during a collision than to threaten your life after driving off a bridge; however, you might be one of those rare rational people trapped under water). Just like the randomness of a sample, the rationality of a decision is determined by the process that produces it. Following the rules is the best one can do. After that, one must live with the result, even if it means drawing 10 successive clubs from a well-shuffled deck, interviewing 75% white males in a supposedly representative survey of U.S. adults, or being one of the responsible unfortunates who drive off bridges. Knowing that one made the best possible choice by following the correct procedure might at least prevent the insult of regret from compounding the injury of one's misfortune.

Two psychological questions are suggested by this model of ideal performance (as well as by the comparable models underlying the research discussed in most of the other chapters in this volume): (a) Do people perform the way that the models claim they should? (b) If not, how can people be helped to improve their performance? Significantly, these have not been equally natural questions for economics, another social science discipline whose heart and soul is human decision making. Rather, economists have traditionally taken it as self-evident that people optimize their decisions. For economists, the underlying assumptions of the rational models are so reasonable that it seems implausible that people should not follow them. As a result, the idea that people optimize when making decisions has the status of a metatheory. Its truth goes without saying. The goal of the empirically minded economist is, therefore, not to test the hypothesis that people optimize, but to determine what it is that people are trying to maximize. Doing so requires considerable ingenuity and technical skill (as well as some additional assumptions about how well informed people are about the world around them and the choices that it offers). If the research is successful, then by carefully observing what decisions people make, one can learn something about the deep-rooted values that motivate them. With additional (macroeconomic) assumptions about how people interact in the marketplace, one can even propose social policies that will give society as a whole more of what it wants. Conversely, one can predict confidently how people will respond to manipulations of various aspects of their environment (e.g., prices, interest rates, taxes).

By allowing economists both to describe and to direct behavior within the same conceptual framework, the rational model provides an enormously powerful tool. This power is enhanced by the fact that the basic model of rationality that is accepted by most economists lends itself readily to the creation of complex models describing what it means to be rational in specific situations. As a result, much economic research is devoted to creating sophisticated mathematical models for figuring out what values have motivated the decisions that people have made in complex situations that already exist or to predict what decisions would be made by people with those motivations in response to complex situations that might be created.

The price paid for this analytic power is the inability to test the metatheory that people are rational. Indeed, rationality is not a theory at all in the sense that it cannot be falsified by any conceivable evidence (Lakatos & Musgrave, 1970; Popper, 1962). Whatever decision a person makes, one can always find some goal that that choice succeeded in optimizing, thereby rescuing the assumption of rationality. Some of the more imaginative fudge factors fall into the categories of *transaction costs*. Decision making itself is seen as incurring such costs, and the process is managed so as to keep those costs down. Thus, a decision that seems to select a suboptimal alternative can be reinterpreted as the result of the decision maker's having worked with a simplified view of the world so as to minimize transaction costs (Simon, 1957).

What one can falsify is local theories regarding what people optimize in particular situations. For example, if one assumes that people both are rational and have all pertinent information, then observing that they sometimes watch news and documentaries allows one to reject the theory that all they want from television is a good time. Note that, in principle, two other kinds of interpretation are possible. One is to accept the theory but reject the auxiliary assumptions regarding how well informed people are. That is, one could argue that people really do just want a good time; however, they erroneously believe that news and documentaries will satisfy that desire. The second alternative is to reject the assumption of rationality. That is, whatever people know and want, they may not optimize their viewing because they have trouble thinking their way through to a good decision.

Faced with a set of competing explanations for an observed choice, it seems reasonable to weigh the evidence and guess which explanation is most likely. For example, one might conclude that the choice of television programs is so simple that viewers probably are quite rational. However, the networks' advertisements showing attractive anchor people mislead viewers into expecting more fun from the news than they actually get. In this light, choosing to watch the news is the best decision given people's beliefs and desires, but it is not the decision they would make if they had perfect information. Of course, there are other interpretations, depending on what one believes about people's beliefs, desires, environment, and decision-making processes.

Why, then, would economists (and psychologists and others [Feather, 1982]) resolutely reject one interpretation (i.e., that the decision-making process is flawed, or irrational)? Their research strategy is perhaps best understood as one response to the inherent difficulty of studying simultaneously the subjective inputs to people's decisions (i.e., their beliefs and values) and the processes by which those inputs are combined to produce an observable output (i.e., the choice among options). All those who study decision making (and, perhaps, any other kind of behavior) face this challenge. As will be seen below, many psychologists meet it by controlling the inputs tightly, hoping thereby to know exactly what their subjects believe about an experimental situation and want to get from it. These investigators can then focus on *how* their subjects combine these facts and values. In doing so, such investigators sacrifice the opportunity to explore the way their subjects interpret situations (identifying the relevant facts and values) in order to get a better look at the way they exploit them.

One reason economists (and others) reject this strategy is that they have a greater interest in the *what* than the *how* of decision making. For example, someone may want to know what can be offered investors (or shoppers or workers or voters or potential lottery participants) that will be attractive to them but not cost much. A second reason is that economists (and others) are interested in real-life situations in which the inputs to decisions cannot be so tightly controlled. For example, it may be important to know the extent to which people suffer from environmental noise in order to decide whether to construct sound barriers along a freeway, to prohibit late-evening airport activity, or to close a foundry in a residential area. Because it is hard (or unethical) to expose people to persistent noise in order to measure their discomfort, environmental economists have attempted to exploit "natural experiments." Namely, they have examined housing prices at various distances from airports on the assumption that people's sensitivity to noise can be gauged by the amount of money they are willing to pay to avoid it. A third reason for ignoring the flaws in human decision making is the enormous analytic power of the rational decision-making models. Taken to the limit, this concept offers a single model to describe all decisions. Its elegance may seem to contrast sharply with the messy methods used by psychologists and the patchwork of psychological processes that those methods often reveal.

What is this powerful model? Its basic logic is straightforward: For any decision, list all feasible courses of action. For each action, enumerate all possible consequences. For each consequence, assess the worth (i.e., attractiveness or aversiveness) of its occurrence, as well as the probability that it will be incurred should the action be taken. Compute the expected worth of each consequence by multiplying its worth by its probability of occurrence. The expected worth of an action is, then, the sum of the expected worths of all possible consequences. Once the calculations are completed, choose the action with the greatest expected worth.

The "how" of this model is the multiplicative procedure for computing expected worth. The "what" is a set of judgments regarding what consequences are worth and how likely they are to be obtained. The rule for combining these considerations when evaluating the expected worth of an individual alternative action is

$$\sum_{i=1}^{n} P_i W_i = P_1 W_1 + P_2 W_2 + \cdots + P_n W_n \qquad (1)$$

In this expression, there are n possible consequences of the action. For a job search decision, they might include regular pay, bonuses, promotion, security, travel, or enjoyable coworkers; W_i is the worth of each if it is obtained; (P_i is the probability that it will be obtained) (if the job is taken). The best jobs would be ones whose sure consequences are good and whose good consequences are sure.

One graphic expression of the decision problem to which such a rule might be applied is shown in Figure 6.1, depicting the situation of a driver pondering whether to wear a seat belt. It begins at the *decision node* with the options and continues through the *event nodes* showing the uncertain contingencies that shape the consequences of each option. A probability is associated with each contingency and a value with each consequence. In this example, the consequences associated with each outcome are lumped together and evaluated as a whole. They range from mildly good (driving unbelted and having no accident) to very bad (driving unbelted and having an accident). This picture could be complicated by listing the different consequences of each outcome separately (e.g., discomfort, thrill, peace of mind, influencing the behavior of others in the car, social approval or disapproval) or by introducing more contingencies (e.g., being stopped by the police in a state with a compulsory seat belt law).

Figure 6.2 pursues both avenues of complication in describing the situation faced by people who have been told that homes in their area might be polluted by radioactive radon emitted by underlying rocks or building materials. First, they must decide whether to learn more about their personal situation. Second, they must decide what to do in response to that information. Each of these 16 action–event–action chains leads to some level of consequence on each of the four factors listed on the right. A good deal is known about how such *decision trees* should be constructed and unraveled in order to identify the best action (Behn & Vaupel, 1982; Raiffa, 1968).

For most economists in the United States, the natural place to look for evidence as to what things are worth is the marketplace. If something is traded directly (e.g., a car, spinach, the right to view a movie), then belief in rationality (along with some strong assumptions about the efficiency of markets) allows one to argue that what people will pay for something represents its true worth. If one can make these arguments and assumptions, the research is easy: One simply looks at the sticker or ticket price. These observed values are often called people's *revealed preferences*, that is, ones that emerge in their actual choices.

The situation becomes much more difficult for the investigator when something is not traded directly. For example, a recurrent question in many recent public policy decisions is, How much is a life worth or, conversely, how much is it worth paying to save a life? An example might be deciding whether to spend $100,000, $1 million, $10 million, or $100 million cleaning up a toxic waste dump, when the expected effect of that action would be preventing one additional death from cancer over the next 20 years.[1] Since the end of slavery, lives have not been bought and sold directly in the United States. Even when they were, the sales price reflected the value of slaves' lives to their owners and not to the slaves themselves. One would no more rely on those prices as an indication of the value of slaves as human beings than one would rely on the amount society currently pays to save

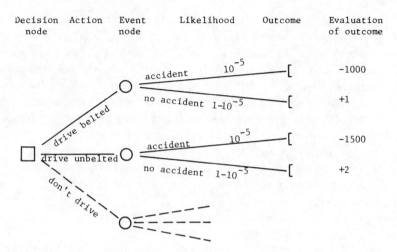

Figure 6.1 Decision tree for using a seat belt on a single auto trip. From Fischhoff, Svenson, and Slovic (1987).

lives as a gauge of the value of its citizens' lives. For example, if society could save the lives of 1,000 child-abuse victims by spending an additional $10 million but is not doing so, one could not conclude that each of those children is worth less than $10,000 (= $10 million/1,000) to society. It could be that society really does not want to pay the money; however, that revealed preference is so immoral and callous that it says nothing about the true worth of children. Or it could be that society would spend the money, but the political leaders responsible for making such decisions have failed to consider the issue seriously enough to realize what the ethical decision is (making the lack of funds a sin of omission rather than one of commission).

A more ethical strategy for evaluating the worth of lives is to look at the compensation people are willing to accept in return for performing riskier jobs. If two jobs were identical in all respects other than risk level, the *safety premium* could be readily calculated. For example, if one job paid $2,000 per year more than another but carried an additional 1 in 1,000 chance of accidental death, one might argue that a single life is worth $2 million (= $2,000 x 1,000). However, identical jobs are scarce when one considers all the factors that can affect wages (e.g., comfort, unionization, security, local unemployment, co-workers, training requirements, predominant sex). A riskier job might even be more poorly paid if it were an entry-level job or in an economically depressed area. Nonetheless, the wages might still be higher than they would be if the risk level of the job were lower. Belief in the rational model described earlier (along with a belief in numerous auxiliary assumptions regarding the accuracy of worker's beliefs and the efficiency of labor markets) allows analysts to try to uncover the value of risk with statistical procedures such as multiple regression. These techniques

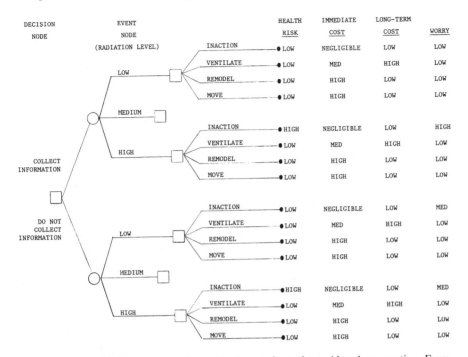

Figure 6.2 The radiation hazard in homes from the residents' perspective. From Svenson and Fischhoff (1985).

involve asking whether knowing the risk level of jobs facilitates the prediction of their pay level if other relevant factors are held constant (Jones-Lee, 1976; Viscusi, 1983).[2]

Such analyses require attention to a great number of technical details, such as the consequences that are included as predictor variables in the regression equation, the correlations among these variables, the ratio of sample size to number of variables, and the reliability with which the variables are measured (e.g., Cohen & Cohen, 1975). Once the analyses have been performed additional care is needed in generalizing their results. Strictly speaking, they pertain only to other items in the same population (with the same intercorrelations, ranges of values, etc.). As one goes farther from that population, the conclusions become less useful. Thus, one might be reluctant to apply conclusions regarding the value of human life based on a study of poorly educated workers in a depressed rural area to university students, to workers in a prosperous suburban area, or to the same rural workers after unionization (Fischhoff & Cox, 1985).

One would qualify those conclusions even further to the extent that the auxiliary assumptions needed for the analysis were not met, for example, if the conditions needed for a free market were violated in such a way that the workers were prevented from obtaining fair compensation for the risks (e.g., if the workers did not know how great the risks were; if refusing hazardous work imperiled their seniority; if the workers did not feel that they had the right to compensation). In this example, the assumption that workers perceive risks accurately seems particularly doubtful (Nelkin & Brown, 1984; Slovic, Fischhoff, & Lichtenstein, 1979, 1981). In other cases, quite different assumptions might be questionable. Indeed, as will be seen from research discussed later, in almost every revealed-preference study, whether conducted by economists or by others, such as the "expectancy-value" theorists working in various areas of psychology (Feather, 1982), there are usually some grounds for doubting either rationality or the auxiliary assumptions that go with it.

Nonetheless, and to the discouragement of skeptics, these models often perform quite well even when their assumptions seem most doubtful. That is, they make decent predictions of people's decisions on the basis of an expected-worth equation [like (1)] that embodies plausible values for the importance of different consequences and the probability of their occurrence. Some of this "suspicious" success can be attributed to the inherently ambiguous nature of the rationality model. Who is to say exactly what consequences should and should not be included in the model or what weight should be attached to each? The research is, after all, designed to find out what people care about; insofar as that is the subjects' own business, any value is conceivable. However, given this freedom, it would seem that, with sufficient ingenuity, the diligent investigator could not help but find some set of values that predicts people's choices well enough that one could say, "This is how they were being rational." An important safeguard against unfairly exploiting the ambiguity of rationality is *replication*: If the equation showing how one group of people is rational also predicts the choices of other people (or of the same people in new situations), than one has confidence that the equation did not work merely by chance.[3]

Unfortunately, however, replication is boring, hard to publish, and surprisingly uncommon. Moreover, concurrent developments in clinical psychology have suggested a rather different interpretation of the predictive success of even those rational models that are replicated. This research has provided additional reasons for believing that the predictive successes were real, along with additional reasons for doubting that such success proves that people are rational.

Clinical judgment

World War II was an important turning point in the development of American psychology. When put to the test, psychologists proved themselves capable of handling a large number of people in a relatively efficient way, using either their clinical skills to diagnose and treat psychological problems or their psychometric tests to identify the best candidates for different jobs. After the war, interest grew in just how effective those efficient decisions were. One focus of this interest was the efficacy of *clinical judgment*. Although the research initially concerned the judgments of psychologists making decisions such as whether clients were "psychotic" or "neurotic," it gradually expanded to include the judgments of radiologists sorting X-rays of ulcers into "benign" or "malignant," of personnel officers choosing the best applicants from a group of candidates, of crisis-center counselors assessing whether callers were serious about their suicide threats, of auditors pondering which loans to classify as "nonperforming," and of brokers weighing which stocks to recommend (Goldberg, 1968, 1970; Kelly & Fiske, 1951; Meehl, 1954; Slovic, 1969). When such judgments are made repeatedly, it is often possible to investigate the strategies that underlie them with a procedure analogous to that used in revealed-preference studies: A large set of judgments is collected, each of which is characterized by those *cues* the judge might have considered. In a study of crisis-center judments, for example, the cues might include sex of caller, time of day, tenor of voice, or history of attempts. Then statistical techniques, such as multiple regression, are used to predict the summary judgments (i.e., suicidal/nonsuicidal).

In a well-known study, Dawes (1971) examined the process by which the Graduate Admissions Committee of the University of Oregon Department of Psychology evaluated 384 applicants for the 1969−70 academic year. Although the committee considered many other cues (e.g., letters of recommendation, full transcripts), their decisions could be predicted very well from three variables: total Graduate Record Examination score (GRE), overall undergraduate grade point average (GPA), and a crude index of the quality of undergraduate institution (QI). The specific equation for predicting the average admissions committee rating was

$$0.0032 \text{ GRE} + 1.02 \text{ GPA} + 0.0791 \text{ QI} \tag{2}$$

Dawes suggested that, if the department actually endorsed this implicit policy, a great deal of time and money could be saved by all parties if prospective applicants were given Formula (2) and discouraged from applying to the department if their score was very low.[4]

In addition to illuminating a specific practical problem, Dawes's study demonstrated some of the basic patterns replicated in dozens of other studies. One is that a rather simple model was able to predict what would seem to be a rather complex process. A second is that the judgmental strategy described by that model did not at all match the strategy the judges involved thought they were following. Not only did the admissions committee members believe that they were considering more variables, but they reported that their evaluation of the three variables GRE, GPA, and QI, involved a more complex process than simple weighting and adding. A commonly asserted form of complexity is called *configural judgment*, in which the diagnostic meaning of one cue depends on the meaning of other cues (e.g., "That tone of voice makes me think 'nonsuicide' unless the call comes at midday").

There are at least three major reasons for this difference between the description of the model and that of the judges themselves. One is that people have difficulty introspecting about their own complex cognitive processes. Particularly when asked to summarize a large set of judgments some time after having made them, people tend to confuse what they did with what they intended to do and with what they believe is generally done in such situations (Ericsson & Simon, 1980; Herrmann, 1982; Nisbett & Wilson, 1977; Smith & Miller, 1978). A second reason for the discrepancy, also supported by concurrent work in cognitive psychology, is that the need to combine an enormous amount of information in one's head overwhelms the computational capacity of anyone but an idiot savant. A judge trying to implement a complex strategy would have difficulty doing so consistently. Indeed, it is difficult to learn and use even a nonconfigural, weighted-sum decision rule when there are many cues or unusual relationships between the cues and predicted variable (Slovic, 1974). Unless they were implemented consistently, more complex strategies would simply cancel one another out when a large set of judgments was studied.

The third reason for the discrepancy was discovered independently by psychologists playing around with their data (Dawes & Corrigan, 1974; Yntema & Torgerson, 1961) and statisticians thinking about the properties of data in general (Wilks, 1938). It is that simple linear equations, like (1) and (2), are extraordinarily powerful predictors. If one can identify and measure the cues that judges consider, one can mimic their summary judgments quite well with simple models that combine those cues in ways that bear no resemblance to the underlying cognitive processes. Indeed, one can often make good predictions with a model assuming that people simply count the number of factors favoring and opposing a particular judgment or decision, giving equal weight to each, and then choose the alternative having the best overall tally (Dawes, 1979).[5]

Because of the similarity of the research methodologies in the two areas, these conclusions from the study of clinical judgment are equally applicable to revealed-preference studies of people's decision making. One chilling implication is that whatever people do will resemble the application of a simple, weighted-sum model like (1) or (2). Such models can reproduce the input−output relations of human behavior without any guarantee of fidelity to the underlying processes. Thus, even if a rational model predicts subjects' behavior, one cannot be certain that they are actually using a rational decision rule. A second implication is that one often cannot take the results of attempts to model specific decisions too literally. If the same simple model makes the same predictions as a variety of complex models, it is difficult to choose the true model from among the candidates.

The source of these problems is *multicollinearity*, the degree of correlation among cues. In a decision-making context, multicollinearity is high when good consequences tend to go together (e.g., well-located apartments also tend to be large); in a judgment context, multicollinearity is high when cues pointing in the same direction are correlated (e.g., students with high GPAs also have high GREs and come from institutions with high QIs). When multicollinearity is high, the weight assigned to a cluster of correlated variables can be distributed among the individual members in varied ways without the overall prediction being seriously affected. For example, the decisions that the admissions committee reached by weighting GRE heavily would be similar to those obtained by weighting GPA heavily. As a result, "best-prediction" weights become unstable and hard to interpret.

In experimental studies, multicollinearity can be eliminated by the creation of stimuli having no correlation among cues. Figure 6.3 shows an example of such stimuli, those used in a study designed to describe how experienced investors evaluate stocks. Because the stimuli are imaginary, all possible combinations of cue variables can be created; this means that a stock's rating in one respect does not tell us how it rates in another. With such stimuli, analysis of variance (ANOVA), a special kind of multiple regression, can be used to evaluate the influence of each cue on judgment, along with the role of configural strategies. A drawback of this solution is that it conflicts with another of the intellectual roots of behavioral decision theory, Egon Brunswik's *probabilistic functionalism* (1952; see also Hammond, 1966). From Brunswik's perspective, the study of behavior involves understanding how people adapt to an uncertain or probabilistic world. Central to that adaptation is learning the natural relationships among cues. A research design that destroys these relationships (e.g., the ANOVA design just described) lacks *ecological validity*. When confronted with such an unnatural stimulus environment, subjects must spontaneously adapt their natural behavior to this unique situation. That adaptation may be quite unrepresentative of real-world behavior.

Another methodological shortcoming of such studies is that subjects are bewildered by the large set of stimuli presenting all possible combinations of values of a set of variables. Because the design of these studies is so transparent and the work is so difficult, there is always the danger that subjects will merely develop some simple rule for putting the cues together. That rule would emerge as systematic behavior, but it would not necessarily reflect the way in which they would respond to a small number of such problems embedded in the confusion of real life.

Thus, the predictive power and the inconclusiveness of linear models are discouraging for those who want to know how people really think (and, in

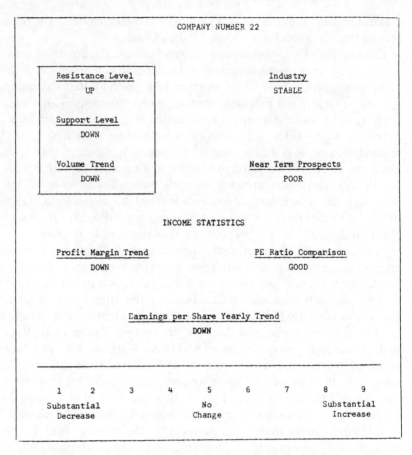

Figure 6.3 Example of a typical stimulus company. From Slovic (1969).

particular, if people actually are rational). They are, however, encouraging for those with more applied purposes. If one is concerned only with predicting people's decisions in order, say, to design a marketing campaign or remuneration scheme, then a rough model may be good enough. Indeed, the models are so powerful that the cause of effective prediction is often served by replacing judges with equations modeling their behavior. Such a *bootstrapped* model[6] can make better predictions than the judges themselves because it is more mechanical and, therefore, more reliable then they are. Equations never have off days, never suffer fatigue, are never distracted by irrelevant cues (e.g., a student's teeth, clothes, accent, or hobbies). Clearly, people know more than what is expressed in such mechanical models of their behavior. However, the research indicates that they cannot exploit this sensitivity to the richness of life's situations in order to make superior predictions.

Dawes's (1971) study produced another result that is common to studies of clinical judgment, namely, another equation produced even better predictions than the one modeling the admission committee's behavior:

$$0.0006 \text{ GRE} + 0.76 \text{ GPA} + 0.2518 \text{ QI} \tag{3}$$

Comparing the weights (or coefficients) in this equation with those in Equation (2), it appears that the admissions committee gave too much weight to GRE and too little to QI.

The observation that intelligent, motivated individuals with a great deal of experience (i.e., the Graduate Admissions Committee) could be outperformed by a relatively unsophisticated statistical procedure was disturbing to many, including some of those intelligent, motivated individuals. The question that evolved in their minds and was addressed by the ensuing research was, How well do people perform as *intuitive statisticians* attempting to discern − and then use − the statistical relationships that they observe in the world around them? The empirical answers to this question suggested that people's statistical intuitions are imperfect. Those answers provoked, in turn, interest in *decision aiding* with the aim of identifying and reducing specific judgmental problems (Kahneman & Tversky, 1979; von Winterfeldt & Edwards, 1986). The pattern of problems that was observed and the difficulty of providing help eventually led to theories that were not so dominated by the formal models and were, some would say, more psychological.

Intuitive statistics

Two seemingly contradictory trends have emerged from studies of people's intuitive processing of statistical information, one suggesting that people do quite well, the other suggesting that they do quite poorly. The difference can be traced to whether their tasks require counting or inference.

In a typical counting study, subjects are exposed to a series of stimuli drawn randomly from a fixed but hidden population. The subjects' task is to estimate some summary statistic describing the population on the basis of the sample. The population might be a hidden urn full of red and blue marbles, the sampling procedure to draw out one marble at a time, and the statistic the proportion of red marbles in the urn. Or the population might be all male undergraduates at a university, the sample procedure to look up the height of each, and the statistic their mean height.

Although the research on such judgments has many interesting nuances (Estes, 1972, 1976; Hintzman, 1976), generally it shows that people do a fairly good job of assessing common measures of the central tendency of what they have just observed (Peterson & Beach, 1967). Those measures would include the mode (or most common observation), the median (the middle value when the observations are ordered from largest to smallest), the mean (or arithmetic average), and proportion (e.g., of red balls among those drawn from an urn). As one might expect, performance on such simple tasks deteriorates some when the subject becomes overloaded, when, for example, there are many colors to keep track of or the set of data becomes very large or the numbers difficult to manage. Such cognitive overload typically adds unsystematic error (or "noise") to subjects' estimates, making them less reliable but not biased in any particular way. One exception might occur with estimates of very small proportions. When these are elicited directly (e.g., .01 red, 1% blue), rather than in ratio form (e.g., 1 in 100), it is easier for the estimates to get larger than smaller (because people tend not to give fractional values). The result will be an artifactual tendency for subjects to overestimate small values and underestimate large ones (Poulton, 1968, 1982).

More interesting problems can arise when more interesting stimuli are used, ones that allow more active involvement with the substance of the stimulus than with a list of heights or group of marbles. For example, Tversky and Kahneman (1973) played subjects two recordings of a speaker reading the names of some famous people (e.g., Richard Nixon, Elizabeth Taylor) and some not so famous ones (e.g., William Fulbright, Lana Turner). On one recording the names of 19 famous men and 20 less famous women were read; on the other the names of 19 famous women and 20 less famous men were read. When asked, 80% of subjects thought that there were more men in the first list and more women in the second, even though the opposite was (marginally) the case. When asked, subjects remembered about 50% more famous names than unfamous ones. Thus, these subjects might have kept a rough running tally in their minds of the number of names of each sex that they had seen, but paid more attention to the more famous names. Or they might not have counted while listening, but uncritically used the number of names they could remember as an indicator of each sex's frequency. The idea of relying on the products of one's memory to guide judgments of frequency was labeled the *availability heuristic* by Tversky and Kahneman (1973). By either of these interpretations, subjects went astray because they attached meaning to the stimuli. What they knew before entering the experiment affected either what attracted their attention or what activated their memories.

The contrast between these flawed frequency judgments and the fine ones observed in studies using artificial stimuli suggests that people can count what they see, but what they see is not necessarily exactly what they are shown. Rather, they interpret what they see, whenever that is even remotely possible. The extent of people's ingenuity in attaching meaning can be seen in a popular variation of the marbles-in-the-urn task. Instead of estimating the proportion of, say, red marbles, subjects guess whether the next marble drawn will be red or blue. In such a task, guessing the color of the marble that appears to be most common is the strategy that would produce the highest expected percentage of correct guesses. Perhaps because that is also a strategy that guarantees a certain number of mistakes, subjects typically prefer to predict each color in proportion to their estimates of its prevalence in the population. For example, if they have seen 70% red marbles, 70% of their predictions will be "red." They could, in principle, be right every time, although that is highly unlikely. In most studies, these prediction percentages are so close to the actual population percentages that such "probability matching" is often taken as establishing people's ability to estimate proportions (Estes, 1972).

Given that people have chosen this prediction strategy, they must find some way to generate a prediction for each marble. One popular strategy is to individuate each marble by the pattern created by the sequence of preceding marbles and predict colors that will extend the sequence in such a way as to make it seem random. Of course, the essence of random sampling is that each event (i.e., marble) is independent of its predecessors. Thus, the attempt to find meaning in the sequence of marbles is a futile effort to discern a signal out of noise. The specific patterns that people like to create suggest further discrepancies between the properties they attribute to random processes and those embodied in statistical theory. For example, they expect fewer and shorter runs than they should, making it seem unduly remote to draw five successive red marbles, give birth to three successive sons, or flip four successive "heads." *Gambler's fallacy* is the name given to the feeling that the next event in such unusual sequences is bound to redress the imbalance (Jarvik, 1951; Tune, 1964).

When subjects engage in such exercises, they are actively interpreting experimental stimuli that were intended (by the experimenter) to be quite meaningless. One reasonable hypothesis is that such interpretation is an automatic and almost unstoppable process. Once they are perceived, stimuli may immediately begin to activate associations with a wide network of related events (Collins & Loftus, 1975). When stimuli are so artificial that there are no memories to activate, subjects' desire to make their task meaningful may encourage them to find some way of interpreting what they have seen (even if it means divining patterns in random sequences).

Conceivably, such insistence on finding meaning has some broad evolutionary utility, in the sense that a thinking organism has a better chance of survival if it always generates some meaningful hypothesis about what is happening in its environment (even if that means interpreting situations where nothing discernible is happening). However intriguing such speculations about the evolutionary value of behavior may be, they are notoriously difficult to test. A behavioral pattern that seems useful in some situations may be useless in others. A strategy that complicates life in the short run may simplify it in the intermediate run and complicate it in new ways in the long run. In general, faulty behavioral patterns that have relatively mild negative consequences are less likely to be detected and corrected than patterns that cause larger, more immediate problems. Determining which patterns take a greater cumulative toll requires aggregating over all situations, time periods, and purposes; this in turn, requires making sweeping generalizations about life and the margin it leaves for error.

A more reasonable aspiration is to identify the local effects of particular biases. For example, the gambler's fallacy may be beneficial if it gives subjects a feeling of control in an otherwise unpredictable experimental task; they may suffer little from making mistakes and feel more gratification from doing something more interesting than, say, always predicting "red." Gambler's fallacy could, however, have disastrous results in serious decision making (e.g., birth planning) or in less benign environments in which this foible could be exploited (e.g., casinos). Automatic interpretation of stimuli can also be useful when it helps one make larger chunks out of diverse bits of information. Indeed, creative interpretation is the secret to mnemonists' phenomenal ability to remember diverse bits of information. However, extraneous knowledge can distort people's perceptions of what they see. For example, a popular diagnostic technique in psychotherapy requires clients to draw a picture of a person. In a survey of practicing therapists, Chapman and Chapman (1971) found that the great majority reported seeing correlations between clinical symptoms and features of the drawings that systematic research had shown did not exist, such as a tendency for clients worried about manliness to draw figures with broad, muscular shoulders or a tendency for suspicious people to draw figures with atypical eyes. One possible reason for clinicians' biased perceptions is that, when these symptoms and features do occur together, they create a highly coherent and memorable package. As a result, when clinicians summarize their experience, these tidy pairs stand out. A second possible reason for this *illusory correlation* is that knowing (or suspecting) a client's diagnosis may increase a clinician's chances of seeing, say, strange eyes if they are there and perhaps even if they are not.

Although the focus of these studies of intuitive statistics is on the direct counting of observed stimuli, few involve simply counting. Some require subjects to make inferences on the basis of what they have seen (e.g., predicting the next marble). Others inadvertently invite interpretation, as subjects attempt to make sense of the stimuli. It is in making these inferences that people seem to have trouble. In studies of statistical judgment that have focused directly on inferential thought processes, potential problems have leaped rather quickly to the foreground (Kahneman, Slovic, & Tversky, 1982).

The conceptual framework for many of these studies has been the Bayesian approach to hypothesis testing, at the core of which is Bayes's theorem, a rule for changing one's beliefs in the light of new evidence (Edwards, Lindman, & Savage, 1963; Fischhoff & Beyth-Marom, 1983). Expressed symbolically, it is

$$\frac{P(H/D)}{P(\bar{H}/D)} = \frac{P(D/H)\ P(H)}{P(D/\bar{H})\ P(\bar{H})} \tag{4}$$

Here, H and $\bar{H}$ are two alternative hypotheses (e.g., loves me/loves me not, suicidal/nonsuicidal, hostile/nonhostile); D is a new bit of information (e.g., an incomplete love letter found in the wastebasket, an agitated phone call at midday, a blip on a NORAD radar screen). The first ratio on the right represents the *prior odds* that H is true rather than $\bar{H}$ in the light of every-thing that is known before D is received. The middle term is the *likelihood ratio*, representing the information value of D for helping one choose be-tween H and $\bar{H}$. If those two terms are multiplied, they give the left-hand term, called the *posterior odds* that H, rather than $\bar{H}$, is true after D is received.

Bayes's theorem is an accepted and central part of probability theory. Bayesian inference is rather more controversial, in large part because it al-lows the use of *subjective probabilities* (Kyburg & Smokler, 1964). That is, people may judge the value of $P(H)$, $P(D/H)$, and so on, without necessar-ily relying on frequency counts, as required in the definition of probability provided by most introductory treatments. Indeed, the Bayesian approach not only allows but requires the exercise of judgment. At the beginning of a marbles-and-urn experiment, before any marbles had been drawn, a fre-quentist could say nothing about the proportion of red marbles; a Bayesian, however, could say, "The proportion of red marbles is probably around 0.5, because that's the way I think psychologists set up experiments, although I admit that it might be anywhere between 0.25 and 0.75." After seeing 300 red marbles in 1,000 draws, both observers would probably agree that the proportion was about 0.3. However, the Bayesian might give another value if, say, it seemed that the experimenter could not be trusted to keep things constant. Although Bayesians can relate to whatever information they want, they cannot give whatever probabilities they want. In this context, at least, subjectivity does not imply a lack of discipline. Specifically, Bayesians' judg-mental probabilities must obey the axioms of probability theory, such as $P(H) + P(\bar{H}) = 1$. If they do not, they are considered *incoherent* and there-fore not probabilities (Lindley, Tversky, & Brown, 1979).

An orderly set of probability judgments need not be a useful one. A well-elaborated delusional system could, in principle, be thoroughly Bayesian (assuming that it admitted of uncertainty). One common way of assessing the extent to which probability judgments correspond to reality is to mea-sure their degree of *calibration*. Over a large set of judgments, probabilities of .*XX* should be associated with true hypotheses *XX*% of the time. A typical calibration study presents subjects with, say, 200 two-alternative statements, such as "Absinthe is (a) a liquor; (b) a precious stone." Subjects' task is to choose the more likely answer and give the probability that it is correct. Figure 6.4a shows some typical results. People's confidence in their answers is related to the truth of those answers, but only moderately so. Overall, there is a tendency toward *overconfidence*. For example, when subjects are 1.00 confident they may have chosen the correct answer only 80% of the time (Fischhoff, Slovic, & Lichtenstein, 1977).

This basic pattern of results has proved so robust that it is hard to acquire much insight into the psychological processes producing it (Lichtenstein, Fischhoff, & Phillips, 1982). One of the few effective manipulations is to force subjects to explain why their chosen answers might be wrong (Koriat, Lichtenstein, & Fischhoff, 1980). That simple instruction seems to prompt recall of contrary reasons that would not normally come to mind given people's natural thought processes, which seem to focus on retrieving reasons that support chosen answers. A second seemingly effective manipulation is to train people intensively with personalized feedback that shows them how well they are calibrated. Figure 6.4b shows the calibration of forecasters working for the United States National Weather Service, which requires them to attach probabilities to precipitation forecasts and reinforces them for accuracy and candor. These forecasters are, in a word, outstanding. The only (mild) criticism one might make is that they say 1.00 too often when it does not rain.

In the terms of learning theory, these forecasters work under nearly perfect conditions. They receive a large quantity of prompt, unambiguous feedback with a clear-cut criterion event (i.e., rain/no rain).[8] Similar opportunities for learning are rare for most people for most kinds of analytic judgments about uncertain events. In that light, it should not be surprising if people − even experts − do not learn how to make such judgments optimally.

Figure 6.5 shows one sign of the limits that exist on the capacity of expertise and experience to improve judgment. Particle physicists' estimates of the value of several physical constants are bracketed by what might be called *confidence intervals*, showing the range of likely values within which the true value should fall, once it is known. Narrower intervals indicate greater confidence. These intervals have shrunk over time, as physicists' knowledge has increased. However, at most points they seem to have been too narrow. Otherwise, the new best estimates would not have fallen so frequently outside the range of what previously seemed plausible. In an absolute sense, the level of knowledge represented here is extremely high and the successive best estimates lie extremely close to one another. However, the confidence intervals define what constitute surprises in terms of current physical theory. Unless the possibility of overconfident judgment is considered, values falling outside the intervals suggest a weakness in the theory. Indeed, the surprising

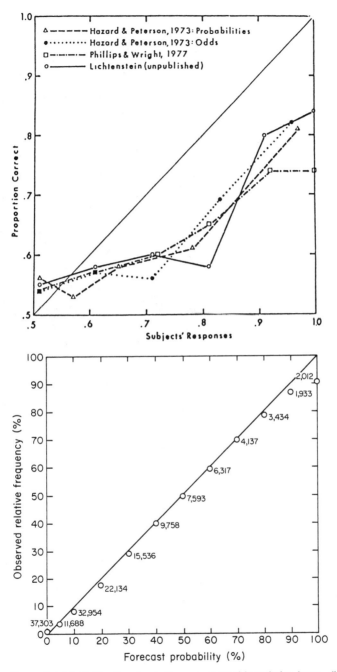

Figure 6.4 (a) Calibration for half-range, general-knowledge items. (b) Reliability diagram for subjective precipitation probability forecasts formulated at 87 National Weather Service offices during the period from April 1977 to March 1979. The number adjacent to each point indicates the number of forecasts with that forecast probability. From Murphy and Winkler (1984).

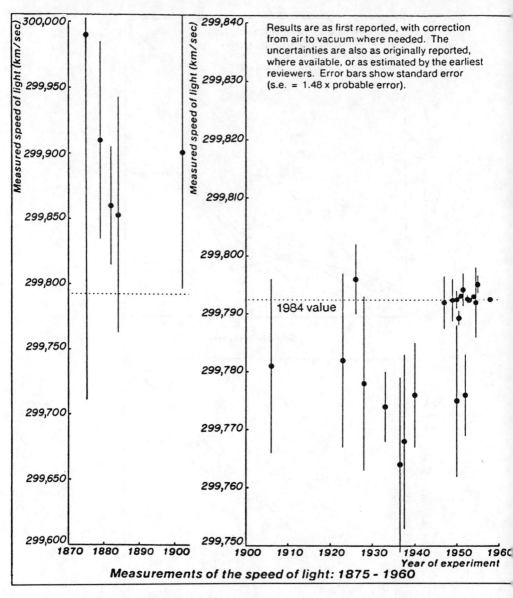

Figure 6.5 Calibration of confidence in estimates of physical constants. From
Henrion and Fischhoff (1986).

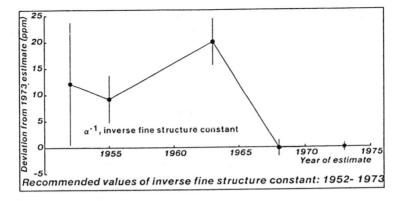

Recommended values of inverse fine structure constant: 1952- 1973

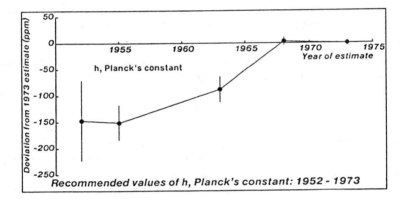

Recommended values of h, Planck's constant: 1952 - 1973

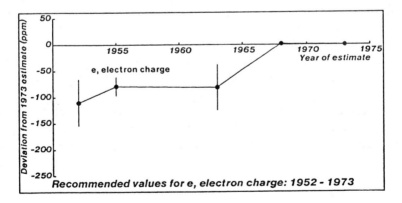

Recommended values for e, electron charge: 1952 - 1973

Figure 6.5 *cont.*

estimates of the speed of light generated in the 1920s and 1930s evoked serious suggestions that it might be increasing or that it varies sinusoidally over time.[9]

From a learning-theory perspective, a psychological account of judgment and decision making would have to restrict itself to processes whose imperfections would not be revealed by experience. In the early 1970s, two Israeli psychologists, Amos Tversky and Daniel Kahneman (1974), proposed a metatheory, implemented by several minitheories, fulfilling this requirement. According to the metatheory, people do not follow laws of statistics when they make intuitive inferences about uncertain events, perhaps because they have never learned those laws (either through training or experience), perhaps because the rules that they do know place excessive demands on their mental computational abilities. Instead, people rely on relatively simple rules of thumb, called *heuristics*, to guide their judgments. These rules have good face validity; that is, they seem to be reasonable rules to follow. They may also have some actual validity, in the sense that they often produce useful judgments. However, they can lead to predictable biases.

The availability heuristic, described earlier, is one of these rules. It seems plausible that events occurring more frequently than others will be more available in memory (and vice versa); hence, there is face validity. Moreover, this is often the case, conferring some actual validity on the rule. However, availability can be affected by factors unrelated to frequency, such as the salience of an event or its timing (e.g., a recent event may be more available in memory than a more distant event). Exaggerating the percentage of famous men's or women's names in the recordings played by Tversky and Kahneman (1973) is an example of a biased judgment attributable to availability. Table 6.1 shows another example, in the form of causes of death whose frequency tended to be over-and underestimated in a study by Lichtenstein, Slovic, Fischhoff, Layman, and Combs (1978). A companion study (Combs & Slovic, 1979) revealed that the overestimated events also tended to be overreported in the news media. In estimating risks of this kind, people seem to do a relatively good job of keeping track of what they see in the paper but a relatively poor job of discerning systematic biases in the choice of events that are reported.

A second heuristic is *representativeness*, reliance on which leads one to judge an event as likely if it "represents" the salient features of the process producing a target event. In a classic study, the underlying process was that creating the individual in the following description:

Tom W. is of high intelligence, although lacking in true creativity. He has a need for order and clarity, and for neat and tidy systems in which every detail finds its appropriate place. His writing is rather dull and mechanical, occasionally enlivened by somewhat corny puns and by flashes of imagination of the sci-fi type. He has a strong drive for competence. He seems to have little feel and little sympathy for other

Table 6.1. *Biased estimates of the frequency of causes of death*

Most overestimated	Most underestimated
1. All accidents	1. Smallpox vaccination
2. Motor vehicle accidents	2. Diabetes
3. Pregnancy, childbirth, abortion	3. Stomach cancer
4. Tornado	4. Lightning
5. Flood	5. Stroke
6. Botulism	6. Tuberculosis
7. All cancer	7. Asthma
8. Fire and flames	8. Emphysema
9. Venomous bite or sting	
10. Homicide	

Source: Lichtenstein, Slovic, Fischhoff, Layman and Combs (1978).

people and does not enjoy interacting with others. Self-centered, he nonetheless has a deep moral sense. (Kahneman & Tversky, 1973, p. 238)

To a group of psychology graduate students who served as experimental subjects, Tom W. seemed so much like a computer scientist that they confidently predicted that computer science was his college major, even though the frequencies of other majors are much higher. Those overall frequencies would determine the *base rate* in Bayes's Theorem [which has a slightly different form than (4) when there are multiple alternative hypotheses, such as different majors]. The informativeness (or *diagnosticity*) of the sketch is captured by the likelihood ratio. Predicting that Tom is a computer scientist requires almost ignoring the prior odds, which is justified only if the information about Tom is very informative. The subjects in this experiment indicated that one could not learn very much from a sketch like the one they were given. However, they relied on the description of Tom almost exclusively, apparently because it is so easy to judge how much Tom resembles the archetype of students taking each major.

Both reliance on representativeness (Kahneman & Tversky, 1972) and neglect of base rates, even in situations not involving representativeness (Bar-Hillel, 1980), have been observed in a variety of settings. For example, Fischhoff and Bar-Hillel (1984a) found a mixture of this strategy and probability matching in a study in which subjects received a set of sketches reportedly drawn from, say, a group of 30 university professors and 70 business executives. When a sketch resembled a professor or an executive, the subjects predicted the associated profession by representativeness; when it did not, they predicted by probability matching, assigning 30% of such neutral sketches to one category and 70% to the other.

Prejudices about biases

The study of judgmental biases stimulated by these and other heuristics has inspired research by psychologists outside the area of judgment (e.g., Nisbett & Ross, 1980) and by investigators outside of psychology (e.g., Eddy, 1982). Like any stimulating topic, it has also engendered much critical comment. Some of this criticism is endemic to all debates among psychologists; some is special to research claiming to show limits to people's performance. Familiarity with the generic claims makes it easier to follow the developments in this field and in others where they recur in slightly different form.

It's not true

Psychologists are adept at picking holes in the design and analysis of experiments. It is, in fact, part of their job to serve as gatekeeepers, preventing research from entering the body of accepted wisdom until it has undergone rigorous scrutiny. The number of criticisms that can be made is very large, however, making it tempting to answer skepticism with counterskepticism.

One way to avoid testing every possible alternative explanation for every empirical result is to ask whether any general statements can be made about the impact of various manipulations. The "unfair tasks" section of Table 6.2 lists some common methodological criticisms – for example, subjects' biases would vanish if one only raised the stakes or clarified the instructions. A review of all studies in which these factors were varied in an attempt to eliminate two biases revealed no evidence of improvement (Fischhoff, 1982a). If this pattern of results were sustained by additional studies considering other biases, the burden of proof might shift to the critics in situations in which neither they nor the defenders of the biases had any specific data.

It's true, but you shouldn't say so

Demonstrations of bias could be construed as exercises in which one very small group of people, the experimenters, makes a very large group of people, everybody else, look stupid. This juxtaposition is not only disingenuous, but also dangerous if it unduly lowers people's self-esteem or the legitimacy of their attempts to make decisions about events affecting their lives.[10] A combative response is that the investigators' responsibility is to report the data accurately, integrate them with extant theory, and surround them with appropriate qualifications. Doing otherwise is not only dishonest, but unfair to the people whose behavior is being described. Giving people too much credit for decision-making prowess can deny them access to needed help, just as giving them too little credit can deny them access to power.

A more conciliatory response is to argue that it is difficult to create a

Table 6.2. *Debiasing methods according to underlying assumptions*

Assumption	Strategies
Faulty tasks	
Unfair tasks	Raise stakes
	Clarify instructions
	Dispell doubts
	Use better response modes
	Discourage second guessing
	Ask fewer questions
Misunderstood tasks	Demonstrate alternative goal
	Demonstrate semantic disagreement
	Demonstrate impossibility of task
	Demonstrate overlooked distinction
Faulty judges	
Perfectible individuals	Warn of problem
	Describe problem
	Provide personalized feedback
	Train extensively
Incorrigible individuals	Replace them
	Recalibrate their responses
	Plan on error
Mismatch between judges and task	
Restructuring	Make knowledge explicit
	Search for discrepant information
	Decompose problem
	Consider alternative situations
	Offer alternative formulations
Reeducation	Rely on experts
	Educate from childhood

Source: Fischhoff (1982a).

balanced summary of the heuristics-and-biases literature. Even the clearest demonstrations of a bias say nothing about its prevalence in life. Making such sweeping generalizations would require a complete theory of what life is like and how the situations that it poses resemble those in the laboratory − hardly work for the timid. Moreover, even if one reports studies accurately, biases make such a good story that they easily become a "figure" overshadowing the "ground" created by the heuristics in routine (and reasonably successful) operation. The danger of such misinterpretation increases as results are reported in secondary and tertiary sources (Berkeley & Humphreys, 1982).

It's true, but it doesn't matter

Many interesting psychological problems have few direct consequences in everyday life. For example, optical illusions reveal important properties of vision without being a major hindrance. A casual way of dismissing judgmental biases as trivial is to argue that somehow experience should have taught people to avoid behavior that is frequently bad for them. A more rigorous way is to show analytically the insensitivity of particular decisions to particular errors. For example, in an analysis that originally focused on the effect of perceptual imperfections on motor behavior, von Winterfeldt and Edwards (1982) showed that, under certain specified conditions, the expected value of decisions with continuous options (e.g., invest X) changes little if one of the probabilities or values in the model is moderately in error.

Such analyses help clarify the relationship between people and their environment. In situations where they show that decisions are insensitive to biases in judgment, they also show that people have little chance to learn more optimal behaviors. That is, if biases do not affect most decisions, there will not be the kind of feedback people need in order to change. As a result, people may be particularly vulnerable to the effects of suboptimal judgment and decision making in those, perhaps few, situations in which accuracy is crucial. Indeed, the difficulties that people experience in thinking their way through to a good decision might be attributed to their great capacity to reach good decisions through trial and error. Unfortunately, this combination makes them vulnerable to error when they need to get things right the first time.

People are doing something quite different − and doing it quite well

In describing behavior as suboptimal, one presumes knowledge of what is optimal. Within decision theory, optimality is defined in terms of what one knows and wants. It would therefore be wrong to claim suboptimality if people act overconfidently in a world that rewards bravado, if a good decision is followed (unfortunately) by a bad outcome, or if people fail to do as well as we might have done in their stead given the benefit of some additional knowledge. The "misunderstood tasks" section in Table 6.2 shows some generic ways in which subject and experimenter might misunderstand one another's perspective on a task. It is to avoid such problems that the study of decision making has retreated to the laboratory, where, in principle, all details can be specified and all extraneous beliefs and distractions can be eliminated. Yet no investigator checks whether each feature is understood exactly as intended. Nor could many subjects absorb a detailed explication of the way they should think about every detail.

When people do seem to have understood the task as intended, they can still be defended against charges of biased behavior by the argument that they subscribe to alternative theories of optimality. Even though the basic definition of rationality described here is widely accepted, some theorists have begun to explore alternative accounts that are more consistent with observed behavior. Time will tell whether this is a case of psychology stimulating philosophy or a case of throwing out the baby (time-honored models of rationality) with the bath water (a few apparently discrepant psychological results).

But look at how well people do other things

The psychological evidence of bias seems strikingly at odds with the fact that planes fly, meals get on the table, and games of enormous complexity (e.g., chess, handball) are played. One easy way to reconcile this conflict is to dismiss the biases as laboratory curiosities. Its converse is to claim that the world is not working all that well and that we would all be better off if we made better decisions. A more complex response is to admit the reality of laboratory results but search for environmental conditions that induce more effective thinking. Table 6.2 lists generic ways of restructuring tasks, several of which have evoked more effective judgments. Perhaps one could argue that life is charitable enough to present problems in ways that enable people to use their minds to best advantage. If that is not a credible hope, such manipulations could become part of training programs (Beyth-Marom, Dekel, Gombo, & Shaked, 1985; Nisbett, Krantz, Jepsen, & Kunda, 1983). Ironically, the very robustness of biases makes it difficult to demonstrate improvement. Often, any intervention that destabilizes the dominant response pattern will tend to reduce the extent of bias, making confusion seem like wisdom (Fischhoff & Bar-Hillel, 1984b). Although confusion is often an intermediate state between holding erroneous beliefs and holding appropriate ones, it can also be an intermediate state between two erroneous beliefs.

Facing the problems

Taking problems seriously opens a number of lines of inquiry. One is understanding why people are so good at some tasks and so poor at others. The prevailing account among behavioral decision theory researchers is that there are no fundamental psychological limitations, beyond information-processing *capacity*, that prevent people from acquiring the skills needed to make better judgments. The barriers are environmental: people receive little training in decision making per se and live in a world that does not provide conditions for learning.

If the problems are real, one can begin doing something serious about them. The "perfectible individuals" section of Table 6.2 lists approaches to training people to make better judgments (which might also incorporate the restructuring options listed). The "incorrigible individuals" lists approaches to living with fallibility. An example of the second entry, recalibration, is the (UK) Central Electricity Generating Board's Policy of doubling engineers' chronic underestimates of the time needed to return units of production before using those estimates in forecasts of power availability (Kidd, 1970).

Finally, taking problems seriously pushes one to develop better theories for predicting how and when they will arise. Perhaps the greatest current need is for theories of the processes by which people choose and apply judgment and decision-making strategies in particular situations (e.g., Payne, 1982). People show such great ingenuity in construing situations that even such apparently straightforward rules as availability could often be interpreted in a variety of ways (e.g., for how long does one produce examples? How are categories defined? What attributes guide the search?). A significant component of such a theory of strategy choice would be an account of the conditions under which people actually choose not to make judgments and decisions deliberately, drawing inferences through the synthesis of available facts. How often does laziness, inattention, or recognition of the difficulty of such decision making lead people to miss the moment of decision or to fill it by reliance on habit, tradition, or some other rule of thumb to guide their behavior?

Notes

1 Some people find the very idea of asking such questions repugnant. Others believe that, because society will not, in fact, pay whatever it takes to save a human life, it should face directly the question of how much it will pay. Still others are willing to ask the question but resent having it cast in dollar terms, which, they believe, cheapens lives and "anaesthetizes moral feelings" (Tribe, 1973). The philosophical implications of the technical question considered in the text evoke some of the significant ethical questions of our day. Discussions and references to further reading can be found in Fischhoff, Lichtenstein, Slovic, Derby, and Keeney (1981), Rhoads (1980), and Schelling (1979).

2 These techniques produce an equation for predicting wages:

$$\text{wages} = a(\text{risk level}) + b(\text{seniority}) - c(\text{local unemployment})$$

The size of a would show how much wages changed with a given change in risk level.

3 In technical terms, replication guards against the danger of *shrinkage*, which occurs when one has looked at a relatively large set of possible variables in order to explain a relatively small set of observations (Cohen & Cohen, 1975). In principle, one can always make the set of variables in a regression equation large enough to achieve any desired degree of correlation with the independent variable. This strategy works by capitalizing on chance relations, in the extreme using a different variable to predict each observation, as though

there were a separate theory for each. The price paid for such ingenious lack of discipline is failure of the rule to work with a new set of observations, which will have its own chance relations. Similar processes seem to be at work when historical events are given elaborate explanations that fail to provide guidance in predicting future events (Fischhoff, 1982b).

4 Dawes (1971, 1979) provides a lively discussion of the ethical implications both of using and of not using such a "dehumanizing" rule for dealing with people.

5 More technical discussions of these issues can be found in Cohen and Cohen (1975), Darlington (1968), Dawes and Corrigan (1974), and Slovic and Lichtenstein (1971).

6 The term comes from the idea of lifting oneself up by one's bootstraps.

7 Although judgments that violated these rules would not be Bayesian probabilities, there are alternative definitions of probability that allow violations of the familiar axioms while imposing other restrictions. For example, it might be possible to leave some probability uncommitted, so that $P(H) + P(\bar{H}) < 1$ until one's feelings of uncertainty are better resolved. These and other possibilities are discussed by Cohen (1981), Dubois and Prade (1986), Shafer (1976), and others. They represent an active area of philosophical research that was prompted, in part, by the psychological evidence that people have difficulty performing in accordance with the familiar axioms.

8 A confounding factor in the interpretation of these data is the fact that the meteorological information provided to forecasters includes computer-generated probabilities. Forecasters' values are better than these probabilities. However, it is unclear to what extent forecasters are aided by their ability to anchor their estimates in the values suggested by the computer.

9 A confounding factor in the interpretation of these data is the fact that physicists are somewhat unclear about the intended meaning of the intervals. The present interpretation assumes that they include all sources of uncertainty, as recommended in the accepted methodological guides. If the intervals are used more narrowly, the evidence of overconfidence is weakened. However, such ambiguity also reduces the opportunity for these scientists to receive clear feedback regarding the appropriateness of their confidence (Henrion & Fischhoff, 1986).

10 Lay people's intellectual competence is, for example, a focal issue in the debate over the proper role of the public in setting society's policy regarding hazardous technologies (Fischhoff, 1985).

References

Bar-Hillel, M. (1980). The base-rate fallacy in probability judgments. *Acta Psychologica, 44*, 211–33.

Beach, B. H., & Beach, L. R. (1982). Expectancy-based decision schemes: Sidesteps toward applications. In N. T. Feather (Ed.), *Expectations and actions: Expectancy-value models in psychology* (pp. 365–394). Hillsdale, NJ: Erlbaum.

Behn, R. D., & Vaupel, J. W. (1982). *Quick analysis for busy decision makers*. New York: Basic.

Berkeley, D., & Humphreys, P. C. (1982). Structuring decision problems and the "bias heuristic." *Acta Psychologica, 50*, 201–52.

Bettman, J. R. (1979). *An information processing theory of consumer choice*. Reading, MA: Addison-Wesley.

Beyth-Marom, R., Dekel, S., Gombo, R., & Shaked, M. (1985). *An elementary approach to thinking under uncertainty* (S. Lichtenstein, B. Marom, & R. Beyth-Marom, Trans.). Hillsdale, NJ: Erlbaum.

Brunswik, E. (1952). *The conceptual framework of psychology*. University of Chicago Press.

Chapman, L. J., & Chapman, J. (1971, November 18–22). Test results are what you think they are. *Psychology Today*, pp. 106–10.

Cohen, J. (1981). Can human irrationality be experimentally demonstrated? *Behavioral and Brain Sciences*, *4*, 317–31.

Cohen, J., & Cohen P. (1975). *Applied multiple regression/correlation analysis for the behavioral sciences*. Hillsdale, NJ: Erlbaum.

Collins, A., & Loftus, E. (1975). A spreading activation model of memory. *Psychological Review*, *82*, 407–28.

Combs, B., & Slovic, P. (1979). Newspaper coverage of causes of death. *Journalism Quarterly*, *56*(4), 837–43, 849.

Coombs, C. H., Dawes, R. M., & Tversky, A. (1970). *Mathematical Psychology*. Englewood Cliffs, NJ: Prentice Hall.

Darlington, R. B. (1968). Multiple regression in psychological research and practice. *Psychological Bulletin*, *69*, 161–82.

Dawes, R. M. (1971). A case study of graduate admissions: Applications of three principles of human decision making. *American Psychologist*, *26*, 180–8.

   (1979). The robust beauty of improper linear models in decision making. *American Psychologist*, *34*, 571–82.

Dawes, R. M., & Corrigan, B. (1974). Linear models in decision making. *Psychological Bulletin*, *81*(2), 95–106.

Dreman, D. (1982). *The new contrarian investment strategy*. New York: Random House.

Dubois, D., & Prade, H. (1986). Recent models of uncertainty and imprecision as a basis for decision theory. In E. Hollnagel, G. Mancini, & D. D. Woods (Eds.), *Intelligent decision aids in process environments* (pp. 3–24). Berlin: Springer-Verlag.

Eddy, D. M. (1982). Probabilistic reasoning in clinical medicine: Problems and opportunities. In D. Kahneman, P. Slovic, & A. Tversky (Eds.), *Judgment under uncertainty: Heuristics and biases* (pp. 249–67). Cambridge University Press.

Edwards, W. (1954). The theory of decision making. *Psychological Bulletin*, *51*, 380–417.

   (1961). Behavioral decision theory. *Annual Review of Psychology*, *12*, 473–98.

Edwards, W., Lindman, H., & Savage, L. J. (1963). Bayesian statistical inference for psychological research. *Psychological Review*, *70*, 193–242.

Elstein, A., Shulman, L., & Sprafka, S. (1978). *Medical problem solving*. Cambridge, MA: Harvard University Press.

Ericsson, A., & Simon, H. A. (1980). Verbal reports as data. *Psychological Review*, *87*, 215–25.

Estes, W. K. (1972). Research and theory on the learning of probabilities. *Journal of the American Statistical Association*, *67*, 81–102.

   (1976). The cognitive side of probability learning. *Psychological Review*, *83*, 37–64.

Feather, N. T. (Ed.) (1982). *Expectations and actions: Expectancy-value models in psychology*. Hillsdale, NJ: Erlbaum.

Fischhoff, B. (1982a). Debiasing. In D. Kahneman, P. Slovic, & A. Tversky (Eds.), *Judgment under uncertainty: Heuristics and biases* (pp. 422–44). Cambridge University Press.

   (1982b). For those condemned to study the past: Heuristics and biases in hindsight. In Kahneman, D., Slovic, P., & Tversky, A. (Eds.), *Judgment under uncertainty: Heuristics and biases* (pp. 335–51). Cambridge University Press.

   (1985a). Managing risk perceptions. *Issues in Science and Technology*, *2*, 83–96.

   (1985b). *Prejudices about bias*. (Report 85-3). Eugene, OR: Decision Research.

Fischhoff, B., & Bar-Hillel, M. (1984a). Diagnosticity and the base-rate effect. *Memory and Cognition*, *12*(4), 402–10.

   (1984b). Focusing techniques: A shortcut to improving probability judgments? *Organizational Behavior and Human Performance*, *34*, 175–94.

Fischhoff, B., & Beyth-Marom, R. (1983). Hypothesis evaluation from a Bayesian perspective. *Psychological Review*, *90*, 239–60.

Fischhoff, B., & Cox, L. A., Jr. (1985). Conceptual framework for regulatory benefits assessment. In J. D. Bentkover, V. T. Covello, & J. Mumpower (Eds.). *Benefits assessment: The state of the art*. Dordrecht, The Netherlands: D. Reidel.

Fischhoff, B., Lichtenstein, S., Slovic, P., Derby, S., & Keeney, R. (1981). *Acceptable Risk*. Cambridge University Press.

Fischhoff, B., Slovic, P., & Lichtenstein, S. (1977). Knowing with certainty: The appropriateness of extreme confidence. *Journal of Experimental Psychology: Human Perception and Performance, 20*, 159–83.

Fischhoff, B., Svenson, O., & Slovic, P. (1987). Active responses to environmental hazards. In D. Stokols & I. Altman (Eds.), *Handbook of environmental psychology*. (pp. 1089–1133). New York: Wiley-Interscience.

Goldberg, L. R. (1968). Simple models or simple processes? Some research on clinical judgments. *American Psychologist, 23*, 483–96.

(1970). Man vs. model of man: A rationale, plus some evidence, for a method of improving on clinical inferences. *Psychological Bulletin, 73*, 422–32.

Hammond, K. R. (Ed.). (1966). *The psychology of Egon Brunswik*. New York: Holt, Rinehart & Winston.

Hazard, T. H., & Peterson, C. R. (1973). *Odds versus probabilities for categorical events* (Tech. Rep., 73 - 2). McLean, VA: Decisions and Designs, Inc.

Henrion, M., & Fischhoff, B. (1986). Uncertainty assessment in the estimation of physical constants. *American Journal of Physics, 54*, 791–8.

Herrmann, D. J. (1982). Know thy memory: The use of questionnaires to assess and study memory. *Psychological Bulletin, 92*(2), 434–52.

Hintzman, D. L. (1976). Repetition and memory. In G. H. Bower (Ed.), *The psychology of learning and motivation: Advances in research and theory*. New York: Academic Press.

Jarvik, M. E. (1951). Probability learning and a negative recency effect in the serial anticipation of alternative symbols. *Journal of Experimental Psychology, 41*, 291–7.

Jones-Lee, M. W. (1976). *The value of life*. University of Chicago Press.

Kahneman, D., Slovic, P., & Tversky, A. (Eds.). (1982). *Judgment under uncertainty: Heuristics and biases*. Cambridge University Press.

Kahneman, D., & Tversky, A. (1972). Subjective probability: A judgment of representativeness. *Cognitive Psychology, 3*, 430–54.

(1973). On the psychology of prediction. *Psychological Review, 80*, 237–51.

(1979). Intuitive predictions: Biases and corrective procedures. *TIMS Studies in Management Science, 12*, 313–27.

Kelly, E. L., & Fiske, D. W. (1951). *The prediction of performance in clinical psychology*. Ann Arbor: University of Michigan Press.

Kidd, J. B. (1970). The utilization of subjective probabilities in production planning. *Acta Psychologica, 34*, 338–47.

Koriat, A., Lichtenstein, S., & Fischhoff, B. (1980). Reasons for confidence. *Journal of Experimental Psychology: Human Learning and Memory, 6*, 107–18.

Kyburg, H. E., Jr., & Smokler, H. W. (1964). *Studies in subjective probability*. New York: Wiley.

Kunreuther, H., Ginsberg, R., Miller, L., Sagi, P., Slovic, P., Borkan, B., & Katz, N. (1978). *Disaster insurance protection: Public policy lessons*. New York: Wiley.

Lakatos, I., & Musgrave, A. (Eds.). (1970). *Criticism and the growth of scientific knowledge*. Cambridge University Press.

Lichtenstein, S., Fischhoff, B., & Phillips, L. D. (1982). Calibration of probabilities: State of the art to 1980. In D. Kahneman, P. Slovic, & A. Tversky (Eds.), *Judgment under uncertainty: Heuristics and biases*. (pp. 306–34). Cambridge University Press.

Lichtenstein, S., Slovic, P., Fischhoff, B., Layman, M., & Combs, B. (1978). Judged frequency of lethal events. *Journal of Experimental Psychology: Human Learning and Memory, 4*, 551–78.

Lindley, D. V., Tversky, A., & Brown, R. W. (1979). On the reconciliation of probability assessments. *Journal of the Royal Statistical Society* (Series A), *142*, (Part 2), 146–80.

Meehl, P. E. (1954). *Clinical versus statistical prediction: A theoretical analysis and a review of the evidence.* Minneapolis: University of Minnesota Press.

Murphy, A. H., & Winkler, R. L. (1984). Probability of precipitation forecasts. *Journal of American Statistical Association*, *79*, 391–400.

Nelkin, D., & Brown, M. S. (1984). *Workers at risk.* University of Chicago Press.

Nisbett, R. E., Krantz, D. H., Jepsen, C., & Kunda, Z. (1983). The use of statistical heuristics in everyday inductive reasoning. *Psychological Review*, *90*, 339–63.

Nisbett, R. E., & Ross, L. (1980). *Human inference: Strategies and shortcomings of social judgment.* Englewood Cliffs, NJ: Prentice-Hall.

Nisbett. R. E., & Wilson, T. D. (1977). Telling more than we can know: Verbal reports on mental processes. *Psychological Review*, *84*, 231–59.

Payne, J. W. (1982). Contingent decision behavior. *Psychological Bulletin*, *92*, 382–401.

Peterson, C. R., & Beach, L. R. (1967). Man as an intuitive statistician. *Psychological Bulletin*, *68*(1), 29–46.

Phillips, L. D., & Wright, G. N. (1977). Cultural differences in viewing and assessing probabilities. In H. Jungermann & G. deZeeuw (Eds.), *Decision making and change in human affairs.* Amsterdam: D. Reidel.

Pitz, G. F., & Sachs, N. J. (1984). Judgment and decision: Theory and application. *Annual Review of Psychology*, *35*, 139–63.

Popper, K. R. (1962). *The logic of scientific discovery.* New York: Oxford University Press. (Clarendon Press).

Poulton, E. C. (1968). The new psychophysics: Six models for magnitude estimation. *Psychological Bulletin*, *69*, 1–19.

   (1982). Biases in quantitative judgments. *Applied Ergonomics*, *13*, 31–42.

Raiffa, H. (1968). *Decision analysis.* Reading, MA: Addison-Wesley.

Rhoads, S. E. (Ed.). (1980). *Valuing life: Public policy dilemmas.* Boulder, CO: Westview.

Schelling, T. (1979). *Micromotives and microbehavior.* New York: Norton.

Shafer, G. (1976). *A mathematical theory of evidence.* Princeton, NJ: Princeton University Press.

Simon, H. A. (1957). *Models of man: Social and rational.* New York: Wiley.

Slovic, P. (1969). Analyzing the expert judge: A descriptive study of a stockbroker's decision processes. *Journal of Applied Psychology*, *79*, 139–45.

   (1974). Hypothesis testing in the learning of positive and negative linear functions. *Organizational Behavior and Human Performance*, *11*, 368–76.

Slovic, P., Fischhoff, B., & Lichtenstein, S. (1977). Behavioral decision theory. *Annual Review of Psychology*, *28*, 1–39.

   (1979). Rating the risks. *Environment*, *21*(3), 14–20, 36–9.

   (1981). Perceived risk: Psychological factors and social implications. In F. Warner & D. H. Slater (Eds.), *The assessment and perception of risk.* (pp. 11–34). London: The Royal Society.

Slovic, P., & Lichtenstein, S. (1971). Comparison of Bayesian and regression approaches to the study of information processing in judgment. *Organizational Behavior and Human Performance*, *6*, 649–744.

Smith, E. R., & Miller, R. S. (1978). Limits on perception of cognitive processes: A reply to Nisbett & Wilson. *Psychological Review*, *85*, 355–62.

Svenson, O., & Fischhoff, B. (1985). Levels of environmental decisions: A case study of radiation in Swedish homes. *Journal of Environmental Psychology*, *5*, 55–85.

Tribe, L. H. (1973). Technology assessment and the fourth discontinuity: The limits of instrumental rationality. *Southern California Law Review*, *46*, 617–60.

Tune, G. S. (1964). Response preferences: A review of some relevant literature. *Psychological Bulletin*, *61*, 286–302.

Tversky, A., & Kahneman, D. (1973). Availability: A heuristic for judging frequency and probability. *Cognitive Psychology*, *5*, 207–32.

    (1974). Judgment under uncertainty: Heuristics and biases. *Science*, *185*, 1124–31.

Viscusi, W. K. (1983). *Risk by choice*. Cambridge, MA: Harvard University Press.

Wilks, S. S. (1938). Weighting systems for linear functions of correlated variables when there is no dependent variable. *Psychometrika*, *8*, 23–40.

von Winterfeldt, D., & Edwards, W. (1982). Costs and payoffs in perceptual research. *Psychological Bulletin*, *91*, 609–22.

    (1986). *Decision making and behavioral research*. Cambridge University Press.

Yntema, D. B., & Torgerson, W. S. (1961). Man–computer cooperation in decisions requiring common sense. *IRE Transactions of the Professional Group on Human Factors in Electronics*, *2*(1), 20–6.

7   Problem solving

Alan Lesgold

Introduction

Problem solving is a major human activity in our high-technology society. Many of the jobs currently available are characterized by the problem solving they require. Doctors have to solve the problem of what is causing their patients' symptoms. Auto mechanics have to determine why cars don't run properly. Counselors often perceive either their role, the client's role, or both as one of solving certain life problems. The political process, on both an international and a domestic level, is driven by the need to solve complex problems. College students have to schedule courses, jobs, and study time. Almost every aspect of daily life seems to involve problem solving.

In this chapter, we are concerned with the theories and empirical knowledge that psychology has amassed about problem solving. We will give primary attention to focused mental activity aimed at achieving specific goals, because that is the kind of problem solving about which we know the most. Where possible, we will try to make links to more popular aspects of problem solving, such as creativity training (Smith, 1985), but not much has been firmly established in that area.

It is a particularly important time for the psychology of problem solving. In reviewing basic school subjects like mathematics, social science, and the natural sciences, teacher and curriculum designer groups have almost universally called for more work on "higher-order thinking skills" (or HOTS), essentially those that involve solving problems: arithmetic word problems, physics problems, social problems, and so on. There is a belief that perhaps HOTS is a topic that merits its own space in the school day. Of course, allocating school time to HOTS would mean decreasing the time given to basic subject matter like reading, writing, and mathematics. So it is important to determine whether there are special problem-solving skills that can be applied to problems of any kind.

This practical consideration is a good starting point in setting the agenda for this chapter. What skills are involved in solving problems? To what extent are these skills general, rather than specific to each subject matter? To what extent should problem solving be treated as something different from doing arithmetic or reading? These questions have practical importance in shaping our decisions about school curricula, training in technical skills such as home appliance repair, and even medical school curricula. Just as important, they represent very basic research issues in the psychology of problem

188

solving. In this chapter, we will consider the mental activity involved in solving problems, concentrating on problems that have clear-cut solutions. We will examine the nature of problem-solving expertise and consider how that expertise is acquired. Finally, we will give some attention to problems with goals that are not obvious, to situations in which an important concern is deciding when the problem has been solved.

Solving problems that have clear goals

From one point of view, many of our daily activities involve problem solving. We decide what to wear, what to eat for breakfast, how to decorate our apartment, what to write in a note to an old friend, how to get to work during a transit strike. Some jobs, like appliance repair or medical diagnosis, consist primarily of problem solving, discovering the faults in a mechanical or human system. One important way of sorting these various activities is to note whether or not we can specify exactly what it means to solve the problem.

For example, the problem we bring to a physician is often characterized by symptoms. I say to my doctor, "I have had bronchitis for two weeks. Please make it go away." In such a case, anyone can figure out whether the doctor has achieved her goal by simply asking me, after a certain amount of time, if I still have bronchitis. Most important, the doctor can check her progress in the same way. The problem of redecorating one's apartment is much different. There is no rule that specifies when the job is done. The same is true of such tasks as designing the 1987 model of an automobile line, getting a good job, or finishing a manuscript. In all of these cases, deciding whether the problem is solved yet is itself a subproblem of the overall problem.

In some cases, an expert will know very clearly when a problem is solved, but a novice may not. For example, when a young child does an arithmetic problem like $1,002 - 99$ and gets the ones' digit of the answer, 3, he may not recognize that even after subtracting 9 from 9 in the tens' place, he still has another 9 (in the hundreds place) to deal with. After some schooling, he learns a rule for deciding when he is finished. (To see how complex such rules can be, try to state the rule exactly.)

For many problems, not only the answer but the set of steps one might follow to find the answer is well defined. In such cases, we can make a graph of the possible actions required to solve the problem. For example, consider the famous missionary–cannibal problem:

Three missionaries and three cannibals are on the left bank of a river. They have a boat that holds two people. If ever the cannibals outnumber the missionaries on either bank, the cannibals will eat the missionaries. How can they all get to the other bank?

We can start graphing the problem by listing all of the possible starting moves. In this case, one cannibal can take the boat to the other side, or two cannibals can take the boat to the other side, or one missionary and one cannibal can go. We can show this pictorially, as in Figure 7.1a or, more concisely, as in Figure 7.1b, where the notation 331, for example, means that the left bank has three missionaries, three cannibals, and the boat. (If we know what is on the left, we can assume that the remaining people are on the right.) If we draw a line from each possible situation code to those representing the result of one additional move, we get the graphical picture shown in Figure 7.2. We call such a graph a depiction of the *problem space*.

A map of the problem space is both a scorecard for specifying how someone attempts to solve the problem and an overview of the entire set of acts that could occur in anyone's solving of the problem. If we think of the problem space as a sort of maze of mental activity through which we must wander, searching for a solution, we have a powerful metaphor for reflecting about the nature of problem solving. Problem solving involves a *search* for a path from the starting situation to the goal state. However, a person solving a problem also has to know what steps are possible – how to *represent* the problem. These two aspects of problem solving, representation and search, are a good start toward understanding problem solving. Notice that for problems with clearly defined solutions and only a small number of possible actions,[1] we can easily specify the complete problem space. As more actions become available or solutions become less recognizable, the problem space grows rapidly beyond our ability to graph it completely.

Recording mental activity

However, it may be possible to graph all the portions of the problem space that are actually reached by people trying to solve the problem. For example, my colleagues and I have studied air force technicians dealing with the problem of fixing a large electronic equipment test apparatus. The apparatus contains about 40 ft^3 of electronic components, thousands of possibilities. When we consider the order in which those components could be tested and the accumulation of evidence that could occur, the possibilities approach infinity. It turns out, however, that the technicians take relatively few solution paths. We have been able to obtain very refined data about both skilled and less skilled technicians by first observing the range of solution approaches taken by a group of technicians of widely varying ability and then building a partial problem space map from our observations. Using this map, we try to figure out the strategies and tactics by which people might reach various points in the problem space. We then test our hypotheses by preparing specific questions to ask a new group of technicians at different points in the problem space.

Our primary method for studying problem solving is watching and listen-

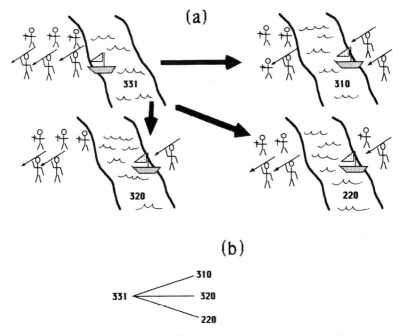

Figure 7.1. Pictorial (a) or graphic (b) representations of the possible first moves in the missionary–cannibal problem.

ing to people as they solve problems. We can simply record the steps of problem solving if it consists of physical behavior, like moving puzzle pieces. In most cases, we ask the problem solver to "think aloud." In the case of the missionary–cannibal problem, as the subject specifies each move to be made as he or she tries to solve the problem, we note the progression of moves, the errors made (e.g., moves that cause missionaries to be eaten), and the impasses (e.g., moves that simply reverse the prior move, such as from State 331 to State 220 back to State 331). As we shall see, this process is more complex than it seems. Some of the thinking activity involved in solving a problem may be unconscious. In such cases, problem solvers not only tell us what they are thinking but also use their personal theories to reconstruct the mental procedures that were not consciously evident to them (Nisbett & Wilson, 1977).

We can also examine the elapsed time (*latency*) between moves. For example, many people, when trying to solve the missionary–cannibal problem, adopt the heuristic[2] of moving as many people from left bank to right and as few from right to left as possible. Such a strategy should produce a long latency before moves that violate the left-to-right principle, such as 110 to 221 (see Figure 7.2), which not only involves moving two people from right to left but also seems at first glance to be an impasse, since the

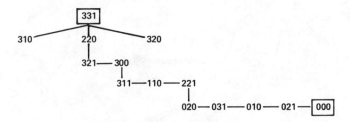

Figure 7.2. Problem space graph for the missionary−cannibal problem.

same configuration, with the boat on the other side, occurred earlier (220 was the likely first move).

To summarize, we can study problem solving by observing it, mapping the problem space, taking transcripts of think-aloud sessions (which we call verbal protocols), and recording latency data. Ericsson and Simon (1984) have argued that the most rigorous theories of problem solving are those that provide the rules from which simulations of the step-by-step problem-solving process can be derived. These simulations can then be compared with verbal protocol data to verify the theory.

Problem-solving methods

We turn now to the issue of representing problem solving − of building simulation models (usually stated as computer programs). If we think about the search process, we see that the procedure required to conclude a successful search (i.e., to solve the problem) can be represented as a series of conditional actions. For example, a veteran missionary−cannibal problem solver might include the following conditional action in his or her problem-solving repertoire:

IF the current state is 110,
THEN move so it becomes 221.

Following the terminology of the logician Post (1943), we call conditional actions *productions*. It can be shown that any process that can be carried out by a conventional computer can instead be specified as a set of productions − a production system. Furthermore, productions have special appeal because they preserve some of the associative character of earlier psychological theory. The idea of a contingent association between a mental state and a mental action is simply an extension of the idea of such a link between a sensory stimulus and a motor response. Of course, it would be trivializing the issue to assert that all a person needs to solve the missionary−cannibal problem is to know beforehand all the steps to be taken (e.g., 110−221). The challenge is to understand how to attack such a problem before we know exactly how to solve it. Following Newell and Simon (1972), we refer to the trivial method of the missionary–cannibal expert as a *strong method*, because it tells us exactly how to proceed most efficiently. Most of our interest is in understanding *weak methods*, which are the methods we use for attacking problems when we do not already know exactly how to proceed, and in understanding the learning processes by which our weak methods enable us to acquire strong methods specific to a particular domain.

There are several weak methods that people seem to rely on heavily in attacking unfamiliar problems. These include *means–end analysis, working forward, working backward,* and *generate and test* (Duncker, 1935/1945; Greeno & Simon, in press; Newell & Simon, 1972). Means–end analysis is a process of trying to move through the problem space using the heuristic of carrying out operations that decrease the distance between one's current location in the problem space and the goal state. For example, trying to get as many people on the right bank as possible and as few on the left is a means–end strategy. Greeno and Simon have used a set of productions to characterize the means–end strategy as follows:

IF the goal is to decrease the difference between the current state and another state,
THEN find an operation that can do this and set the goal of applying it.

IF the goal is to apply an operation O and a condition C is unsatisfied,
THEN set the goal of decreasing the difference between the current state and one
   which satisfies C.

IF the goal is to apply an operation O to the current state,
THEN do this.

IF there is a disparity between the current state and the goal state,
THEN set the goal of decreasing this disparity.

IF there is no disparity between the current state and the goal state,
THEN you are done.

To understand the means–end production system, one must know its *execution discipline*. When a mental procedure is specified as a list of productions, some assumptions must be made concerning the structural limitations on human thinking capability. In the case of the means–end production system, Greeno and Simon assumed, implicitly, that only one production could be active at a time. If the conditions for two productions are satisfied at the same time, the one listed earlier is the one that is executed. For example, at the beginning, the first production to have its condition satisfied happens to be the fourth in the list. Then, in the next time interval, the first production will "fire."[3] Only when there are no pending goals to satisfy and no differences between the current state and the final goal state will the fifth production fire. What actually happens, then, is that a difference between the current and goal state is identified and an effort is made to remove that difference. Sometimes further conditions must be satisfied before the difference-removing operation takes place. In these cases, one sets a subgoal of trying to achieve satisfaction of these special conditions and this becomes the target of difference-reducing activity until it is achieved.

One can focus on something other than the difference between the current and the goal state. This change of focus is necessary whenever it is not possible to know how close one is to a solution. For example, a comic detective trying to solve a murder may be right next to a clue and not realize it. In more general terms, means–end analysis depends on having enough expertise to know when one is getting closer to a solution. This is not always possible. When insufficient knowledge is available, we need some other general strategy to guide our efforts. There are two other general strategies that Newell and Simon (1972) explored: *working forward* and *working backward*. The working-forward strategy involves considering the actions that are possible and selecting the best one, observing what happens and repeating the process. Working backward is a bit more complex. It involves breaking a large problem into smaller problems. For example, the detective might say to herself, "If I knew a motive and had some fingerprints, I could probably figure out who the killer was; so, I'll look for motive information and for fingerprints."

The final weak method is *generate and test*. In essence, this strategy is one of unmotivated selection of possible actions, carrying each out until progress is apparent, and then reevaluating the problem situation. For example, if you were trapped in a cave with a small number of mountaineering tools, you might simply try one tool after another, hoping to find a way to use one in order to get out. Clearly, this is the least focused of all strategies. However, it can be adequate under some circumstances. For example, if you do not know which drawer of your desk has your pipe in it, you might systematically try one after another until you find the pipe. What makes the generate-and-test approach work in that case is that the set of choices is small and there is a systematic way of ensuring that each is tried only once.

An important point to be made about the weak methods we have characterized is that they do not depend on the field, but they do depend on specific knowledge for specifying differences and for the goal-directed operations they invoke (Greeno & Simon, in press). Basically, they impose order on the process of using what one knows about the problem domain to try to solve a problem. Put another way, they impose a strategy or plan on the problem-solving activity, even if it is only the simplest generate-and-test plan of trying different things until something works.

Plans can have many different levels of detail. A general, when planning, thinks in terms of broad troop movements. A sergeant plans in terms of getting all of his men to the right place at the right time. An individual soldier, for the most part, simply plans the specific action he is to carry out. In the section on learning to solve problems, we shall see that problem solving involves developing the capability to carry out the details automatically so that planning can take place at a higher level of abstraction.

What makes problems hard to solve? Limits on human capability

Although we can formally represent the problem space, at least for simple problems, the formal representation does not capture everything of importance about the problem. In fact, Hayes and Simon (1974) published an extensive account of differences in the degree of difficulty of solving a set of problems. The problems had the same structure but tended to produce different mental representations in subjects. This distinction between problem structure and problem representation is an important one. The problem structure is a formal abstraction. If two problems have isomorphic problem spaces, they have the same structure – we can translate every situation and every possible problem-solving action on one problem into a related situation or action on the other.

Consider the problem shown in Figure 7.3a. Two players are to take turns picking up single cards. When a player holds three cards that sum to exactly 15, he or she puts them down and is declared the winner. This problem is isomorphic in structure to the familiar game of tic-tac-toe, but we tend to represent the two games differently. When we think about tic-tac-toe, we think about lines, sides, corners, and the center. When we think about the first game, we think about needing three odd numbers or two evens and an odd, or perhaps we think about needing two numbers that sum to 10, plus the 5. Our mental representations are different, and this often leads us to notice only some of the constraints in the problem as posed.

Kotovsky, Hayes, and Simon (1985) published an extensive series of studies examining why two isomorphic problems can differ in difficulty. They demonstrated that limitations on temporary memory were a primary source of difficulty and that some problem representations help us circumvent this limitation more than others do. Three sources of aid are provided by the best representations:

> Good representations allow us to represent blocks of planned moves as a single "chunk" of memory.
>
> Good representations allow us to represent the rules of the game easily and to ascertain whether a move is legal and productive.
>
> Good representations allow us to represent our position in the problem space efficiently.

Each of these possibilities is illustrated in the comparison of the number-pickup game with tic-tac-toe. With tic-tac-toe, we can immediately see possible goals: the corners, the center, a line of three. With the number-pickup representation, we are forced into more cumbersome thinking that requires continual mental arithmetic. Similarly, in tic-tac-toe we can more easily assess whether, according to the rules of the game, a potential move will produce a win; we simply look for three marks in a row. Finally, we can see the threats we face more quickly looking at a Tic-Tac-Toe board than looking at the numbers in our hand and on the table, even though the abstract infor-

(a) Players take turns choosing cards. First with three that sum to 15 wins.

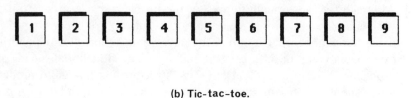

(b) Tic-tac-toe.

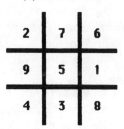

Figure 7.3. Isomorphic problems usually represented differently by subjects.

mation content is identical in the two cases. Expressing game states and rules with simple visual representations seems to be a particularly powerful way to make a problem easier.

More on production systems

So far in our discussion of production-system models of problem-solving activity, we have considered only the program, the set of productions. In order to consider differences in problem-solving ability, our next topic, we must first discuss the processor that will run these programs – the human mind. For the most part, we use Anderson's (1982, 1983) ACT*[4] theory of thinking and learning. In Anderson's theory, memory and goal structures play a critical role, so we discuss each of these briefly.

Basically, Anderson's theory asserts that mental activity consists of productions being executed. Productions are pieces of programs, and memory is the data on which those programs operate. When the *condition* part of a production matches a memory pattern, the production can execute its *action* part (we say it "fires"). The *action* part often produces changes in memory, which have the effect of changing or combining memory patterns.

Memory. This view renders memory very critical to mental activity, an intuition that is consistent with our common sense. For Anderson, memory consists of nodes and relations – it is an associative structure. Nodes correspond to nouns, verbs, qualifiers, and other concepts. Each idea in our memory can be represented by some nodes and some connections among them and between them and other memory structures. For example (see

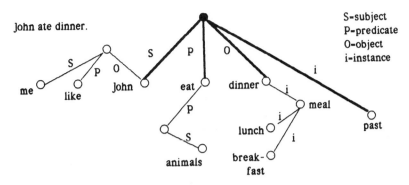

Figure 7.4. Memory structure (somewhat simplified) for *John ate dinner*.

Figure 7.4), if we read and understand a sentence like *John ate dinner*, this means we have added a new memory structure (shown in Figure 7.4 as the black nodes and links) to some structure we will assume was already there as a result of earlier experience or reading of an earlier sentence in the text. From the *eat* node, there would be a *subject* link, or relation, to the *John* node, a *time* link to the concept *past*, and an *object* link to the *dinner* node. Note that this idea, encoded in this way into memory, now has connections to every other idea about *John*, because they all have links to the *John* node, too.

We often have the experience of one piece of information about a person or situation prompting us to recall other, related information. Anderson provided for this contingency by including in his theory a process called *memory activation*. When new information is added to memory, it has a high activation level. Activation spreads from node to node through relations, or links. Memory that is active is in our consciousness, and paying attention to an idea is equivalent to keeping it activated. Activation spreads from concepts to which attention is currently being paid, that is, to which activation has been applied. As activation is split among an increasing number of alternate paths that fan out from the various nodes, it decreases. Furthermore, activation throughout the network is continually decaying.

The conditions of productions. The conditions of production, their *IF* side, are relational structures of the same form as those in memory. For a production's conditions to be satisfied, a segment of memory corresponding to the structure in its conditions must reach a high enough level of activation. Hence, productions are mental actions made in response to mental states, where those states amount to patterns of memory activation. A special case arises when we consider sensory input. Sensory input also activates special memory node structures that are permanently connected to our sensory systems. Such nodes might correspond to the simple pattern detectors for lines and angles that have been demonstrated in the visual system. Perception, then, consists of the automatic execution of productions that determine the meaning of the sensations. At the same time, higher-order cognitive productions operate on our overall pattern of current thoughts, sensations, and goals.

Goals. We have discussed thoughts and sensations, which correspond to memory activation patterns; we now must consider goals. Anderson has suggested that very special memory structures and some special processing rules are needed to represent goals. The basic scheme is that there is a hierarchical goal structure. Productions generally have a special condition naming the goal(s) for which they are to be applied. In order to fire, a production must match the current goal state as well as some activated subset of memory corresponding to its other conditions. This matching imposes considerable structure and consistency on thinking. It eliminates, or at least weakens, the possibility of some production totally unrelated to the current pattern of thought suddenly executing just because its conditions accidentally match currently active memory.[5]

Anderson proposes a specific kind of goal structure − a hierarchical goal structure. Some of our problem-solving productions act by splitting major goals into several subgoals that are easier to achieve. He suggests that we have the mental apparatus to organize complex tasks in this way and to keep track of our position in the goal structure. Dialing a telephone number is a good example. Researchers at Bell Laboratories studied the number of digits a person could dial correctly immediately after hearing a phone number and concluded that if more than four digits were attempted at once, errors would occur. So they introduced the convention of dividing phone numbers into smaller groups. For example, if my goal is to dial the information operator in Pasadena, I set two subgoals: to dial the area code and then to dial the local number; I then split the task of dialing the local number into two subsubgoals. By splitting the phone number into segments, we are able to attempt each group of three or four separately, as a separate subgoal.

Declarative knowledge. It will be useful to pause for a moment to consider the two types of knowledge we have been discussing. One is the knowledge embodied by productions. We call this procedural knowledge − knowledge for carrying out mental activities, knowing *how*. The other kind of knowledge is that in the memory network, which we call declarative knowledge, knowing *what*. Given this distinction, consider what happens when a teacher tells a student how to solve some type of problem and then assigns a set of problems of that type as homework. The knowledge that is acquired from listening to the teacher and memorizing what he or she said is *declarative knowledge*. By itself, this knowledge does not help a student solve a homework problem. The student must be able to activate his or her memory of the teacher's comments at the right time and then interpret them – turn them into mental acts.

Students face this problem particularly in courses like geometry. They are asked to write proofs, but they do not know how to do so. They search their memories for examples or incidents in class that might be relevant, and sometimes they find some. Applying what they remember from class, they make many mistakes. Only after considerable practice and advice from the teacher on the use of appropriate tactics are they able to prove geometry problems reliably. Some students never receive this coaching and advice and never learn how to generate proofs. The same thing can happen in courses like organic chemistry. Students are not always given strategies for determining the identity of an unknown substance, so they must rely on memorization and later recall of declarative knowledge that is not organized into efficient problem-solving procedures. This form of problem solving is based on rote memorization, but it could also be taught in such a way that students could make use of practiced skills of problem solving.

Anderson tells us that our capability for interpreting and carrying out verbal instructions is quite limited. Computers have the same problem. In order to work efficiently, they must be given programs written in their procedural language, sometimes called machine language. When we write a program that we want to run efficiently, we *compile* it into machine language. Computers often have interpreters that can carry out programs stated in more human-like language, a source language. When they are operating in this interpretive mode, they are substantially slower than when they are carrying out machine-language instructions. Furthermore, the interpreter itself is a program, and it must be available on the computer or the language cannot be interpreted at all.

A "dedicated" computer can solve one specialized kind of problem very well and very rapidly. A general-purpose computer can solve many kinds of problems, but it is much slower at any specific task, because it does not have the same degree of specialization as a computer built for a single type of problem. However, we can make it more expert (faster) by supplying it with compiled programs it can execute quickly, or even adding new automatic instructions called microcode. In this respect, human beings resemble a general-purpose computer. They can learn to do many different things well, but they start out somewhat inefficiently and slowly. The initial inefficiency is the price paid for adaptability. This brings us to our next topic – the characteristics of expertise and the differences between experts and novices.

Characteristics of expert and novice problem solvers

As we have seen, the way in which a problem is represented influences the ease with which it can be solved. Declarative knowledge is less reliably and less quickly executed than procedural knowledge. Furthermore, productions can execute only when their conditions are activated in memory. This activation requires both that the needed declarative structure be present and that the structural dynamics of memory match the productions that are available. For example, if memory decays quickly, a procedure cannot "light up" a memory structure too far in advance of the point at which it must cue a particular production. Finally, the goal structure of a procedure has much to do with how well it executes. Procedures that are not adequately orchestrated do not work together well on complex problems.

These hypotheses lead us to an interesting view of problem-solving expertise: Experts are people whose problem-solving procedures and representations of problems overcome the three limitations discussed earlier:

> Their procedures are compiled.
> The load their procedures place on temporary memory activation is consistent with the limitations on memory dynamics. Because of their organizational structures of memory, the needed activation sequences will occur with greater reliability.
> Their procedures are organized around an efficient strategy that can be driven by the goal-structuring apparatus.

Understanding expertise is difficult because experts' cognitive performances result from a set of production rules that they themselves have difficulty verbalizing directly. So we must look at many different forms of expertise from many different views if we are to have more than the experts' verbal theories about why they solve problems with such facility.

The chess master. Much of our understanding of expertise began with the study of skill in chess (Chase & Simon, 1973; de Groot, 1965, 1966; Simon & Chase, 1973). Several things became apparent once chess expertise was seen from the right viewpoint. For example, de Groot interviewed chess players about what they were doing and asked them to think aloud while planning their next moves. Until that time, it had been widely believed that expertise in chess consisted in being able to think ahead more moves than the average person could. From this point of view, chess expertise seemed to be a special, perhaps inborn talent, not an acquired set of procedural skills. However, de Groot found that, although advanced chess players think ahead quite a few moves and novices do not, the real masters are similar to novices in that they do not explicitly review all of the possible move sequences from their current position. An immediate explanation for this comes to mind: Experts do not have to work through long move sequences because they already know from experience the correct move for many board positions.

A series of experiments by de Groot and by Chase and Simon tended to confirm this viewpoint. They showed that the master chess player has a large repertoire of specific patterns that can be accessed in memory and quickly recognized. The experimental methods these investigators used were quite imaginative. They asked people to look at the positions of chess pieces on a chessboard and reconstruct them either immediately or after the original display was removed. The size of perceptual "chunks" was shown to vary with expertise. The master chess players noticed more pieces in each glance and, when recalling board positions, tended to put down larger "bursts" of pieces between pauses. That is, the experimenters recorded the time that elapsed between the placement of one piece on the reconstructed board and the placement of the next piece. The number of pieces the masters placed between relatively long pauses was greater than the number placed by novices. Also, the pieces within an advanced player's "chunk" were related by knowledge about chess – they were pieces related by mutual defense, proximity, attack possibilities, and so on. This superiority of the advanced chess players applied only to board arrangements from real games. When the boards were arranged randomly, there were no longer any differences between novice and more advanced players in perceptual efficiency or completeness of recall.[6]

Chess experts' problem solving, then, is based on rapid recognition processes that tap acquired knowledge rather than exclusively on conscious analytical thinking processes. Chess masters recognize the board situation they confront and know what to do about it. They do not excel by thinking ahead dozens of moves, as we once thought; indeed, they think ahead fewer moves than advanced players who are not yet at the master level. Chess masters also seem to have an ability to construct a mental representation of board positions in terms of play-relevant features that they can immediately recognize and to which they can immediately respond (Chase & Chi, 1981).

The physics expert. In more traditional school subjects, such as physics, a similar phenomenon has been observed: Highly competent performers are better than others at developing a good initial representation of the problem space (Larkin, McDermott, Simon, and Simon, 1980; Simon & Simon, 1978). Good representation skills enable the knowledgeable physicist to solve routine problems rapidly and without much conscious deliberation. When asked to sort problems into groups that belong together, experts organized physics problems according to the principles of physics they involve, whereas novices attended to more peripheral information, such as the mention of ramps or pulleys (Chi, Feltovich, & Glaser, 1981).

This finding has been demonstrated in several ways. For example, if one records the activity of people solving textbook problems in basic physics, one notes several differences between the performance of experts and that of novices. For example, experts do not simply choose an equation for solving the problem and then do the algebra. This is a novice approach. Experts spend a proportionately greater amount of problem-solving time than novices in building a representation of the problem in terms of basic physics principles, before they carry out a solution plan. Novices quickly start trying to retrieve from their declarative knowledge an equation that will take them from the quantities given to the quantity needed to answer the problem. Novices use means–end analysis when they search memory for a likely equation; experts have learned that it is worth understanding the situation before choosing the best solution path.

The knowledge of experts and the mental representations they construct include information about the application of what they know. In contrast, novices' knowledge structure may be more loosely organized, containing information that is most centrally relevant to the problem as stated but lacking any information about related principles and their application. For this reason, novices may have more difficulty making inferences from the literal problem statement. Their problem-solving difficulties may be attributed to the inadequacy of their knowledge base rather than to any limitations on their capacity to carry out processes.

In general, competent individuals can be described as having knowledge that is organized into a fast-access pattern recognition or encoding system that greatly reduces their reliance on the vagaries of declarative knowledge. These acquired knowledge patterns enable them to form an appropriate representation of the problem situation.

The expert radiologist. Physics and chess are areas that rely heavily on abstract reasoning. To get a sense of expertise in other areas, my colleagues and I have studied radiologists, whose expertise lies largely in their ability to perceive complicated patterns in very noisy visual displays (Lesgold et al., in press), and electronics technicians, non-college-trained experts who have to fix complex equipment (Glaser, Lesgold, & Lajoie, in press). The picture we built from this extension of expertise research into visual and practical areas matches the view of researchers studying chess and physics fairly well, although we obtained a few novel results.

In the work with radiologists, we studied residents and senior hospital staff. The residents had completed a premedical college program, medical school, and an internship in a hospital (generally involving experience with perhaps 10,000 X-ray pictures). The staff physicians had had at least 10 years of postresidency experience and generally had dealt with perhaps 500,000 X-ray pictures each. So we were studying people with well-learned skills. We gave them some very difficult cases to solve and analyzed their diagnoses, their defense of their diagnoses, their ability to incorporate new evidence (laboratory test data) into diagnoses to which they were already committed, and even their ability to outline, on the X-ray film, the abnormalities they claimed to see. The following were our key findings:

1. *Experts build a thorough representation of the patient's anatomy.* Like expert physicists, expert radiologists spend proportionately more of their problem-solving time generating a representation of the situation posed by a problem than do novices. When they talk about an X-ray film, they use more anatomy terms and speak in greater detail, and they use fewer spatial terms referring to film locations than residents do. They also have more elaborate general plans for dealing with different types of disease situations that enable them to describe more precisely the situation that seems to be present, and their general plans (psychologists call them *schemata*) contain specific procedures for verifying whether they fit the case and for finding unaccounted for features that might signal pathology (e.g., "This looks like a normal young female chest, except there's a funny blob in the apex of the left lung").

2. *Experts quickly begin executing pertinent general plans.* In looking at a film, they quickly mention a diagnostic category, which we take to indicate the invocation of a general plan, or schema, and then examine and discuss the film in the context of that schema, mentioning more findings that relate to it and fewer that are irrelevant to it than residents would.

3. *Experts exhibit flexibility and tuning of schemata.* Not only do experts test their choice of schema more completely; they also are more capable of adapting to the range of normal variation in human anatomy and radiographic technique. They are likely to mention aspects of the film that are inconsistent with the schema they have invoked, but they are also likely to find a model of anatomical variation that makes the apparent abnormality consistent with the schema. For example, in one case, one of our experts, looking at a collapsed-lung film, remarked that he could not see the edge of the upper lung lobe in the position it ought to be occupying. Then he reasoned that it would not be apparent because of the patient's position while the film was made. (The patient was in bed, rather than standing, and not quite straight; the radiologist could determine this from looking at skeletal structure.)

4. *Experts can analyze several objects that overlap in a film.* In one of the films, there was a large, clearly visible abnormality. Residents tended to see various normal structures extending into the region of this abnormality and "used up" most of the abnormality that way. As a result, they "saw" only a small abnormality, which they misdiagnosed. For them, X-ray pictures are much like embedded-figure tests, in which the extensions of other contours "invade" features that might otherwise be recognized. (Try to find the 4 in the embedded-figure item shown in Figure 7.5; it may be difficult even though you certainly know a 4 when you see one.)

5. *Experts are opportunistic in the face of new evidence.* One of the films in our study was that of a healthy person who, 20 years earlier, had undergone surgery for removal of a lobe of her lung. Because of the air pressure dynamics of the chest, when something is removed the remaining organs shift to occupy the extra space. In this case, when the heart shifted, it turned so that it appeared to be wider than normal (see Figure 7.6). Many residents mistook that appearance for an enlarged heart, a sign of congestive heart failure, a disabling condition; so did some experts. However, when the experts were told to reexamine the film after learning that the patient had been found perfectly healthy in a recent physical examination and had undergone surgery a number of years before, they quickly solved the case, whereas the residents who had made the congestive heart failure diagnosis still insisted that the patient was just about in the coffin.

6. *Not all learning is monotone; sometimes practice produces worse performance.* On some cases, new residents did almost as well as senior staff

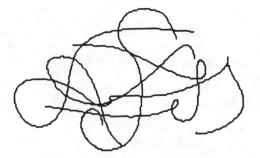

Figure 7.5. Embedded figure: Try to find the 4.

and better than third-and fourth-year residents. In fact, in a few cases the same person, looking at the same film, made the correct diagnosis in his first year but the wrong one in his third year. When we examined this result in detail, it became apparent that the new residents had been successful initially because the films were classic, almost textbook examples of particular diseases. Such films can be tricky, because the basic features that stand out, although classic indicators of one disease, may also be consistent with several others. New residents seemed to have little ability to consider critically the less likely alternatives, so they made the most likely choice. After additional training, they knew that the alternatives had to be considered, but they still did not have the capability of choosing definitively among them. As a result, they sometimes chose a less likely alternative that they did not know enought to rule out. Other studies of medical education suggest that this explanation is reasonable. For example, given a small set of symptoms, middle-level medical trainees will consider many more diagnoses than either beginners or experts and will often settle on the wrong choice.

The promising technician. We turn briefly to work done, not on experts, but on relatively new technician trainees and on the emergence of bits of expertise. We investigated an enlisted specialty in the air force that involves using noncomputerized test facilities to troubleshoot certain electronic components of F-15 fighter planes. The people doing this work receive several months of technical school training and then receive a job assignment in a repair squadron at a base. During the next few years, they are given more responsibility as quickly as they can handle it. We studied people who had been in the air force less than three years and compared the performance of those who were making the most progress (i.e., who could perform the most difficult repair tasks reliably) with the performance of those making less progress.

Among the many detailed findings of this work, perhaps the most important is that high- and low-ability people do not differ either in their knowledge of weak problem-solving methods or in their general knowledge of electrical and electronics principles. The differences lie exclusively in strategies and tactics that are specific to the kinds of troubleshooting they must do and in declarative knowledge relating to the specific levels of components

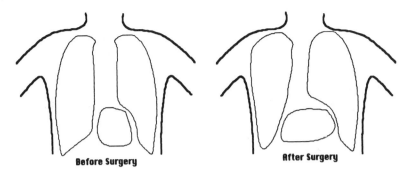

Figure 7.6. Outline of chest organs before and after removal of lung lobe.

about which they must make decisions. If they are asked how a resistor works, their replies, though not uniformly correct, are no worse for the low-ability group than for the high-ability group. Similarly, they all use subgoaling strategies; that is, they split complex problems into several subproblems that can be considered in turn. However, they vary greatly in their ability to develop the specific plan types that produce efficient solutions to the problems they face.

One way of interpreting this difference is to say that they are all on the same path of acquiring the necessary procedural and declarative knowledge to support their performances, but that the high-ability group is simply farther along. Although this interpretation seems valid, it is important to note that airmen assigned to this specialty have to meet rather strict aptitude test requirements that probably ensure that they are, as a group, very similar in their general learning capabilities. Nonetheless, our results at least support the general view that expertise is based mainly on one's store of knowledge that is very specific to the tasks one faces and not primarily on general aptitude, knowledge of weak methods, or structural dynamics of memory and cognition.

Learning to solve problems

We turn now to a fundamental psychological question, How do people learn to solve problems? In one sense, problem-solving expertise mainly involves learning specific information and methods that vary from one domain to another, so it should be acquired by the same laws of learning that apply to any other capabilities. From another point of view, however, the essence of problem solving is being able to deal with novel situations, or problems one has not been specifically trained to solve. Although psychological theory is not as well developed in this respect, there are some interesting possibilities to consider. First we deal with training in solving specific types of problems.

Anderson's learning theory applied to problem solving

The aspects of Anderson's (1982, 1983) theory already discussed lay the foundation for his learning theory. Cognitive capabilities result primarily from the development of procedures for carrying them out. The units of those procedures are productions. The condition side of productions must match activated memory and the currently active subgoal in order for the action side to be executed. Learning, then, must include the development and refinement of productions and of the declarative knowledge base that supports them.

Anderson's learning theory is a stage theory, in which the character of competence and the circumstances that can produce learning undergo qualitative changes with learning. Anderson proposes three stages of learning:

1. *The declarative knowledge stage.* In this stage, weak procedures rely on declarative knowledge to drive problem solving. That is, we apply very simple, domain-independent methods that simply search our declarative knowledge for relevant information and then try to act on it. For example, when we read a recipe for a dish we have never cooked, say a soufflé, we acquire declarative knowledge.

2. *The procedural knowledge stage.* With practice, successful sequences of activity that are produced by the application of weak methods to declarative knowledge are compiled into domain-specific new productions. Compilation results from two effects of practice – *proceduralization* and *composition.* Proceduralization is a process that notices repeated occurrences of a particular mental action shortly after a particular declarative memory and subgoal activation pattern and generates a production corresponding to the repeated correlation of pattern and action. Composition eliminates unnecessary steps from a sequence of productions. When we practice making soufflés, we are eventually able to make them automatically, without having to read the recipe.

3. *The tuned procedures stage.* Once knowledge is procedural, there remains the problem of tuning it. Three processes are involved in tuning: *strengthening, generalization,* and *discrimination.* Every production has a strength. When several productions match currently active memory and subgoal, it often is not possible to execute them all simultaneously. In such cases, the stronger productions will generally prevail. Productions are strengthened when they are used successfully. Productions are generalized by the replacement of some of their condition patterns with variables. For example, we may initially learn that if we fire a water pistol at a target and hit it too low, we should raise our arm. This fact might generalize to a production that says that any time we are shooting at a target, we should aim high. Discrimination occurs when a production results in an impasse or cannot execute. For example, at close range, it is unwise to aim high. The errant production is weakened relative to productions with similar conditions that have been more successful. Following our soufflé example, we learn how to make any kind of soufflé – cheese, chocolate, or liqueur-flavored – with perfect results. The tuning process is illustrated in the following comment by someone who was reflecting on his experiences in learning to play the piano: "I was busy watching my hands and the terrain of the keyboard to see that

they did not get into trouble; or I was looking at the keyboard in order to find places to take my fingers, so that instructional work was occurring as a form of guidance in which my looking was very much implicated. Then my look became preoccupied in more subtle ways, party to a kind of imaginary conceiving of various aspects of the territory in which I was moving" (Sudnow, 1978, p. 1).

Anderson's learning theory makes an immediate prediction of great importance. Practice is necessary if learning is to occur. Furthermore, because the procedures one wants to develop and refine are procedures for solving problems and not procedures for memorizing texts, one should invest one's effort in problem solving, not just in listening to a teacher talk about it or in reading about it. Also, how-to-do-it information generally prevails over how-it-works information (Pirolli & Anderson, 1984). The best instruction involves the student in actual problem solving, with the instructor making the process more efficient by preventing the student from pursuing wild goose chases and providing hints if no progress is being made (Anderson & Reiser, 1985).

Why is this? Cutting off wild goose chases is probably effective because once students have gone far enough to know what path they have been following, there is no point in their going farther if it is the wrong one. Trying to optimize successful problem-solving time is likely to be effective for the same reason: It maximizes the opportunity for proceduralization and tuning and makes it less likely that wrong productions will execute and be strengthened.

There remains, however, the problem of generality, of preparing students to deal with novel situations. We know little about this, except that the best preparation for dealing with novel situations may be a great deal of experience with problems in related situations. To pursue the matter of learning problem solving in novel domains a bit farther, we shall take a somewhat different approach. So far, we have dealt with a coherent theory that has substantial support and is being extended continually. When we talk about general problem-solving skill, we do not have such a validated theory. What we do have are ideas and efficacy testing. That is, we formulate ideas about teaching problem solving that intuitively make sense to us, and test them in almost the same way we test drugs like aspirin. If they work, we accept them, just as we accepted aspirin decades before we had any theoretical understanding of *how* it works.

Improving problem-solving capabilities

In this section we consider suggestions made in a recent practical book on improving problem-solving skills (Whimbey & Lochhead, 1981). Whimbey and Lochhead (1981) first endorse the importance of practice as a means of improving problem solving. They then point out the following things to avoid while practicing:

> Failure to observe and use all the relevant data
> Jumping to conclusions without checking them
> Failure to spell out relationships fully
> Being sloppy and inaccurate

Later in their book, they offer the following aspects of good problem solving:

> Positive attitude
> Concern for accuracy
> Breaking of the problem into parts
> Avoidance of guessing
> More mental activity

The most striking thing about this book is that almost all of it is devoted to specific sequences for specific types of problems. Implicitly, the authors have accepted Anderson's fundamental assertion, that domain-specific practice is the source of (relatively) domain-specific problem-solving skill. The rest of the suggestions involve overcoming certain school-produced habits that can compete with successful problem solving. Working alone, we are bound to reach impasses in our problem-solving practice from time to time. From formal schooling, we learn that a certain level of effort invested in trying to solve problems will pay off (in terms of passing courses, etc.), whereas any significant effort beyond that point will not produce much more reward. Even worse, we learn that if we have worked for a while without success, the best thing to do, with respect to getting a good grade without suffering excessively, is to guess the answer and go on. This may not be the way to optimize learning to solve problems.

To learn to solve problems, one has to solve some problems successfully. At points of impasse, several strategies may help to ensure that this success occurs. The problem representation may be incorrect or incomplete. If one reexamines the problem and checks the details of one's understanding, a memory pattern may be activated that triggers useful productions; thus, checking one's understanding and trying to avoid inaccuracy will have the effect of increasing the probability that the right approach will be triggered if one has already learned something appropriate. Similarly, elaborating one's understanding ("spelling out relationships") also increases the likelihood of activating either a useable production that should be generalized or some declarative memory on which a weak method can operate interpretively.

Having a positive attitude and being thorough may be keys to moving from the novice state of responding to superficial characteristics of a problem to the expert stage of correctly dealing with all apparent possibilities. As we noted in our discussion of radiological expertise, people seem to go through intermediate stages of learning in which they can, if they persist, notice or mentally represent the full range of issues they must confront to ensure a correct solution but in which they may or may not actually succeed in dealing with those issues. Someone who always makes a "quick and dirty" decision presumably never practices and consequently never develops a more refined problem-solving capability.

Much of what we know about problem solving seems to be good old-fashioned common sense: Work hard, be thorough, take heart and do not give up, monitor your performance, and watch for errors. In addition, people like Anderson, who develop rich theories and then apply those theories to the practical question of how to learn, tell us this: Practice solving the kinds of problems you would like to be able to solve more readily. Instead of merely reading books or listening to lectures about problem solving, try to solve problems. A teacher can be extremely helpful in guiding one's practice if he or she understands how to increase the odds that one will do approximately the right thing while noticing the circumstances under which one did it:

People seek teachers and teaching in order to find something that they do not know already. In reality, however, teachers and teachings exist to help people to apply and practice, not to amuse or give experience that must be new. (Shah, 1971, p. 108)

Creativity

We conclude with a brief discussion of a different aspect of problem-solving skill — creativity. This is an area in which much is said but little is well understood. We do not yet have theories of creativity that are as robust as our theories of problem solving and expertise. Our everyday experience tells us that people occasionally have powerful insights that seem to differ from the results of step-by-step thinking.

A generation ago, psychologists spent considerable time trying to understand insights. They studied famous thinkers, both historical and contemporary, in an attempt to figure out the processes by which they conceived their ideas. For example, Wertheimer (1945/1959) studied Gauss and Einstein, among others. Although those psychologists provided good descriptions of insightful problem solving, or creativity, they were unable to formulate a theory that was both empirically supported and practical. So as methods for studying solutions of well-structured problems arose, most psychologists gave up the study of creativity and other less-constrained problem solving.

The same expertise that produces high-quality mental representations of a well-structured problem is probably similar to that involved in the creative process. Let us take as an example Einstein's development of the theory of relativity (Wertheimer, 1945/1959). Einstein thought about aspects of the problem for decades. Most of the mathematics necessary for understanding

the consequences of light having constant velocity had already been produced by others. Einstein's breakthrough consisted in the radical step of
making the constancy of the speed of light a central principle of physics
rather than an anomaly to be explained by other principles.

Let us look at Wertheimer's account of Einstein's work (see Table 7.1).
Several things are apparent. First, Einstein engaged in recurrent activity of a
sort undertaken by many kinds of experts: He constructed a representation,
then tested it, applying both weak and strong methods. For example, Lorenz
provided an explanation of the Michelson experiment, in which it appeared
that the velocity of light was constant, but Einstein found it unacceptable.
Why? Because it treated this situation as a specal case. The constancy of
light velocity is not interconnected with other important physical principles.
Experts have knowledge that is generally redundant; the principles they
know are interconnected, not isolated from related issues.

Second, Einstein oscillated between intensely focused problem solving,
trying, for example, to understand simultaneity, and temporary abandon-
ment of pieces of the problem for which no partial solution path was present. Because experts know what to do in most cases, they have the capacity
to decide whether they can solve a problem given their current resources or
whether they need new information or methodology. It has sometimes been
said that the trick to getting a Nobel Prize is knowing which problems are
not yet "ripe" for solution and thus not wasting time on them.

Moreover, Einstein made an effort to restate new ideas and new experimental results in everyday terms — he performed "thought experiments."
Here again, the effect was to force the generalization of ideas, from laboratory situations to everyday events, like a ride on the trolley, to mental trips
on stars through the heavens. Again, this seems to have been an extension
of the representation testing idea, which matches well with work on less
creative problem solving.

The one component of Einstein's efforts that seem most in need of more
explanation is the apparent value of moving between focused, intense activity and a retreat from this intensity. Psychologists know a bit about the
effects of focusing on a task. Basically, as one's arousal increases, as one
works harder, one pays more attention to the most central features of the
situation at hand and less to more peripheral features (Easterbrook, 1959;
Kahneman, 1973). One becomes faster and more efficient, but only at following the clearest, most obvious path. Because creativity is partly the discovery of new paths, it must require some periods of decreased intensity, of
relaxation, of musing rather than struggling.

One way to interpret this change of focus is to see it as a change in the decay
rate of memory activation. When attention is focused, we more strongly
activate representations of the obvious at the expense of ignoring the barely
present. Put another way, only memory and sensory patterns that are strongly

Table 7.1. *Steps in Einstein's thinking*

Einstein wonders as a child what would happen if he chased a beam of light.

Einstein doubts whether the velocity of light depends on the movement of the observer.

Einstein tries to understand the relationship between the velocity of light and basic principles of movement (mechanics).

Michelson's experiment suggests the constancy of the velocity of light.

Lorenz provides an explanation for the results of Michelson's experiment, but it seems ad hoc to Einstein.

Einstein reflects on the fact that velocity involves time and time involves simultaneity. What would happen if the same experiment were performed under two different movement conditions, but simultaneously?

Einstein wonders what would happen if one started from the assumption that the velocity of light is not like all other velocities, but is fixed.

Einstein formulates and tests both rapid thought experiments and detailed confirmatory experiments to make certain he is right.

activated are noticed – faster decay prevents much spread of activation. In such situations, productions that have few conditions will be favored, because few memory nodes will be activated at any time. Also, we can interpret focus of attention as increasing the possibility that, even if more than one production matches a current memory state, only the strongest one will be able to execute – mental activity falls into a rut.

Einstein's genius, then, lay partly in his having the right combination of powerful focused thinking ability and expert understanding of physics and partly in his ability to back off and muse for a while. One final way to view this aspect of creativity is to conceive of the possibility of inhibiting the execution of productions and simply letting activation patterns and the spread of activation dominate our thinking. Practical experience and anecdote, along with Eastern philosophy, tell us that this path can produce good outcomes if combined with period of intense, focused expert procedural activity. The exact mechanisms involved have yet to be identified – we still need a few brilliant creative psychologists.

Notes

1 For example, a boat can contain a missionary, a cannibal, two of either, or one of each, and it can be going from left bank to right or vice versa, so there are 2×5, or 10 possible operations, or actions; half are ruled out because it is known which bank the boat is on, and others are ruled out because they leave the missionaries in vulnerable positions.

2 By *heuristic*, we mean a procedure that often works but is not guaranteed to work all the time.

3 We use the term *fire* essentially in the way it is used to describe the behavior of a neuron. A production fires if its condition is satisfied and it has priority in the execution discipline over other productions with satisfied conditions.

4 Pronounced "act-star."

5 A characteristic of the conversational patterns of some schizophrenics is that they hop from topic to topic, driven by all sorts of accidental associations, without any overriding purpose in their remarks. Their behavior operates without strong maintenance of a goal structure. Furthermore, our everyday belief that there is some overlap between being creative and being crazy may make more sense if we think of creativity as involving, in at least some phases, a relaxation of strong goal-structuring discipline, so that new approaches can come to mind.

6 Miller (1956) demonstrated that the number of chunks of information we can retain briefly is approximately seven. The Chase and Simon data showed that this was also true for chess players of all levels. What differed was that the better chess players could rapidly encode larger chunks, if the display was a board from a real game.

References

Anderson, J. R. (1982). Acquisition of cognitive skill. *Psychological Review, 89,* 396–406.
    (1983). *The architecture of cognition.* Cambridge, MA: Harvard University Press.
    (1985). *Skill acquisition: Compilation of weak-method problem solutions.* Pittsburgh: Carnegie-Mellon University.
Anderson, J. R., & Reiser, B. J. (1985). The LISP tutor. *Byte, 10,* 159–75.
Chase, W. G., & Chi, M. T. H. (1981). Cognitive skill: Implications for spatial skill in large-scale environment. In J. Harvey (Ed.), *Cognition, social behaviors, and the environment* (pp. 111–36). Hillsdale, NJ: Erlbaum.
Chase, W. G., & Simon, H. A. (1973). Perception in chess. *Cognitive Psychology, 4,* 55–81.
Chi, M. T. H., Feltovich, P., & Glaser, R. (1981). Categorization and representation of physics problems by experts and novices. *Cognitive Science, 5,* 121–52.
de Groot, A. D. (1965). *Thought and choice in chess.* The Hague: Mouton.
    (1966). Perception and memory versus thought: Some old ideas and recent findings. In B. Kleinmuntz (Ed.), *Problem solving: Research, method, and theory* (pp. 19–49). New York: Wiley.
Duncker, K. (1945). On problem solving. *Psychological Monographs, 58,* Whole No. 70. (Original German version published 1935.)
Easterbrook, J. A. (1959). The effect of emotion on cue utilization and the organization of behavior. *Psychological Review, 66,* 183–201.
Ericsson, K. A., & Simon, H. A. (1984). *Protocol analysis: Verbal reports as data.* Cambridge, MA: MIT Press.
Glaser, R., Lesgold, A., & Lajoie, S. (in press). Toward a cognitive theory for the measurement of achievement. In J. Glover (Ed.), *The influence of cognitive psychology on testing and measurement.* Hillsdale, NJ: Erlbaum.
Greeno, J. G., & Simon, H. A. (in press). Problem solving and reasoning. In R. C. Atkinson, R. Herrnstein, G. Lindzey, & R. D. Luce (Eds.) *Stevens' handbook of experimental psychology* (rev. ed.). New York: Wiley.
Hayes, J. R. & Simon, H. A. (1974). Understanding written instruction. In L. W. Gregg (Eds.), *Knowledge and cognition* (pp. 167–200). Hillsdale, NJ: Erlbaum.
Kahneman, D. (1973). *Attention and effort.* Englewood Cliffs, NJ: Prentice-Hall.
Kotovsky, K., Hayes, J. R., & Simon, H. A. (1985). Why are some problems hard? Evidence from the tower of Hanoi. *Cognitive Psychology, 17,* 248–94.
Larkin, J. H., McDermott, J., Simon, D. P., & Simon, H. A. (1980). Expert and novice performance in solving physics problems. *Science, 208,* 1335–42.
Lesgold, A., Rubinson, H., Feltovich, P., Glaser, R., Klopfer, D., & Wang, Y. (in press). Expertise in a complex skill: Diagnosing X-ray pictures. In M. T. H. Chi, R. Glaser, & M. Farr (Eds.), *The nature of expertise.* Hillsdale, NJ: Erlbaum.
Miller, G. A. (1956). The magical number seven, plus or minus two: Some limits on our capacity for processing information. *Psychological Review, 63,* 81–97.

Newell, A., & Simon, H. A. (1972). *Human problem solving.* Englewood Cliffs, NJ: Prentice-Hall.

Nisbett, R. E., & Wilson, T. D. (1977). Telling more than we know: Verbal reports on mental processes. *Psychological Review, 84,* 231–59.

Pirolli, P. L., & Anderson, J. R. (1984, November). *The role of mental models in learning to program.* Paper presented at the twenty-fifth meeting of the Psychonomic Society, San Antonio, Texas.

Post, E. L. (1943). Formal reductions of the general combinatorial problem. *American Journal of Mathematics, 65,* 197–268.

Shah, I. (1971). *Thinkers of the East.* Harmondsworth: Penguin Books.

Simon, H. A., & Chase, W. G. (1973). Skill in chess. *American Scientist, 61,* 394–403.

Simon, D. P., & Simon, H. A. (1978). Individual differences in solving physics problems. In R. S. Siegler (Ed.), *Children's thinking: What develops?* (pp. 325–48). Hillsdale, NJ: Erlbaum.

Smith, E. T. (1985, September 30). Are you creative? *Business Week,* 80–4.

Sudnow, D. (1978). *Ways of the hand.* Cambridge, MA: Harvard University Press.

Wertheimer, M. (1959). *Productive thinking.* New York: Harper & Row. (Enlarged edition of a book published in 1945.)

Whimbey, A., & Lochhead, J. (1981). *Problem solving and comprehension: A short course in analytical reasoning.* Philadelphia: Franklin Institute Press.

8   Language and thought

Sam Glucksberg
Introduction

What sets people apart from the rest of the animal kingdom? Language, of course, plays a central role in socal interaction, social perception, and cultural transmission. Does language also play a central role, perhaps a determining one, in human mentality − human thought and reasoning? The special place of language in human mentality is reflected in Roger Brown's clear denial of human language and therefore human mentality in nonhuman species:

I grant a mind to every human being, to each a full stock of feelings, thoughts, motives and meanings. I hope they grant as much to me. How much of this mentality that we allow one another ought we to allow the monkey, the sparrow, the goldfish, the ant? Hadn't we better reserve something for ourselves alone, perhaps consciousness or self-consciousness, possibly linguistic reference?

Most people are determined to hold the line against animals . . . man alone can use language to make reference. There is a qualitative difference of mentality separating us from the animals. (Brown, 1968, p. 1550)

A similar point of view had been expressed by Ivan Pavlov (1941), the discoverer of the conditioned reflex: "It is nothing other than words which has made us human" (p. 179).

Brown and Pavlov clearly imply a deep connection between mentality and language. Such a connection can operate in at least two different ways. The first is not very controversial: Our minds have evolved in such a way as to make language possible, if not inevitable, in every human being. The second has excited both interest and controversy: The human mind is special not because it makes language possible. Instead, it is language itself that shapes the mind. Language sets us apart from other animal species not only because it reflects the complexity and richness of human thought, but because it makes certain forms of thought possible. This claim can be extended even further to entail differences among languages. The particular language that we speak may not merely reflect thought, but directly control how we think and what we can think about.

This recognition of a deep connection between language and thinking has

This chapter was completed while the author was a fellow at the Center for Advanced Study in the Behavioral Sciences. I am grateful for financial support provided by National Science Foundation Grant BNS 84-11738. The research was supported in part by NSF Grant BNS 85-19462 to Princeton University. I thank Kay Deaux for her insightful and cogent criticism and suggestions.

existed since Aristotle. In North America, the identification of thought as language was revived by developments in two separate domains: the radical behaviorism of the early 1900s in American psychology (see Watson, 1913, 1925) and the cultural anthropology and descriptive linguistics of the same era (see Sapir, 1921, 1968).

In this chapter, we examine the various forms that this general claim — that thought and language are intrinsically related to one another — has taken. The following questions are examined in detail. Can there be thought without language? Do different languages reflect different ways of thinking? Even more interesting, do different languages *cause* differences in the ways people think?

One of the early proponents of the idea that thinking is nothing more than language behavior was John Watson, the founder of radical American behaviorism in the early 1900s. For Watson, unobservable events and processes such as thinking were to be ruled out as objects of scientific study. How, then, could one reconcile a science of psychology with the undeniable fact of human thought? Watson's solution was simple: Thought is nothing more than speech. As children, we think aloud by speaking. Gradually, the overt thinking-aloud speech of children becomes covert, and for Watson this covert speech *is* thought: "Thought processes are really motor habits in the larynx" (1913, p. 174). Here Watson is echoing a Russian psychologist who had earlier proposed that thought in children is mediated by speech or whispers (Sechenov, 1863). Some hundred years later, Luria characterized the development of thinking in children as "the process in which functions previously shared between two persons gradually change into the complicated functional systems in the mind which form the essence of higher mental activity" (Luria, 1961, p. 18).

For Sechenov and Luria, the developmental role of speech was critical; its role in adult cognition was not particularly important. For Watson, however, it was the role of the actual motor movements of speech that was crucial. Because a behaviorist could study only observable behavior, thinking could be studied if and only if thinking *was* observable. Implicit speech could not, of course, be directly observed, but its existence could be inferred from electromyographic records of muscle activity in the speech organs. When sensitive electronic sensors are placed on a person's throat and the person is asked to think, we do indeed find that thinking is often accompanied by covert, silent speech (Jacobsen, 1932). When the same kind of experiment is done with nonhearing people who use American Sign Language, implicit motor movements are detected in the muscles that control hand and finger movements (Max, 1937). At the very least, then, thinking is often accompanied by speech-associated muscle activity. Is such activity a *necessary* component of thought? Can people think *without* implicit speech?

To answer this question, Smith, Brown, Tomas, and Goodman (1947) used a curare-like drug that completely paralyzes the striate (voluntary) muscles of the body. The only muscle tissues not affected are the smooth muscles, such as the heart and the digestive system. Smith himself ingested the drug, breathed via artificial respiration, and while in this state was given problems to think about. When the drug wore off, he could describe the problems he had been given, and he also reported that he had been able to think quite clearly while completely paralyzed. This finding means that speech-associated muscle movements are not necessary for adult thought, even adult verbal thought.

However, even though people can think without implicit speech, language itself may be necessary for thought, and different languages may lead people to think differently. Do people who speak totally different languages think in totally different ways?

At about the time that Watson was arguing for his radical behaviorism, cultural anthropologists and linguistics, such as Edward Sapir (1921), were making contact with languages that were strikingly different from those they had studied before. They examined the languages of American Indians of the Southwest, such as Hopi and Navaho, intensively in an effort to record and analyze them fully before they perchance disappeared. These languages differed from Indo-European languages in such fundamental ways that they seemed to reflect completely different means of conceptualizing the world. For example, in the Nootka language, studied by Benjamin Lee Whorf (1940/1956), nouns and verbs are not distinguished as they are in the English language. Whorf thus suggested that the Nootka people did not partition nature into two classes, things and actions, *because* the grammar of their language did not differentiate between the two. This general idea is known as the Whorfian hypothesis, or linguistic relativity: People who speak different languages think differently *because* of the difference between the languages. Whorf's teacher, Edward Sapir, put it in this way:

Human beings do not live in the objective world alone, nor alone in the world of social activity as ordinarily understood, but are very much at the mercy of the particular language which has become the medium of expression for their society. It is quite an illusion to imagine that one adjusts to reality essentially without the use of language and that language is merely an incidental means of solving specific problems of communication or reflection. The fact of the matter is that the "real world" is to a large extent unconsciously built upon the language habits of the group . . . we see and hear and otherwise experience very largely as we do because the language habits of our community predispose certain choices of interpretation. (Sapir, 1968, p. 162)

There are actually two parts to this proposal. The first can be called *linguistic determinism*: The nature of human language determines the nature of human mentality and thought. The second part, and by far the more controversial, is *linguistic relativity*. This goes beyond general linguistic determinism because it is an assertion that differences in languages cause differences in thinking. The greater the difference between two languages, the greater will be the difference between the speakers of those two languages in their conceptualization of the world. How close is the relationship between language and thought? Can we think independently of language in general? Independently of the particular language we speak?

Linguistic determinism: thought without language?

Concepts

One common argument for linguistic relativity is the observation that different people have different words for the same thing. The Inuit of the far north (commonly called eskimos) are said to have many words for snow, whereas people in the United States generally have only one or two such words (unless one is a dedicated skier). It is possible to have a concept without labeling it?

Consider the concept *corpse of a dead plant.* For some people, this is like one of our concepts labeled by a single word, *mulch.* For people who are not interested in gardening, the remains of dead plants do not have a single-word name. Yet we have no trouble picturing this concept in our minds. Similarly, we have one-word labels for the following concepts: *floor, walls, ceiling, windows, doors.* We do not, in English, have a single-word label for the combination of these five concepts, the *interior surfaces of a room.* This concept, easily apprehended by anyone, has not been *lexicalized,* that is, given a single-word name.

Why are some concepts lexicalized and others not? The most likely reason is that some concepts are frequently referred to in a culture, whereas others are rarely or never brought up in conversation. When we want to talk about something for which no word exists, we usually use a descriptive phrase. If we want to talk about a concept fairly often, we will coin a new word. When television first came on the scene, we coined the word *television,* meaning "vision at a distance" (*tele-*). With repeated usage, such words are often shortened, as in *TV* or the *tube.* Often, instead of coining a new word, we will borrow an old one to refer to a new concept. When small cars were first offered for sale in the United States, they were referred to as *compact cars,* and this label was later shortened to *compacts.* Before this happened, the term *compact* usually referred to a small make-up case that held face powder and a mirror — and it still does. Our language is full of words that mean more than one thing (*port, lead, cast,* etc.), but we can easily discern the intended meaning of a word from the context in which it is used. So the use of *compact* to refer to both a face-powder case and a small car poses no problems.

Many coined phrases are metaphorical extensions, as is often the case among young children when they want to talk about something but have not yet learned the appropriate word or words. Upon seeing her father's bald spot for the first time, a two-year-old exlaimed, "Daddy has a hole in his hair." Chukovsky (1963) provides numerous examples of this kind of language behavior in children, where the meaning of a word is extended to cover a related concept.

The process of metaphorical extension is used in a more sophisticated form for developing ways of talking about abstract concepts that are not directly perceptible or tangible, such as the concept of time. People conceive of time as one-dimensional, running from behind us (the past) and going ahead of us (the future; see Clark, 1973). As our language develops, we borrow words that refer to the spatial concept of a single dimension (a line) to refer to time. It is interesting that virtually all English words that refer to time are either spatial terms, such as *before* and *after*, or terms that now refer exclusively to time but were originally spatial location terms, such as *then* (from *thence*), *when* (from *whence*) or *past* (from *passed*). As in other domains, we use analogy both to understand and to talk about new and unfamiliar concepts, thereby rendering those concepts familiar (Gentner, 1982). A language community develops such useful analogies and abstract terms in the long run; individual children and adults do the same when the need arises in the short run. The basic process is the same. First a concept is developed, either with or without a multiword description. Then, if there is frequent reference to that concept, it is lexicalized (Carroll, 1985; Krauss & Glucksberg, 1977). Linguistic determinism does not seem to operate at the level of individual concepts. We can have concepts without names.

Mental operations

Do we need language to perform operations on concepts? Most psychologists would agree that thinking can proceed in terms of specific words but that it need not be confined to verbal codes. People can think in concrete imagery, or in modes that seem not to be identifiable with any single perceptual or verbal code. An example is *incubation*, the sudden appearance of a problem solution in consciousness. This way of unconsciously arriving at a solution is quite common and applies to everyday problems, such as crossword puzzles, as well as to major inventions, such as Gutenberg's invention of the printing press (Koestler, 1964).

Another form of nonverbal thinking inolves imagery, such as visual imagery. Consider the following problem:

Imagine a rectangle that is three times as high as it is wide. Next, imagine drawing two lines parallel to the base so that the rectangle is divided into three equal parts. Now draw (in your mind) two diagonals, one from each corner of the original rectangle to the opposite corner. How many segments are now in the rectangle?

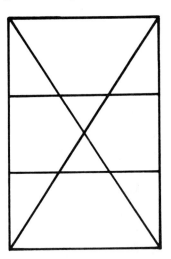

Figure 8.1. How many segments are produced in the imaginary drawing? See text for a statement of the problem.

People report that they solve this problem by mentally inspecting the figure they imagine and counting the number of segments that they "see" (see Figure 8.1).

We can easily construct such mental images and then manipulate them. A classic demonstration of mental transformation of visual images was provided by Shepard and Metzler (1971). People judged whether two geometric shapes (as in Figure 8.2) were the same or different. The time it took to judge that they were the same was directly related to the difference in orientation between the two shapes. This is exactly what we would expect if people mentally rotated one shape until it was aligned with the other and then inspected the two to see if they matched. The greater the angle of mental rotation, the longer it takes to come to such a decision.

Although such laboratory demonstrations seem far removed from daily life, they do demonstrate processes that people use every day. Consider how you would answer the following question (after Kosslyn, 1983). Do the ears of each of the following dogs stick up above the head? German shepherd; beagle; cocker spaniel; fox terrier. Most people can answer the question very easily, and most report that they do it by visualizing the dog and then "seeing" how the ears appear relative to the head. Such problems are not solved verbally; it is highly unlikely that anyone has ever memorized a list such as shepherd−up; beagle−down; and so on. Similarly, people seem to rely on imagery to decide whether any given upper-case letter of the alphabet is formed from only straight lines or has at least one curve. For example, which of the following lower-case letters have at least one curve in their

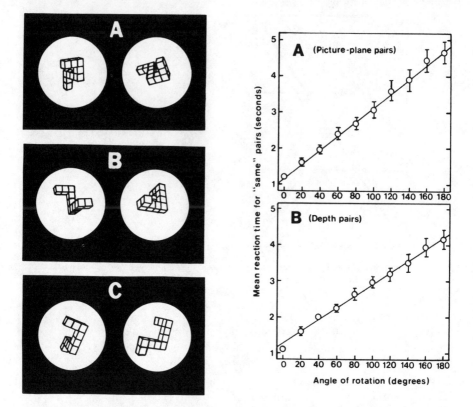

Figure 8.2. Examples of pairs of perspective drawings used by Shepard and Metzler (1971) to demonstrate mental rotation of visual images.

upper-case versions? a, d, e, g, m, r, t. People report that they use imagery for this task. It is not surprising that people with certain kinds of brain damage that produce selective impairments in visual imagery abilities have difficulty performing such tasks (Kosslyn, Holtzman, Farah, & Gazzaniga, 1985).

Thinking can also be done in abstract codes that are neither verbal nor visual. These *propositional* codes probably underlie our knowledge of the grammar of our language, of basic arithmetic, and even of such mundane things as whether or not camels have livers. Such forms of knowledge also enable us to translate freely and quickly between other modes of thought. For example, pictures of objects and the names of those objects represent the same concepts. Both the word *table* and a picture (or image) of a table represent our concept of the natural category *table*. One indication that pictures and words represent the same underlying concepts is our ability to read rebus sentences without any apparent difficulty. A rebus sentence is one in which one or more words are replaced by a picture, as in Figure 8.3. When people are asked to read such sentences quickly, they do just as well with the rebus sentences as with ordinary sentences, suggesting that the pic-

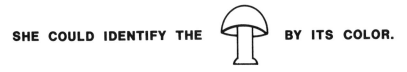

SHE COULD IDENTIFY THE   **BY ITS COLOR.**

Figure 8.3. A rebus sentence. How easily can such sentences be read?

tures do not have to be translated into a verbal code before being understood. Instead, they are understood directly and immediately as words are (Potter, Kroll, Yachzel, Carpenter, & Sherman, 1986). Similarly, if a person knows the name for, say, *table* in three different languages, then those three different words are different verbal codes for the same underlying concept of *table* (Glucksberg, 1984; Snodgrass, 1984).

These convergent lines of evidence make it clear that neither the content nor the processes of thought need be verbal. As George Miller (1972) put it, "Thinking can proceed in terms of relatively specific words or in abstract or concrete imagery" (p. 379). Words are one form of concrete imagery, visual images another. Abstract imagery refers to the propositional code that has been called the *language of thought* (Anderson, 1980).

Effects of language perception on memory, judgment, and thought

We have argued that thinking need not proceed in words, but this does not mean that the particular language we use to describe and to think about events and situations has no effects on the way we think or what we think about. Under the appropriate circumstances, the ways we use language can affect such basic cognitive functions as perception, memory, judgment, reasoning, and problem solving.

Perception and memory

The way we describe an object or event can affect both perception and memory. Figure 8.4 is deliberately ambiguous. If it is labeled *part of a beaded curtain* people tend to see it that way. If it is labeled as *a bear cub climbing the far side of a tree*, people tend to see it that way instead. Perhaps a more dramatic demonstration of the effect of a label on perception is illustrated in Figure 8.5. At first, people do not see any recognizable pattern at all. However, as soon as they are told that it is a picture of a knight on horseback, they tend to see it immediately and will continue to see it that way from then on. The seemingly meaningless pattern is now organized and stable.

Labels can also affect memory, even when they do not directly affect perception. When people are shown ambiguous line drawings such as those illustrated in Figure 8.6, their later recall of the drawings clearly show the

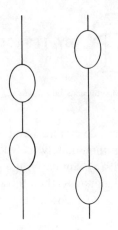

Figure 8.4. What is this? See text for an explanation.

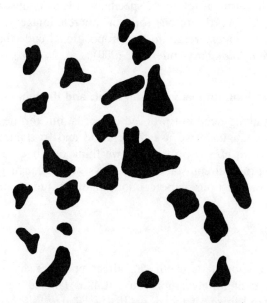

Figure 8.5. What is this? See text for an explanation.

effects of the labels originally attached to the drawings. In a classic study, Carmichael, Hogan, and Walter (1932) showed such pictures to people, along with one label or another. For example, the first picture in Figure 8.6 could be shown with either the label *bottle* or the label *stirrup*. Later, drawings of the picture from memory were systematically influenced by the label, as illustrated in Figure 8.6. Such effects of labels on perceptual memory are limited to reproduction memory; recognition memory is far more resistant

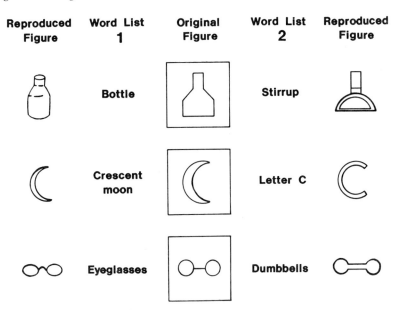

Reproduced Figure	Word List 1	Original Figure	Word List 2	Reproduced Figure

Figure 8.6. Effect of labels on reproduction memory. The original figures, when drawn from memory, tended to be distorted in the direction of the labels associated with them.

to such influences, as we might expect. Few of us could accurately draw specific objects from memory, yet we can easily recognize and distinguish something we have seen from something completely new to us.

Problem solving

The way we describe a situation can often have a powerful effect on the way we later deal with that situation. In some cases, the use of language can be critical to the solution of a problem. Nonverbal animals, such as chimpanzees, have inordinate difficulty performing tasks that involve matching or making comparisons among different sensory modalities. For example, if a chimpanzee learns to discriminate between a bright and a dim light, it cannot transfer this learning in order to discriminate between a loud and a soft sound. Before acquiring language, young children also have difficulty. Young children become much better at solving problems of this kind when they learn how to use language. One such problem is the far transposition test. A child is taught to look under the smaller of two small boxes to find a hidden toy. Then the child has to choose the smaller of two much larger boxes. Children who were unable to express the original problem solution in words, that is, "Pick the smaller one of the two," had difficulty with the new task of picking the smaller of two very large boxes. In contrast, children who

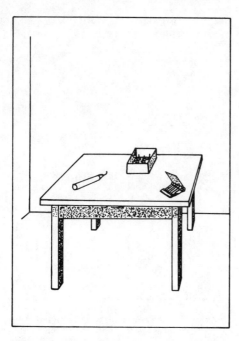

Figure 8.7. The candle problem. If only the materials on the table are used, how can the candle be mounted on the wall?

could describe the answer to the first problem generally succeeded on the second (Kuenne, 1946).

Sometimes adults' success in solving a problem also depends on the way they describe, or represent, the problem. Consider the problem illustrated in Figure 8.7. Given the materials shown − a candle, matches, and a box of thumbtacks − how can the candle be mounted on the wall so that it burns freely and does not drip wax on the table? More than half the people given the problem in this form failed to solve it in the 20 minutes allotted (Dunker, 1945; Glucksberg, 1962). However, when the tack box is presented empty, with the tacks loose on the table, the solution is obvious: Tack the box to the wall and use it as a candleholder. This form of presentation makes the box psychologically available.

Language can be used to accomplish the same thing, namely, to produce a psychological separation between the tack box and its contents. If the box is explicitly labeled *box* and all the other materials are also labeled separately and appropriately, everyone solves the problem in less than a minute (Glucksberg & Weisberg, 1966).

Of course, mere labeling is not the important factor here. What is impor-

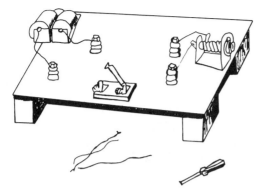

Figure 8.8. The circuit problem. There is not enough wire; how can the circuit be completed?

tant is that the labeling led to an appropriate problem representation. In a somewhat different problem, such labeling is not necessarily helpful. For example, people are instructed to complete a circuit, as illustrated in Figure 8.8. After working on the problem for a few minutes, they discover that there is not enough wire. As in the candle problem, people often fail to notice that one of the objects available – the screwdriver blade – can be used as a wire substitute. Labeling the screwdriver *screwdriver* does not help because it merely reinforces the original representation of the problem. However, labeling the appropriate screwdriver part, the blade, is helpful (Glucksberg & Danks, 1968). More interesting, giving the objects nonsense names also helps. If the screwdriver and other objects in the problem are referred to as *beems*, *peems*, and *jods*, the problem becomes significantly easier. Apparently, the novel names make it easier to imagine novel uses, perhaps by releasing the inhibitory effect of the habitual name. The screwdriver, in a sense, became a doohickey or a *gadget*, a "contrivance, object or device for doing something" (*Webster's New Collegiate Dictionary*, 1949). When the name of that something is left open, the possibilities for using the device seem also to remain open.

Decision making

How a particular situation is stated, or *framed*, can have a significant biasing effect on decision making. Assume that you have just entered a theater lobby and discover that you have lost your ticket, which had cost you $45. Would you buy a second ticket for $45 to see the show? Many people say that they would not because the show is not worth $90. However, if this situation is described in a slightly different way, people tend to buy the ticket. The objective situation is exactly the same, except that instead of having lost a $45 *ticket*, you arrive at the theater box office and discover that you have lost $45 in *cash*. Would you then still buy a ticket (assuming that you have the money with you)?

In the latter case, people tend to say yes, presumably because the ticket costs only what they had expected to pay, namely, $45. The way the language is used in this case is analogous to the way it is used in the functional-fixedness problems described above. One way of describing the candle-and-tacks problem makes the tacks and box one unit, and so makes the problem more difficult. One way of describing the theater-ticket situation makes the two tickets one unit costing $90. This makes it difficult to buy the second ticket. The second way of describing the situation separates the ticket price from the $45 cash loss, and so the idea of spending $45 to buy one ticket is more palatable.

The same mechanism is at work in the following problem:

A man buys a horse for $10, then sells it for $20. The next day he realizes that he wanted the horse after all, so he buys it back for $30. After a while he decides to sell it and does so for $40. What is the net profit or loss from this series of transactions?

Many people judge that the man came out even, with neither a net profit nor a loss. However, the situation can be described in a slightly different way:

A man buys a horse for $10, then sells it for $20. The next day he buys a cow for $30 and after a while sells it for $40. What is the net profit or loss from this series of transactions?

Now, virtually everyone correctly says that the net profit is $20, or $10 from each of the two sales. But notice that this is exactly analogous to the first case. The first way of describing the problem links the two sets of transactions by involving the same object, a single horse. The second description clearly separates the two transactions because it involves two different objects, a horse and a cow. This, of course, makes no real difference. In both cases, an object was sold at $10 profit on two separate occasions (see Kahneman & Tversky, 1982, for more detailed analyses of such framing effects).

In these examples, the way language is used to represent situations clearly influences people's decision making. Do different languages predispose people to think in certain ways about things by influencing certain ways of representing the world?

Linguistic relativity

Languages differ in two major ways: lexically and grammatically. The lexicon of a language is the set of words that are used in that language. The grammar of the language consists of the rules for putting words together (syntax) as well as the rules for expressing such semantic concepts as singular − plural, possession, and tense. Do such differences have demonstrable effects on thought?

Lexical differences

One language will have a word for a particular concept; another will not. One language will have many different words for different varieties of a concept; others only one or two. For example, the nomadic peoples of the North African deserts have more than 20 words for camel; we have only one. Native Peruvian Indians have more than 50 words for different varieties of potatoes; we have only one (albeit appropriately modified to differentiate among baking potatoes, new potatoes, Red Bliss potatoes, Idaho potatoes, etc.).

The possibility that differences in lexicon cause differences in thinking is very difficult to test, because usually it is not possible to separate language and culture. At the least, however, the linguistic relativity hypothesis requires that differences in lexicons be *accompanied by* differences in conceptualizations. One such area of potential differences is the semantic domain of color terms. People of different cultures can have very different ways of naming colors. Gleason (1961) pointed out that not only the number of color terms, but the way those terms are mapped onto the visible spectrum could vary substantively among different language groups (Figure 8.9). For example, whereas in English we refer to three colors by three color names, *purple*, *orange*, and *red*, in Shona these terms are referred by the same name. Are such labeling differences associated with conceptual differences as well? If so, are those conceptual differences caused by the lexical differences?

More specifically, what are the behavioral and cognitive effects of differences in color terminology? At the simplest level, we would expect that the richer the color vocabulary the easier it would be to talk about and communicate about colors. At a somewhat more complex level, our memory for colors might be influenced by our color vocabulary, because if we have different names for different colors, then naming them might help us remember them. A third possibility is that our ability to perceive and discriminate among colors could be related to our color vocabulary. Might a richer vocabulary aid perception and perceptual discrimination? Finally, the most interesting question concerns the relation between our color vocabulary and our conceptualization of the semantic domain of color. Do people with a fairly restricted color vocabulary have, as a consequence, a restricted conceptualization of the color domain?

The ease with which a topic can be communicated or talked about is related to the kind of vocabulary that is available. Until new words are coined,

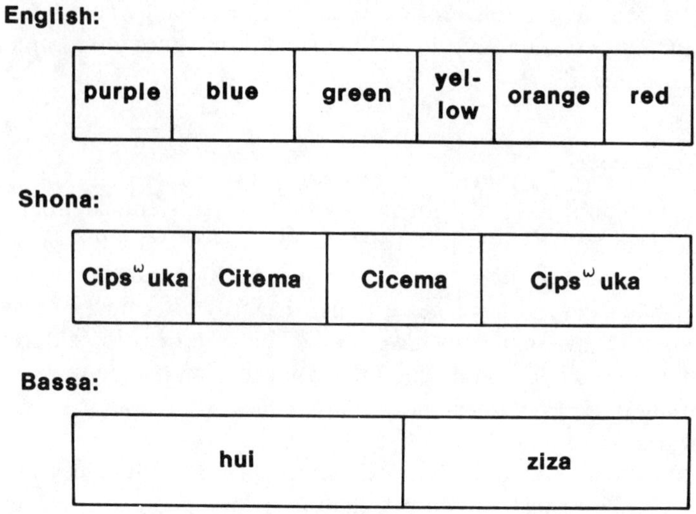

English:

purple	blue	green	yel-low	orange	red

Shona:

Cips$^{\omega}$uka	Citema	Cicema	Cips$^{\omega}$uka

Bassa:

hui	ziza

Figure 8.9. Three ways to categorize the rainbow. Shona and Bassa are languages spoken in Africa. After Gleason (1961).

people have difficulty talking about things for which no words are available (Carroll, 1985). The same should hold true for colors. Languages differ in their color lexicons, and even within a given language, colors differ in their *codability* − if a color has an agreed-upon short name, it is a high-codability color (Brown & Lenneberg, 1954). Examples in English would be *red*, *sky blue*, and *orange*. Low-codability colors are those we tend to describe analogically, such as the *mustardy brown translucent muck of the smog over Manhattan*.

When people are asked to communicate with one another about different colors, color codablity affects their accuracy and efficiency. In one communication task, a speaker tries to tell a listener which color to select from an array of colors. Colors that can be described with short names, such as *red*, *green*, or *blue*, are easy to identify on the basis of verbal descriptions. Colors that have longer (and usually less agreed upon) names, such as *blueberry cream* or *greenish taupe*, are more difficult to identify (Lantz & Stefflre, 1964; Stefflre, Castillo Vales, & Morley, 1966). This is not surprising, and it does not necessarily imply that people who speak different languages conceptualize colors in different ways. Furthermore, the ease of talking about any color depends not only on the availability of a color name, such as *red*, but also on the set of alternatives involved. If an array of colored chips contains, say, 10 different reds, then knowing the word *red* is not enough; the particular red that is intended must now be chosen by the use of appropriate modifiers, such as *fire-engine red* or *cherry red*. In some trades and professions people often discriminate and describe many colors that closely resemble one another; to facilitate communication, an enriched color vocabulary is developed. Interior decorators, painters, and artists are among those who have developed rich color vocabularies.

Memory for colors can also be affected by codability (Brown & Lenneberg, 1954). If you were shown a colored chip that could be described as *bluish green* and then some time later shown a set of three colored chips, each of them describable as *bluish green*, you might have difficulty remembering which one of the three was the original color. If the three colored chips had different names, the task would be much easier, even though the three colors in question would not differ physically any more widely than the bluish green ones. To the extent that verbal coding can help recognition memory, the codability of colors can affect recognition memory for colors. Again, codability can be context dependent. A bluish green in an array of colors that cannot be decribed as bluish green would be a high-codable color in that context. The same color in an array of blues and greens would be a low-codable color. Are there colors that are high-codable irrespective of context? Namely, is there a set of primary or basic colors that are universally high-codable?

Until recently, color naming was considered to be relatively arbitrary (see, e.g., Gleason, 1961; Lenneberg, 1967). According to this view, the visible spectrum (the colors of the rainbow from purples at one end to red at the other) is a uniformly graded continuum that can be partitioned arbitrarily to suit any given language community. Color names can be assigned without physical or psychological constraints. In addition, the number of color categories is unconstrained, and even the boundaries between color categories can vary freely from language to language. So, as Gleason argued (see Figure 8.9), not only will different languages contain different numbers of color terms but the category boundaries will vary as well.

The alternative view is that color perception and color conceptualization are cognitive universals whose properties are determined by the physiological properties of the human visual system (Bornstein, 1975). According to this view, there are four psychologically primary hues: red, yellow, green, and blue. If we added black and white, we would have six primary colors and so would need a minimum of six color terms in order to refer to any possible set of contrasts. This view has five testable implications (Miller & Glucksberg, in press):

1. All people should perceive and conceptualize color relationships in the same way. That is, the organization of the color domain should be universal and should conform to the standard three-dimensional color solid (Figure 8.10).
2. When languages differ in the number of color terms that they have, it should be possible to translate into any of the languages that have the full (minimal) set of six terms. Furthermore, when a language has only two color terms, that pair should reflect one of the three primary contrasts.

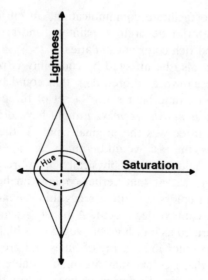

COORDINATES OF THE COLOR SOLID

Figure 8.10. Coordinates of the color solid. Brightness is represented by the vertical dimension. The hues are arranged in a circle, with saturation at a minimum at the outer edges.

Therefore, a two-term system should not contrast, say, orange versus yellow, or purple versus red.
3. The four primary hue terms (*red*, *green*, *blue*, *yellow*) should be sufficient to name all possible chromatic colors.
4. A color that is prototypical of its category (e.g., red) in one language community should also be the prototypical example in any other language community.
5. Color category boundaries should be universal, even in infants who have yet to learn any language at all.

Each of these implications seems to be true. The color space for English speakers conforms to the color solid illustrated in Figure 8.10. Color name space also conforms to this space. Fillenbaum and Rapoport (1971) asked American college students to rate the similarities among 15 common color names and then subjected those ratings to a nonmetric multidimensional scaling analysis. The obtained color *name* space closely resembled the color space itself, at least with respect to the circular arrangement of hues. The six spectral hues − red, orange, yellow, green, blue, and violet − were appropriately ordered in the color circle. Would the same color space be obtained from people with much more restricted color vocabulary?

Heider and Olivier (1972) obtained color similarity data from a West New Guinea people called the Dani. The Dani color vocabulary has only two color names: *mili* and *mola*. *Mili* refers to dark, cold colors; *mola* to light, warm colors. A group of Dani and a group of Americans were given a recognition memory task involving a set of 40 colors. A sample color was briefly shown; then a half-minute later the sample had to be selected from the full set of 40 colors. As might be expected, the American group, with a far richer color vocabulary, made fewer recognition errors than did the Dani. However, the *kinds* of errors that each group made were very similar. The colors that the American group tended to confuse with one another were the same as those the Dani confused.

These confusion errors can be treated as an index of color similarity; similar colors tend to be confused with one another. When these errors were subjected to a multidimensional scaling analysis, the resulting color spaces for the two groups − American and Dani − were highly similar. The Dani color space, despite the Dani color vocabulary, turned out to be the universal three-dimensional color solid (Figure 8.10). Hue, brightness, and saturation characterized both the Dani color space and the American color space. So despite the striking difference in color vocabulary, the Dani's conception of color relationships is no different than ours.

The two terms that the Dani use are consistent with our second expectation, namely, that terms do provide a basic contrast. In this case, it is between dark and light, consistent with Berlin and Kay's (1969) observation that (a) every language known to date has at least two basic color terms, and (b) if there are only two, they do provide for a black−white or dark−light contrast. If a language has three color terms, the most likely third term will be a name for red. When there are more than three terms, yellow, green, and blue are labeled before such nonprimary colors as brown, pink, violet, and orange. The ethnographic evidence is generally consistent with the notion that the color terms *white*, *black*, *red*, *yellow*, *green*, and *blue* are primary and that these terms form a minimal contrastive set of color names.

Additional evidence on this point comes from studies of the minimum number of terms people need to describe all possible chromatic colors. Jameson and Hurvich (1959) asked American students to describe monochromatic lights sampled from the entire visible spectrum. However, the students were allowed to use only four color terms: *red*, *yellow*, *green*, and *blue*. The students had no trouble with this limitation. They described orange hues as mixtures of red and yellow, purple as a mixture of red and blue, and so on. When one of these four color terms, such as *yellow*, is not available, people cannot describe all possible colors adequately (Sternheim & Boynton, 1966).

The fourth aspect of the universality of color perception and conceptualization concerns the location of color category boundaries and the choice of those colors that best exemplify each category. These colors were called *focal points* by Berlin and Kay (1969), who found that speakers of diverse languages picked the same best examples of the basic color terms in their language from an array of colored chips. Any color that was selected as the best or prototypical example of a term in one language tended to be the best example of the analogous color term in English. Heider and Olivier (1972) found that the Dani of New Guinea, with their two basic color terms, remembered focal colors better than nonfocal ones and could learn names for focal colors more easily than those for nonfocal colors.

Further evidence that color perception is indeed independent of naming comes from yet another source – young children. Heider (1971) found that three-year-old American children preferred focal colors to nonfocal ones, even before they had a full set of color names. Bornstein, studying preverbal infants, showed that the color categories used by adults are present very early in life, before the first year (Bornstein, 1975).

The weight of evidence, at least for the domain of color and color terminology, is very clear. Lexical differences among peoples do not lead to perceptual or conceptual differences. Whether the linguistic relativity hypothesis would fare better with a more suitable semantic domain is not yet known because the work to date has concentrated almost exclusively on the domain of color terms. Unfortunately this domain may have been the worst place to look for linguistic effects. The structure of color space is universal; it is constrained by the neurophysiology of the human color vision system. Might better evidence for the linguistic relativity hypothesis be found in the area of grammar or syntax?

Grammatical differences

The grammar of a language severely constrains people's expression of various ideas and concepts. For example, every language provides for a distinction between singular and plural. This means that people must specify numerosity. With the exception of such words as *sheep*, which take the same form for one and more than one (one sheep, nine sheep), English speakers must specify the distinction between one and more than one. In English, as in all languages known to date, this minimum singular–plural distinction is *obligatory*.

However, languages can and do differ with respect to other distinctions that may be obligatory versus those that are optional. For example, distinctions among noun genders are obligatory in such languages as French and German but are optional in English. In French, common nouns such as the words for pen and window are masculine and feminine, respectively. Accordingly, a French speaker would use the masculine article for pen (*le stylo*) and the feminine for window (*la fenêtre*). In German, a threefold distinction is made among masculine, feminine, and neuter, as reflected in the three definite articles *der*, *die*, *das*. In English, such distinctions are optional, and we make them only when we use pronouns such as *he*, *she*, or *it*. Thus, we can refer to a ship as either *she* or *it*, but not as *he*. Such things as radios and filing cabinets can be referred to only as *it*. The rule in English seems to be that *she* is used only for things that can be personified and so can also be spoken of with some affect. Thus, cars, ships, and tropical storms can be referred to as *she* or *her* (as in "Spring brings with her a hint of summer"). A smaller number of things can be referred to as masculine (as in "Winter brings his harsh winds"). Everything else is essentially neuter, taking the pronoun *it*. We cannot make such distinctions in the plural form.

Gender distinctions are only one example of the way languages may differ. Form of address is another. French is one language that makes the distinction between informal and formal forms of address obligatory. Whereas in English we would say *you*, in French one would have to choose between the formal *vous* and the informal *tu*. Japanese speakers are even more constrained; level of formality must be specified in verb and noun inflections (e.g., suffixes). These examples demonstrate that what may seem basic and indispensable in one language may not even exist in another. For example, Russian provides no grammatical device for specifying definite versus indefinite reference. In English, we are obligated to specify this distinction, as in *a* house versus *the* house.

Do such differences in obligatory versus optional distinctions cause differences in conceptualization? The causality question is, as noted earlier, difficult to answer. However, we can begin by asking whether differences in grammatical form are accompanied by differences in thought. The logic of this approach is straightforward. The first step is to identify a grammatical difference between two languages. The second is to identify an aspect of conceptualization or thinking that is directly related to this specific grammatical difference. The third step is to determine whether people in the two different language communities think differently in ways that are related to this grammatical difference. Only after we find such a clear and specific relationship can the question of which came first — the language or the thought — be considered.

This is the essential logic behind Whorf's arguments about the differences between English and some American Indian languages and the different ways of thinking that these languages might entail:

Our Indian languages show that with a suitable grammar we may have intelligent sentences that cannot be broken into subjects and predicates. Any attempted breakup is a breakup of some English translation or paraphrase of the sentence, not of the Indian sentence itself. . . . When we come to Nootka, the sentence without subject or predicate is the only type. The term "predication" is used, but it means "sentence." Nootka has no parts of speech; the simplest utterance is a sentence, treating of some event or event-complex. . . .

The English technique of talking depends on the contrast of two artificial classes, substantives and verbs, and on the bipartitioned ideology of nature. . . . . Our normal sentence, unless imperative, must have some substantive before its verb, a requirement that corresponds to the philosophical and also naive notion of an actor who produces an action. This last might not have been so if English had had thousands of verbs like 'hold,' denoting positions. But most of our verbs follow a type of segmentation that isolates from nature what we call "actions," that is, moving outlines.

   Following majority rule, we therefore read action into every sentence, even into 'I hold it.' A moment's reflection will show that 'hold' is no action but a state of relative positions. Yet we think of it and even see it as an action because language formulates it in the same way as it formulates more numerous expressions, like, 'I strike it,' which deal with movements and changes. (Whorf, 1940/1956, pp. 242–3)

   Whorf's claim is crystal clear. He has identified a difference in the grammars of two languages, English and Nootka. English has nouns and verbs; Nootka apparently does not. He has thus completed the first step in testing the linguistic relativity hypothesis. He has also identified an aspect of thinking that might be related to this linguistic difference, namely, the conceptual dichotomy between objects and actions. This completes the second step. However, the third step – demonstrating that English speakers and Nootka speakers think differently – has yet to be taken. We do not know whether the Nootka draw a conceptual contrast that is different from ours. Whorf's inference about the Nootka world view is based entirely on his identification of Nootka thinking with a literal English translation of the Nootka language.

   If we did this with other languages, we would be forced to conclude that people who speak French or German must think very differently than we do. The French phrase *Comment ça va?* is literally translated "How it goes?" It is intended to mean "How are things" or "How are you?" Just because French and English speakers use different words to express the same general intention does not necessarily mean that French and English speakers differ in their conceptions of interpersonal relations. Similarly, German sentence construction differs from that of English. Mark Twain, in a speech to the Vienna Press Club in 1897, remarked on this difference:

I am indeed the truest Friend of the German language – not only now, but from long since – yes, before twenty years already. . . . I would only some changes effect. I would only the language method – the luxurious, elaborate construction compress, the eternal parenthesis suppress, do away with, annihilate; the introduction of more than thirteen subjects in one sentence forbid; the verb so far to the front pull that one it without a telescope discover can. With one word, my gentlemen, when you her for prayer need, One her yonder-up understands.

   . . . I might gladly the separable verb also a little bit reform. I might none let do what Schiller did: he has the whole history of the Thirty Years' War between the two members of a separate verb in-pushed. That has even Germany itself aroused, and one has Schiller the permission refused the History of the Hundred Years' War to compose – God be it thanked! After all these reforms established be will, will the German language the noblest and the prettiest on the world be. (Twain, 1910, pp. 45–9)

   If people really think exactly as they speak, we must surely think differently than German speakers. Do we because of the languages that we speak so differently think? The difficulty of using literal English translations to infer conceptual differences between speakers of different languages is illustrated very well by an example brought to my attention by Harris Savin (personal communication). Consider the river people described in a recent novel:

> The speech of the river people posed philosophical as well as linguistic problems. For example, since they had no regular system of plurals but only an elaborate system of altered numerals for denoting specific numbers of given objects, the problem of the particular versus the universal did not exist and the word 'man' stood for 'all men'. This had a profound effect on ther societisation. The tenses divided time into two great chunks, a simple past and a continuous present. A future tense was created by adding various suffixes indicating hope, intention and varying degrees of probability and possibility to the present stem. (Carter, 1972, p. 91)

The river people's language does seem strange, and our first inclination is to agree that these people do think differently than we do. For example, because their language has no simple future tense, they must have no concept of the future as a simple counterpart or opposite of the past. But if this is true, do they really think differently than English speakers? If English grammar reflects the way we think about the future, we are just like the river people. English, like their language, has no future tense per se. We are obligated to use modal auxiliaries when we refer to the future, and these auxiliaries express "hope, intention and varying degrees of probability and possibility": "I *might* walk," "I *shall* walk," "I *will* walk," "I *should* walk." It is not obligatory in English to express such hopes and intentions for the present or past tenses − for example, "I am walking," "I walked." Nor is it obligatory in French to express such hopes and intentions for past, present, *or* future; French has a "proper" future tense. Do we therefore think about time differently than French speakers?

Whether we do or do not can be determined only independently of our languages. Most people would agree that English speakers have a clear conception of the future uncontaminated by the expressions of hopes, intentions, and possibilities that are forced on us by our grammar. Similarly, the Nootka may very well dichotomize nature into objects and actions, just as we do, even though their language does not make this distinction in the form of nouns and verbs.

What we need is a demonstration of conceptual differences independent of language. Whenever a demonstration of this sort has been attempted, the evidence has generally been negative. Differences in grammar do not seem to be related to differences in thinking. In one of the early attempts to discover such differences, Joseph Casagrande (as reported in Carroll & Casagrande, 1958) noticed a potentially interesting difference between Navaho and English. Navaho, like English, has obligatory tense marking. In addition, Navaho has obligatory shape marking; the form of the verb depends on the shape of the object that one is talking about. The verb form must agree with the object shape, so the verb for *picking up* a ball (round), *picking up* a stick (long and thin), and *picking up* a sheet of paper (flat and flexible) would take different forms. Does this characteristic of the language affect the relative saliency of shape for Navaho speakers? To answer this question, Casagrande compared the shape preferences of English- and Navaho-speaking children. In general, young children tend to group objects by color before they group them by shape (Brian & Goodenough, 1929). Since Navaho children learn to use these shape-specific verbs quite early, will they therefore categorize objects by shape rather than color at an earlier age than do English-speaking children? If they do, perhaps the verb forms have influenced the development of their classification schemes.

Casagrande found that Navaho-speaking children from a particular reservation classified objects according to shape more than did English-speaking Navaho children from the same reservation. This result is consistent with the linguistic relativity hypothesis. However, the performance of English-speaking white children from the Boston area more closely resembled that of the Navaho-speaking children than that of the English-speaking Navaho children. Casagrande tried to explain this anomaly by appealing to the possibility that middle-class children from Boston develop more rapidly than do Navaho children. Although this explanation is consistent with other data indicating that middle-class children do shift from color to form classification earlier than do lower-class children (Honkavaara, 1958), the effects of language still seem to be minimal here.

A more recent study, this time of a difference between English and Chinese, seemed to provide evidence for a language-related difference in thinking. Bloom (1981) noted that the Chinese language has no grammatical device for indicating the counterfactual. A counterfactual statement is one that describes a state of affairs that did *not* happen but might have happened if something else had been true, as in "If Whorf had been correct, then English and Chinese speakers would think differently." Most English speakers would interpret this sentence to mean that Whorf was *not* correct and that English and Chinese speakers do *not* think differently. More prosaic examples are "If I had gone to the library, I would have met Susan," and "If I had baked a cake, I would have had enough for dinner."

In English, the counterfactual can be marked by use of the past perfect form of the verb (*had gone*) and form *would have* or *might have* or *could have*, for example, "Had the Hindenburg not exploded we might have zeppelin travel today." In Chinese, there is no such explicit way of signaling the counterfactual. Whereas in English one could say, "If I were the president, I would think before I spoke," in Chinese one would say, "If I am the president, then I will think before I speak" (Au, 1983). Chinese, unlike English, does not have a distinctive grammatical form for distinguishing between implicational statements and counterfactual statements: Both kinds of statement use the *if—then* form without the distinguishing verb forms that are used in English.

Bloom (1981) noticed this grammatical difference and suggested that there might be a related conceptual difference. Because Chinese does not differentiate grammatically between implication *if—then* statements and counterfactual *if—then* statements, Bloom thought that Chinese speakers would have trouble understanding and possibly using the counterfactual. Bloom tested this idea in a series of experiments that compared English- and Chinese-speaking people's understanding of counterfactual statements. Bloom used, among other materials, a story about a European philosopher named Bier who was interested in principles of the universe. During the course of the story, a counterfactual statement occurs: "Bier could not read Chinese, but if he had been able to read Chinese, he would have discovered that . . . Chinese philosophical works were relevant to his own investigations." Later in the story, we discover that had Bier read Chinese, he would have done a number of other things. In the Engish version of this story, people can use the signals of the counterfactual condition, that is, "If . . . had been able . . . would have." The Chinese version, of course, could not have such signals.

American readers, by and large, understood the counterfactual, as indicated by their correct choice on a multiple-choice question (54 of 55 correct). In contrast, Chinese readers seemed to miss the counterfactual: Only 8 of a group of 120 native Chinese speakers made the correct (counterfactual) choice after reading a Chinese translation of the English story. A linguistic difference, then, seemed to be accompanied by a conceptual difference: the relative ability to reason counterfactually. From this and similar results, Bloom concluded that the form of a language can influence the way people think. Perhaps more important, Bloom (1981) suggested that speakers of different languages would have serious difficulties in understanding one another because of such cognitive differences:

By intervening in highly abstract realms of thought to shape their speakers' cognitive lives, languages act to insure the maintenance across generations of the most complex cognitive attainments of the human race and of the most complex cognitive attainments of its individual cultures. But, ironically, these same cognitive contributions act to separate their speakers cognitively from speakers of other languages—to create and perpetuate significant cognitive barriers to cross-linguistic communication and understanding. The barriers are certainly not impenetrable. But to penetrate them one cannot rely simply on a translation equivalent or a convenient paraphrase. Here, in highly abstract realms of thought, translation depends on, and provides the direction for, cognitive growth. (p. 86)

This means that for a Chinese speaker to understand counterfactual reasoning, he or she must learn an abstract thinking pattern that is not provided for in Chinese. This conclusion, as well as the original conclusion concerning differences between Chinese and English counterfactual reasoning, was questioned by a native Chinese speaker, Terry Kit-Fong Au, at Harvard University. Au (1983) repeated Bloom's experiments and, in general, found

that Chinese–English bilinguals had no difficulty in understanding the counterfactual, either in English or in Chinese. Au argued that Bloom's original
Chinese translations were not adequately idiomatic for Chinese readers. To
show that a nonidiomatic translation can lead to poor understanding, Au
asked Chinese bilinguals to translate an idiomatic Chinese version of the
philosopher story into English. These translations were judged to be similar
to the original in content but distinctly less idiomatic for English readers.
When American high school students read the nonidiomatic versions in English, only 60% appeared to understand the counterfactual, compared with
97% of the monolingual Chinese who were given an idiomatic Chinese
version.

The difficulty of understanding a nonidiomatic English translation is apparent from the version used by Au (1983, pp. 186–7):

Bier was a German philosopher in the 18th century. To study about the theory of the
Great Harmony and the laws of nature was his greatest interest. In those days, the
communication between China and Europe had already developed to some extent.
Chinese works could be found in Europe but the translations of them were still not
available. If Bier had known about the technique to master the Chinese language, he
would certainly discover the different attitudes between the Chinese philosophers
and the European philosophers when describing the natural phenomena: the Chinese
stressed the interrelationships among these aspects while the European ignored them
and studies each aspect separately. Suppose Bier had learnt about Chinese philosophy, he would certainly develop his own theory, which included not only a thorough
study about the nature of natural phenomena, but also a clear explanation of the
relations among various natural aspects. Such theory not only patched up the disadvantages of the Western philosophy, but also influenced deeply and furthered the
development of philosophy in Germany, France, and Holland towards science.

From the above article, what new influence had Bier brought to the West?
Please choose one or more of the following answers:

(1) Awakened the consciousness of the Western philosophers about the nature of
     natural phenomena.
(2) Awakened the consciousness of the Western philosophers about the interrela-
     tionships among the natural phenomena.
(3) Pushed the European philosophy a step towards science.
(4) Pushed the Western philosphy a step towards Chinese philosophy.
(5) None of the above (Please explain your opinion briefly).

The correct answer, of course, is (5) – none of the above. Clearly, Bloom's
original finding reflected the language materials that he used, not a difference in cognition between Americans and Chinese. As intriguing as the notion might be, we have yet to find convincing evidence that linguistic differences are even related to cognitive differences, let along causally related.

This conclusion can be extended to include a form of language that was,
until recently, considered to be rudimentary and primitive, namely, the sign
language of the deaf. In his masterful book *When the Mind Hears: A History
of the Deaf* (1984), Harlan Lane describes how sign came to be used in
eighteenth century France to educate the deaf. Sign was used to teach not
only communication but also reading and writing, and once these conceptual

skills were mastered, the skills of the deaf were indistinguishable from those of the hearing (see Groce, 1984, for a description of a fully integrated hearing-and-deaf community on Martha's Vineyard, which flourished for 250 years until 1952, when the last nonhearing person in this community died).

What the literature on sign language and the cognitive accomplishments of the deaf tells us is that a "language" may indeed be necessary for complex human cognition but that the "language" itself is not restricted to spoken speech, or for that matter any particular form or modality. What seems crucial is some system of symbols that permits two indispensable and crucial activities: communicating with others and manipulating symbolic information. It may turn out that Watson was right after all − thought is speech − but it is the speech of the mind, not of the tongue, that matters.

References

Anderson, J. R. (1980). *Cognitive psychology and its implications*. New York: Freeman.

Au, T. Kit-Fong (1983). Chinese and English counterfactuals: The Sapir–Whorf hypothesis revisited. *Cognition, 15*, 155−87.

Berlin, B., & Kay, P. (1969). *Basic color terms: Their universality and evolution*. Berkeley & Los Angeles: University of California Press.

Bloom, A. (1981). *The linguistic shaping of thought: A study in the impact of language on thinking in China and the West*. Hillsdale, NJ: Erlbaum.

Bornstein, M. H. (1975). Qualities of color vision in infancy. *Journal of Experimental Child Psychology, 19*, 401−19.

Brian, C. R., & Goodenough, F. L. (1929). The relative potency of color and form perception at various ages. *Journal of Experimental Psychology, 12*, 197−213.

Brown, R. (1968). *Words and things*. New York: Free Press.

Brown, R., & Lenneberg, E. H. (1954). A study in language and cognition. *Journal of Abnormal and Social Psychology, 49*, 454−62.

Carmichael, L., Hogan, H. P., & Walter, A. A. (1932). An experimental study of the effect of language on the representation of visually perceived form. *Journal of Experimental Psychology, 15*, 73−86.

Carroll, J. B., & Casagrande, J. B. (1958). The function of language classification in behavior. In E. E. Maccoby, T. Newcomb, & E. L. Hartley (Eds.), *Readings in social psychology* (3rd ed., pp. 18−31). New York: Holt, Rinehart & Winston.

Carroll, J. M. (1985). *What's in a name? An essay in the psychology of reference*. New York: Freeman.

Carter, S. (1972). *The infernal desire machine of Doctor Hoffman*. London: Rupert-Hart-Davis.

Chukovsky, K. (1963). *From two to five* (M. Morton, Trans.). Berkeley & Los Angeles: University of California Press.

Clark, H. H. (1973). Space, time, semantics and the child. In T. E. Moore (Ed.), *Cognitive development and the acquisition of language* (pp. 27−64). New York: Academic Press.

Dunker, K. (1945). On problem solving. *Psychological Monographs, 58*, Whole No. 279.

Fillenbaum, S., & Rapoport, A. (1971). *Structures in the subjective lexicon*. New York: Academic Press.

Gentner, D. (1982). Are scientific analogies metaphors? In D. S. Miall (Ed.), *Metaphor: Problems and perspectives* (pp. 106−32). Brighton, Sussex: Harvester Press.

Gleason, H. A. (1961). *An introduction to descriptive linguistics* (rev. ed.). New York: Holt, Rinehart & Winston.

Glucksberg, S. (1962). The influence of strength of drive on functional fixedness and perceptual recognition. *Journal of Experimental Psychology*, *63*, 36–41.

——— (1984). Commentary: The functional equivalence of common and multiple codes. *Journal of Verbal Learning and Verbal Behavior*, *23*, 100–4.

Glucksberg, S., & Danks, J. H. (1968). Effects of discriminative labels and of nonsense labels upon availability of novel function. *Journal of Verbal Learning and Verbal Behavior*, *7*, 72–6.

Glucksberg, S., & Weisberg, R. W. (1966). Verbal behavior and problem solving: Some effects of labeling in a functional fixedness problem. *Journal of Experimental Psychology*, *71*, 659–64.

Groce, N. E. (1984). *Everyone here spoke sign language: Hereditary deafness on Martha's Vineyard*. Cambridge, MA: Harvard University Press.

Heider, E. R. (1971). "Focal" color areas and the development of color names. *Developmental Psychology*, *4*, 447–55.

Heider, E. R., & Olivier, D. C. (1972). The structure of color space in naming and memory for two languages. *Cognitive Psychology*, *3*, 337–54.

Honkavaara, S. (1958). A critical re-evaluation of the color and form reaction, and disproving of the hypotheses connected with it. *Journal of Psychology*, *45*, 25–36.

Jacobsen, E. (1932). The electrophysiology of mental activities. *American Journal of Psychology*, *44*, 677–94.

Jameson, D., & Hurvich, L. M. (1959). Perceived color and its dependence on focal, surrounding and preceding stimulus variables. *Journal of the Optical Society of America*, *49*, 890–8.

Kahneman, D., & Tversky, A. (1982). The psychology of preferences. *Scientific American*, *246*, 160–73.

Koestler, A. (1964). *The act of creation*. New York: Macmillan.

Kosslyn, S. M. (1983). *Ghosts in the mind's machine*. New York: Norton.

Kosslyn, S. M., Holtzman, J. D., Farah, M. J., & Gazzaniga, M. S. (1985). A computational analysis of mental image generation: Evidence from functional dissociations in split-brain patients. *Journal of Experimental Psychology: General*, *114*, 311–41.

Krauss, R. M., & Glucksberg, S. (1977). Social and nonsocial speech. *Scientific American*, *236*, 100–5.

Kuenne, M. R. (1946). Experimental investigation of the relation of language to transposition behavior in young children. *Journal of Experimental Psychology*, *36*, 471–90.

Lane, H. (1984). *When the mind hears: A history of the deaf*. New York: Random House.

Lantz, D., & Stefflre, V. (1964). Language and cognition revisited. *Journal of Abnormal and Social Psychology*, *69*, 472–81.

Lenneberg, E. H. (1967). *Biological foundations of language*. New York: Wiley.

Luria, A. R. (1961). *The role of speech in the regulation of normal and abnormal behavior*. New York: Liveright.

Max, L. W. (1937). An experimental study of the motor theory of consciousness: 4. Action curve responses in the deaf during awakening, kinaesthetic imagery and abstract thinking. *Journal of Comparative Psychology*, *24*, 301–34.

Miller, G. A. (1972). English verbs of motion: A case study in semantics and lexical memory. In A. W. Melton & E. Martin (Eds.), *Coding processes in human memory* (pp. 335–72). Washington, DC: Winston.

Miller, G. A., & Glucksberg, S. (in press). Psycholinguistic aspects of pragmatics and semantics. In R. D. Luce, R. A. Atkinson, & R. Herrnstein (Eds.), *Steven's handbook of experimental psychology* (2nd ed.). New York: Wiley.

Pavlov, I. P. (1941). Lectures on conditioned reflexes. In *Conditioned reflexes and psychiatry* (Vol. 2; W. H. Gantt, trans.). New York: International.

Potter, M. C., Kroll, J. F., Yachzel, B., Carpenter, E., & Sherman, J. (1986). Pictures in sentences: Understanding without words. *Journal of Experimental Psychology: General*, *115*, 281–94.

Sapir, E. (1921). *Language: An introduction to the study of speech*. New York: Harcourt, Brace.

(1968). Language and environment. In D. G. Mandelbaum (Ed.), *Selected writings of Edward Sapir in language, culture and personality*. Berkeley & Los Angeles: University of California Press.

Sechenov, I. M. (1863). Releksy golovnogo mozga (Reflexes of the brain). *Meditsinskiy Vestnik, 3*, 461–4, 493–512. Cited in D. I. Slobin, *Psycholinguistics*. Glenview, IL: Scott Foresman, 1971.

Shepard, R. N., & Metzler, J. (1971). Mental rotation of three-dimensional objects. *Science, 171*, 701–3.

Smith, S. M., Brown, H. O., Tomas, J. E. P., & Goodman, L. S. (1947). The lack of cerebral effects of *d*-tubocurarine. *Anesthesiology, 8*, 1–14.

Snodgrass, J. G. (1984). Concepts and their surface representations. *Journal of Verbal Learning and Verbal Behavior, 23*, 3–22.

Stefflre, V., Castillo Vales, V., & Morley, L. (1966). Language and cognition in Yucatan: A cross cultural replication. *Journal of Personality and Social Psychology, 4*, 112–15.

Sternheim, C. E., & Boynton, R. M. (1966). Uniqueness of perceived hues investigated with a continuous judgment technique. *Journal of Experimental Psychology, 72*, 770–6.

Twain, M. (1910). The horrors of the German language: Address to the Vienna Press Club, November 21, 1897. In *Mark Twain's speeches* (pp. 43–51). New York: Harper & Bros.

Watson, J. B. (1913). Psychology as the behaviorist views it. *Psychological Review, 20*, 158–77.

(1925). *Behaviorism*. New York: Norton.

Webster's new collegiate dictionary. (1949). Springfield, MA: Merriam.

Whorf, B. L. (1956). Languages and logic. In J. B. Carroll (Ed.), *Language, thought and reality: Selected writings of Benjamin Lee Whorf* (pp. 233–45). Cambridge, MA: MIT Press. (Original work published 1940.)

9 Text comprehension

Richard J. Gerrig

Roughly 11,000 years ago the earliest precursor of writing was invented, giving readers their first texts to comprehend (Schmandt-Besserat, 1978). As writing systems improved over the millennia, so did their expressive power: Early writing systems were specialized for functions such as agricultural record keeping; modern writing systems allow for communication of an unlimited range of topics. As readers in the modern era, we are challenged to understand texts that describe thoughts and opinions, historical and current events, and fanciful and fictional worlds.

In day-to-day life, we meet this challenge with deceptive ease. Rarely are we conscious of the complex processes and representations that underlie our comprehension ability. Nonetheless, they *are* complex. Theories of text comprehension have dual goals: to document these complexities and to specify how the illusion of ease is achieved. This chapter reports the progress that has been made in achieving these goals. We begin by reviewing researchers' motives for studying text comprehension.

Why study text comprehension?

Consider this description of an event:

Years ago, a child in a tree with a small caliber rifle bushwhacked a piano through the open summer windows of a neighbor's living room. . . . Dragged from the tree by the piano's owner, his rifle smashed upon a rock and flung, he was held by the neck in the living room and obliged to view the piano point blank, to dig into its interior and see the cut strings, the splintered holes that let slender shafts of light ignite small circles of dark inside the piano.

There are many different circumstances in which one might have encountered such a story: One may have been present when the event happened; one may have heard the story from a friend who was a witness; one may have read the account as the opening lines of Thomas McGuane's novel *The Bushwhacked Piano*; one may have had a friend recount the opening scene of McGuane's novel; one may have read another novel in which one of the characters describes this opening scene.

Preparation of this chapter was supported in part by BRSG SO7-RR07015 from the Biomedical Research Grant Program, Division of Research Resources, National Institutes of Health. I thank Janet Davidson and Robert Sternberg for helpful comments on earlier drafts.

242

From the standpoint of cognitive psychology, we would predict some commonalities across these situations. First, we would expect many similarities in the *mental processes* that would enable us to extract information from the different instantiations of the story. In each case, we would make use of information stored in our memory to understand the story. Furthermore, we would implicitly attempt to answer the same sorts of questions – for example, "Why did the boy bushwhack the piano?" and "Why does the owner want the boy to view the damage?" Second, we would expect similarities in the structure and content of the *representations* we create in memory. This equivalence would be manifested by correspondences among the summaries we would offer in each instance or in the accessibility of different details.

Thus, one reason for studying text comprehension is the pervasiveness of *narrative* experiences – witnessed, heard, or read – in our lives. Text versions of these experiences provide a convenient means for psychologists to study common processes and representations. A similar concordance exists between other types of text and other types of life experience. We read *expository* prose that instructs and informs us; we can witness a demonstration or attend a lecture that subsumes the same function. We read *persuasive* prose that intends to change our attitudes or behaviors; we can be shown evidence or hear arguments in service of the same goal. In each genre, researchers consider texts to be invaluable models of the broader spectrum of experiences.

Texts do, of course, have some special features of their own, which provide another reason for their study. Consider the opening paragraph of Franz Kafka's story "The Metamorphosis":

As Gregor Samsa awoke one morning from uneasy dreams he found himself transformed in his bed into a gigantic insect. He was lying on his hard, as it were armorplated, back and when he lifted his head a little he could see his domelike brown belly divided into stiff arched segments on top of which the bed quilt could hardly keep in position and was about to slide off completely. His numerous legs, which were pitifully thin compared to the rest of his bulk, waved helplessly before his eyes.

We know from the opening sentence that this story could not have taken place in our everyday world. Researchers must explicate how we establish fictional worlds – how we can imagine what it would be like for someone to turn into a gigantic insect and how we prevent this imaginary occurrence from influencing our thinking about the everyday world.

Expository and persuasive texts also raise special issues. Some of these are related to the lack of interaction between writer and reader: We cannot question or challenge the writers of these texts as we could if speakers were present to provide the same information. Thus, educators have been concerned with the form instructional texts should take for optimal learning. Essayists have been concerned with the structure that arguments should assume to accomplish maximal persuasion.

With these motives in mind, we now review theories and experimentation relevant to text comprehension. We begin by examining several topics on narrative texts, because researchers have most thoroughly explicated the processes and representations underlying this type of comprehension.

Narrative texts

In this section, we consider several theories and experimental results that are related to narrative texts. We describe the types of information readers retrieve from memory to aid comprehension, the representations they create when they understand text, and the difficulties they have in navigating fictional worlds. Much of the discussion is related, at least by implication, to the wide range of situations in which people comprehend narrative accounts. For ease of communication, however, *reader* will stand as the name for the person who assumes a variety of roles, such as witness, hearer, and reader.

The uses of memory structures: plot

Incomplete knowledge is a primary obstacle readers must overcome to understand texts. For example, in the excerpt from *The Bushwhacked Piano* we simply do not know enough about the child to understand why he shot the piano. He may have wanted merely to be destructive; he may have been aiming at the owner and missed; he may have been trying to get himself arrested. This missing knowledge is related to a fairly abstract level of understanding. Note that we *can* comprehend the meaning of each of the sentences of the passage, and we can even create a coherent image of the scene. What we cannot do is provide a unique, meaningful explanation of the character's motives — his goals and the plans he has developed to satisfy those goals.

Because this excerpt opens the novel, we must await further information from McGuane before we can overcome this obstacle to understanding. In most cases of comprehension — when a speaker or author has not purposefully denied us knowledge — we are able to fill in missing information by virtue of preexisting structures stored in memory. For example, we can infer a motive for the *owner's* behavior because many of us have been in a similar situation. The owner's goal is to make the child appreciate the consequences of his destructive behavior. Nor are we particularly confused by the references to *strings* and *holes* in the passage, because we know something about the composition of pianos and the products of bullets.

To make these inferences, a reader must be able to deploy knowledge stored in memory. Theorists have coined the term *schemata* to refer to the memory structures that incorporate clusters of information relevant to comprehension (see Alba & Hasher, 1983; Bartlett, 1932; Brewer & Nakamura, 1984; Mandler, 1984; Rumelhart, 1980a; Rumelhart & Ortony, 1977; see also Minsky, 1975). A primary insight of schema theories is that we do not just have isolated facts in memory. Information is gathered together into meaningful, functional units. For example, the knowledge we have about *offices* is stored in memory so that when someone mentions visiting a professor's office, we are readily prepared to interpret comments about bookshelves or desks (Brewer & Treyens, 1981).

We have schemata for almost everything we have encountered (e.g., offices, chairs, and accountants) and everything we have done (e.g., playing baseball, attending concerts, and folding laundry). The information stored in a schema is abstracted over many different instances (all the chairs we have seen) or occasions (all the times we have played baseball). For example, a schema for common American coins includes the abstracted information that they must have *some* president's picture on the "heads" side (Rubin & Kontis, 1983). The identity of the president is a variable that is instantiated differently for each coin. Because of our coin schema, if we were shown the "tails" side of an unfamiliar coin, we would be able to make highly accurate inferences about the types of things that would be found on the other side. In comprehension, we are faced with an analogous situation. We are given only partial information and use schematic knowledge to make highly accurate inferences about what has been left unstated.

Scripts. To illustrate this process, we turn to a well-documented type of schema known as a *script* (Abelson, 1981; Schank & Abelson, 1977). A script is a memory structure that specifies a list of actions that people carry out in stereotypical situations. When asked to describe the sequence of actions in scenarios like *attending a lecture, grocery shopping,* and *visiting a doctor,* individuals largely agree on what takes place (Bower, Black, & Turner, 1979; Graesser, Gordon, & Sawyer, 1979). The following are the actions most commonly listed in a *going to a restaurant* script (Bower et al., 1979):

> Be seated.
> Look at menu.
> Order meal.
> Eat food.
> Pay bill.
> Leave.

When we encounter a scripted situation in a story, we can immediately generate a number of *expectations* about the activities that will follow. The simple statement that "Laurie has been seated at a restaurant" suggests to us that she will look at a menu, order a meal, and so on. When reading a story, we also use our scripts to make *inferences* about unstated activities. Consider this short text:

Laurie went to a restaurant. She ordered the one vegetarian dish on the menu. She signaled for the waitress. She ate the food quickly and hurried back to her office.

Because of our scripted knowledge, we infer that Laurie sat down while she was in the restaurant and that she paid her bill before she left. A short time after reading a story of this type, individuals often find it difficult to discriminate between statements that they actually read and those that they simply inferred from the script. For example, when asked to identify which of a series of sentences were actually present in a script-based story, readers often falsely asserted that they had actually read inferred sentences like "Laurie paid her bill" (Bower et al., 1979).

Scripts incorporate more, however, than lists of actions. When a script is invoked, readers also retrieve associated characters and objects from memory (Sanford & Garrod, 1981; Schank & Abelson, 1977). Because of this stored information, we were not surprised by the mention of *a menu* and *a waitress* when we read about Laurie. They are already part of our representation of the story. Thus, as with plot actions, readers will falsely assert, on the basis of inferences, that they have read words related to the script, particularly when the words are of central importance to the activity, such as *waitress* or *meal* (Walker & Yekovich, 1984). Scripts also help us, even while we are reading a story, to generate expectations about the words we will be likely to see: Words related to a script, like *candles* in a children's party scenario, are processed more swiftly than are irrelevant words (Sharkey & Mitchell, 1985).

We have been concerned so far with the *content* of scripts. Researchers have also been interested in their structure: How are scripts represented in memory? An answer to this question has emerged as the result of a continuous interplay of theory and research. In their original theoretical conception, scripts were thought to be structures that encoded the complete story of a stereotypical situation (Schank & Abelson, 1977). That is, when we read a text about visiting a dentist's office, an entire *visit to the dentist* script was retrieved from memory and used as a framework for understanding the text. Stories about similar but distinct events – visiting a doctor or a chiropractor – would evoke entirely different scripts. However, experimentation suggested that readers confused the events in similar scripts (Bower et al., 1979). For example, reading three similar stories – *dentist, doctor*, and *chiropractor* – rather than just one increased the likelihood that readers would falsely assert they had read some statement that was actually absent from one of the stories. Theorists were led to the conclusion that scripts with common actions made use of some shared memory representation (Bower et al., 1979; Schank, 1982). A revised theory suggests that scripts are constructed from smaller units known as *memory organization packets*, or MOPs (Schank, 1982). The *dentist visit* and *doctor visit* scripts share the MOPs that specify the overlapping aspects of office visits. Experimentalists have now provided further support for the existence of smaller, MOP-like units (Abbott, Black, & Smith, 1985; Galambos & Rips, 1982). Thus, theory and research have converged on a consistent representation of scripts.

Story grammars and story schemata. Starting at an early age, we are exposed to a great number of stories. Theorists have suggested that, as in most other domains, through repeated exposure we abstract the common features of these stories and develop two mental structures: a *story grammar* and a *story schema* (Johnson & Mandler, 1980; Mandler, 1984; Mandler & Johnson, 1977; Rumelhart, 1975, 1977; Stein & Glenn, 1979; Thorndyke, 1977). A *story grammar* is defined by analogy to a linguistic grammar: Just as the grammar of a languge specifies units (e.g., nouns and verbs) and the order in which the units may appear in a sentence (e.g., in a canonical English sentence, a noun phrase precedes the verb phrase), a story grammar specifies the units (e.g., attempts and outcomes) and the order of units in a story (e.g., in a canonical story, setting information precedes the episodes). A *story schema* shares the properties of other schemata: It enables comprehenders to generate expectations about the abstract types of information they are likely to encounter as they proceed through a simple story.

These related concepts have been the subject of a number of empirical investigations designed to test their validity as memory structures (see Mandler, 1984, for a review). For example, if readers use story grammars to guide comprehension, normal processing should be disrupted when the constituents of stories are written in an unusual order (Mandler & Goodman, 1982). In the following story, the *beginning* event has been moved from its normal location preceding the *reaction* to it (Mandler, 1984):

There was a penguin who lived on a floating iceberg. The penguin lived by himself in a cozy little igloo. The penguin was truly sorry his friends had no home [reaction], since one day a storm destroyed all the other igloos [beginning]. He decided he must share his igloo with his friends. (p. 60)

Although this story excerpt is comprehensible, it takes much longer for readers to understand the *beginning* statement than it would if that statement preceded the *reaction* (Mandler & Goodman, 1982). This result and others suggest that abstract knowledge of story structure guides readers' comprehension.

Despite this empirical support, story grammars and schemata have proved to be controversial theoretical constructs (e.g., Coots, 1982). One source of criticism has been the lack of true correspondence between the properties of story grammars and linguistic grammars (e.g., Black & Bower, 1980; Black & Wilensky, 1979; de Beaugrande, 1982). For example, linguistic grammars enable one to discriminate between strings of words that are acceptable sentences of a language and those that are not; story grammars do not enable one to discriminate between acceptable and unacceptable stories (Black & Bower, 1980; Meehan, 1982). Proponents of story grammars have argued, however, that they adopted the notation only for the sake of convenience, without intending to borrow the other theoretical underpinnings of a grammar (Mandler, 1984; Rumelhart, 1980b).

Perhaps more telling criticisms are aimed at the general usefulness of story grammars and story schemata. These structures characterize only a small range of "stories from the oral tradition" — folktales, fables, and myths (Johnson & Mandler, 1980; Mandler, 1984; Mandler & Johnson, 1977). Thus, they have limited applicability to the bulk of the stories readers encounter. This, in itself, is not a major concern if these story structures are unambiguously intended to be used in this limited set of circumstances. Researchers from other theoretical traditions, however, have argued that structures inferred for more general classes of stories are of primary importance even in the comprehension of these simple stories (Black & Bower, 1980; Black & Wilensky, 1979; Brewer & Lichtenstein, 1982). Empirical evidence suggests that readers do have story-grammar knowledge stored in memory. At issue is whether this knowledge is ordinarily put to use. In a later section we review the evidence for a different approach, which suggests that goals and plans are more important than structure.

Other Schemata. Schematic information other than scripts and story schemata also facilitates text comprehension. Consider, for example, the following pair of sentences (Haviland & Clark, 1974):

We checked the picnic supplies. The beer was warm.

Because *beer* (or *beverages*) is part of our schematic knowledge of *picnic supplies*, we can draw an appropriate inference to bridge these two sentences (Clark & Haviland, 1977). In most instances, new entities, like *beer*, must be introduced into a text with an indefinite article, like *a*, or pronoun, like *some*. This is a signal that a reader should establish a representation of the entity in memory:

Robin bought *a* new car. The car had gold racing stripes.

Lee was planting *some* flowers. They were daisies and violets.

However, when the entity is an element of schematic knowledge, as *beer* is for *picnic supplies*, it is already an incipient part of the memory representation and so need not be introduced by the indefinite article. The invocation of the schema for *picnic supplies* facilitates later comprehension by making information about other entities, such as *beer, potato chips*, and *hot dogs*, readily available in memory. In every domain, schemata are essential for comprehension.

Schemata, text interpretation, and memory. Often schematic information is needed to bring coherence to a text. Researchers have dramatically demonstrated the wide-ranging effects of schemata in the laboratory. Consider the following paragraph (Dooling & Lachman, 1971):

With hocked gems financing him, our hero bravely defied all scornful laughter that tried to prevent his scheme. "Your eyes deceive," he had said. "An egg, not a table, correctly typifies this unexplored planet." Now three sturdy sisters sought proof.

Forging along, sometimes through calm vastness, yet more often over turbulent peaks and valleys, days became weeks as many doubters spread fearful rumors about the edge. At last, from nowhere, welcome winged creatures appeared signifiying momentous success. (p. 217)

Without appropriate information from memory, it is almost impossible to draw this paragraph into a coherent tale. However, if we know the title, "Christopher Columbus Discovering America," we find it much easier to interpret the passage. We can now use what we already know about Christopher Columbus to organize the information. Schematic information often makes difficult texts comprehensible (Bransford & Johnson, 1973; Dooling, & Lachman, 1971).

Schematic information can also alter our recollection of texts. In one of the best-known experiments in cognitive psychology, Bartlett (1932) asked English readers to recall a story taken from the oral literary tradition of Canadian Indians, called "The War of the Ghosts." Barlett reported that his readers systematically altered the story in recall to conform to their own schematic information; they distorted the story to fit their own cultural stereotypes. For example, a reference to "hunting seals" in the original text became "fishing" in one individual's recall. Inconsistent information within a story can also prompt readers to "recall" information that is at odds with what was actually present. For example, when faced with a story in which two individuals got married despite a major obstacle (the two vehemently disagreed on whether they ought to have children), readers invented material to explain the discrepancy (Spiro, 1980). The readers created sentences that were entirely absent from the original story, such as "They separated but realized after discussing the matter that their love mattered more" (p. 91). Schematic information in memory has a powerful influence on our understanding and recall of the texts we read.

Memory for nonschematic information. Schemata provide us with a ready-made method for understanding the ordinary events and objects around us. Simultaneously, they serve as a background against which we notice unusual things; by encoding what is standard, schemata make evident what is nonstandard. Note that *nonstandard* does not mean bizarre: Many aspects of objects or situations are unusual − in the sense that they are not common enough to have become part of schematized knowledge − without being genuinely strange. For example, students would not be shocked if a professor sipped a cup of coffee during a lecture, even though that activity is not part of the *lecture* script (Nakamura, Graesser, Zimmerman, & Riha, 1985).

When information is not schematized, it receives special treatment in processing, the consequence of which is differential memorability (Graesser, 1981; Graesser et al., 1979; Graesser & Nakamura, 1982; Nakamura, Graesser, Zimmerman, & Riha, 1985). For example, in one experiment, students were present at one of two versions of a lecture in which a professor performed some scripted activities (e.g., "sitting on a corner of a table" in version A and "erasing a sentence off the blackboard" in version B) and some nonscripted activities (e.g., "wiping off glasses" in version A and "picking up a pencil off the floor" in version B). When faced with a subsequent recognition test ("Did you see this action?"), the students found it very difficult to discriminate among the possible scripted actions but could readily say which nonscripted actions they had seen (Nakamura et al., 1985). Because the scripted activities could be assimilated to the generic structure in memory, students took little notice of which of these activities actually took place. Conversely, nonscripted activities necessarily received special attention. These considerations explain the memory results. Note, once again, that the nonscripted activities were relatively mundane (e.g., "wiping off glasses"). Memorability relied not on bizarreness, but on whether an action was included in the script.

The uses of memory structures: plans and goals

Let us return briefly to our difficulty with the excerpt from *The Bushwhacked Piano*: We could not infer a unique motive for the child's behavior. Readers are particularly uncomfortable when they lack motive or goal information. Several theorists have suggested that text comprehension is guided by an appreciation of the way actions follow as a consequence of characters' goals (e.g., Black & Bower, 1980; Bower, 1982; Lichtenstein & Brewer, 1980; Schank & Abelson, 1977). When we know what goals characters have in mind, we can make sense of what they say and do. We can understand a text by tracing the causes and consequences of characters' behaviors (e.g., Schank, 1975; Stein & Trabasso, 1982; Trabasso, Secco, & van den Broek, 1984; Trabasso, Stein, & Johnson, 1981). These analyses suggest that we have structures in memory comparable to the schemata we have already encountered, but at a more abstract level: Rather than filling in plot details, these memory structures help us to understand and predict the characters' motivations.

Consider the following paragraph (Schank & Abelson, 1977):

John knew that his wife's operation would be very expensive. There was always Uncle Harry. . . . He reached for the suburban phone book. (p. 70)

When we read this brief story, we sense immediately why Uncle Harry is relevant to the situation (i.e., he must be rich) and why John needs the phone book (i.e., he wants to call Uncle Harry). As we read the story, we infer pairs of goals and plans:

Goal: John needs to raise money.
Plan: John will get the money from Uncle Harry.
Goal: John needs to contact Uncle Harry.
Plan: John will call him on the phone.

None of these goals or plans is stated explicitly in the text. In each case, they are inferred because we have appropriate structures in memory to fill in the missing information. In general, we are very adept at extracting goals and plans from text and in deciding how actions are related to them.

Researchers have tried to characterize the abstract structures that enable us to make these plan and goal inferences (Schank & Abelson, 1977; Wilensky, 1982). Here the idea is to characterize what situations are "ready-analyzed" in memory: What are the basic relationships between goals and plans and plans and actions that we have abstracted from repeated exposure to narratives and the world? Theorists have identified a number of goals that recur in our lives, like *get money* and *get food*. Consider, for example, this pair of sentences (Schank & Abelson, 1977, p. 71):

Willa was hungry. She took out the Michelin Guide.

Our *get food* plan schema enables us to infer the link between these two sentences: Willa is looking in the *Michelin Guide* to find a place to eat. To understand most stories, however, we have to be able to recognize more complicated goal structures. Consider this brief story (Wilensky, 1982):

John wanted to marry Mary. He also wanted to marry Sue. John took Mary out and proposed to her. She agreed. Later, John called Sue and told her he wouldn't be seeing her anymore. (p. 360)

In this story, John has conflicting goals – he wants to marry two people at once. To understand the story, we must first recognize the goal conflict; then we can appreciate the way in which the remainder of the story spells out the resolution. The inferences we make suggest that we have abstract knowledge about the way goals may interact (Wilensky, 1982).

Goal and plan inferences. Researchers have provided direct evidence that we make goal and plan inferences while reading (Seifert, Robertson, & Black, 1985). In line with the results for scripts, readers are often unable to discriminate between goal and plan statements that they have actually read and those that they have inferred. Consider the following story (adapted from Seifert et al., 1985):

Provo is a picturesque kingdom in France. Corman was heir to the throne of Provo. He wanted to be king *[goal]*. He was so tired of waiting. He decided to poison the king *[plan]*. He thought arsenic would work well. Corman went to the storeroom. There was arsenic in the storeroom *[state]*. He hid the arsenic in his coat. The king was looking out the window. His cup was on the table near the door. The king fell ill after drinking. Corman knew he would soon be king. (p. 420)

In an experiment, some students read this story with the *goal* sentence and the *plan* sentence included. Others read a version with one of the two sentences missing. Later, students reported with nearly equal confidence that they had seen each of these sentences whether or not they were actually present in the story. That is, most of these readers were unable to distinguish inferred from stated goals and plans. This result suggests that making goal and plan inferences is a regular part of text comprehension. In contrast, readers correctly asserted that they had not seen the *state* sentence, "There was arsenic in the storeroom," when it was not present in the story. Readers thus do not automatically make all the inferences they could.

In general, there are a large number of inferences that we could draw from any passage. The difficulty is that it is not feasible to make all possible inferences in the small amount of time we take to comprehend texts (Rieger, 1975). We limit our inferences to those that are most important for our ultimate understanding; in most cases these are inferences in service of plans and goals.

Goals and plans in text interpretation. Knowledge of a character's goal or motivation will often radically alter our experience of a text. Consider the following account (Owens, Bower, & Black, 1979):

Nancy arrived at the cocktail party. She looked around the room to see who was there. She went to talk to her professor. She felt she had to talk to him but was a little nervous about just what to say. A group of people started to play charades. Nancy went over and had some refreshments. The hors d'oeuvres were good but she wasn't interested in talking to the rest of the people at the party. After a while she decided she'd had enough and left the party. (p. 186)

The text seems rather mundane, but it takes on new meaning if it is reread with the following introduction:

Nancy woke up feeling sick again and she wondered if she really were pregnant. How would she tell the professor she had been seeing? And the money was another problem.

When this passage was read in an experimental setting, the presence or absence of the introduction had a sizable effect on comprehension. When asked to recall the story, students who had read the introduction included many ideas related to Nancy's pregnancy that were not present in the text. Armed with knowledge of Nancy's motives, the students stamped their own interpretation on the actual text (Owens, et al., 1979).

Readers also bring their own goal and plan perspectives to their interpretation of a text. In one series of experiments, subjects were asked to read a passage describing a home and to take the perspective of either a homebuyer or a burglar (Anderson & Pichert, 1978; Pichert & Anderson, 1977). Many facts in the passage were important for one perspective but not the other (e.g., a leaky roof for a homebuyer, a color television for a burglar). When later asked to recall the text, the patterns of recall reflected the difference in perspective: "Burglar" readers recalled more "burglar" facts; "homebuyers" more "homebuyer" facts. However, the readers had not simply ignored the information in the story irrelevant to their perspective. When asked to recall the text again, adopting the alternative perspective, they were able to produce new, appropriate information (Anderson & Pichert, 1978). This result suggests that perspective guides both comprehension and recollection of a text.

Causal analysis in text comprehension. One theory of text comprehension suggests that the ultimate product of understanding is a *causal network* that represents the causal relationships among events in a story (Stein & Trabasso, 1982; Trabasso & van den Broek, 1985; Trabasso et al., 1984; Trabasso & Sperry, 1985; Trabasso et al., 1981; see also, Black & Bower, 1980; Omanson, 1982). As readers proceed through a text, they find the underlying causal links between events and, in particular, they form the *causal chain*: the sequence of causally important events that gives shape to the story. Consider the following story (adapted from Trabasso et al., 1984):

Judy's grandmother knew that she really wanted a hammer and saw for her birthday. She decided to get them for her because she knew that when Judy grows up and becomes a woman she will have to fix things when they break. Judy's grandmother went out that very day and bought the tools. (p. 91)

Even this brief narrative contains some statements that are causally important and some that are not. We are offered a pair of causal explanations for why Judy's grandmother buys the tools: Judy wants the tools; her grandmother believes that Judy will benefit from having them. Conversely, there is nothing causally important about knowing the *content* of the grandmother's reason (i.e., that Judy someday will have to fix things) — only that she has one. From the standpoint of casual analysis this content is a *dead end* (Schank, 1975). Causal analysis thus differentiates the causally important (causal-chain) and dead-end information in a story. These categories of information are differentially remembered (Stein & Glenn, 1979; Trabasso et al., 1984). When fifth-grade children were asked to recall short stories, they were much more likely to report causal-chain events than dead-end events. Furthermore, they had greater recall for stories with a larger proportion of events belonging to the causal chain (and thus a smaller proportion of dead ends). These results lend support to the theory that readers are differentially attuned to causally important story information.

Types of representations in text comprehension

When readers approach a text they must carry out several comprehension tasks. They must determine the meanings of individual words, of sentences, of groups of sentences, and of the text as a whole. Theorists have suggested that readers create representations at different levels of specificity, from single words to whole texts. We now discuss some of these representations and the evidence for them.

Propositions. Readers begin text comprehension by extracting basic units of meaning, or *propositions* (Clark & Clark, 1977; Kintsch, 1974). Propositions generally consist of a *predicate* plus one or more *arguments*. Thus, the proposition *sings (Michael)* encodes the information that *Michael sings. Love (John, Mary)* encodes the information *John loves Mary.* Complex sentences generally contain a number of propositions. Consider, for example, the following sentence (Kintsch, 1978):

The governor asked the detective to prevent drinking. (p. 61)

The sentence contains three major propositions, each of which is embedded in another. First, there is *drink(someone)*, which asserts that there are people who drink. Next, *prevent(detective, drink(someone))* asserts that the detective should prevent someone from drinking. Finally, *ask(governor, detective, prevent (detective, drink(someone))* asserts the whole sentence.

The importance of propositions in text comprehension has been thoroughly documented (for reviews, see Kintsch, 1974, 1978). For example, if two words in a sentence belong to the same proposition, they will be represented together in memory irrespective of their proximity in the actual text (Ratcliff & McKoon, 1978). Consider the following sentence (Ratcliff & McKoon, 1978):

The mausoleum that enshrined the tzar overlooked the square. (p. 406)

There are two main propositions in the sentence: *enshrined(tzar, mausoleum)* and *overlooked(mausoleum, square)*. Thus, although *mausoleum* and *square* appear at opposite ends of the sentence, they belong to a common proposition. After reading a small number of sentences like this one, the subjects in an experiment were given a list of words and asked to indicate whether each word had been in one of the sentences they studied. Sometimes these lists contained consecutive words from the same proposition (e.g., chauffeur, *square, mausoleum*, truck, . . .), and sometimes there were consecutive words from the same sentence but from different propositions (e.g., chauffeur, *square, tzar*, truck, . . .). When a word, like *mausoleum*, came directly after a word from the *same* proposition, like *square*, it took subjects reliably less time to say that the word had been in a sentence than when the word came directly after a word from a *different* proposition, like *tzar* (Ratcliff & McKoon, 1978). Confirming the presence of the first word from the proposition makes it easier to verify the second word. This suggests that members of the same proposition are stored together in memory.

Macrostructures. A second type of representation, at a more abstract level than propositions, is the *macrostructure*, made up of *macropropositions* (Kintsch & van Dijk, 1978; van Dijk, 1977, 1980). The theory of macrostructures suggests that, as readers make their way through a text, they unify sequences of propositions into more abstract structures that capture the gist of, or important ideas in, the text. For example, consider the following excerpt from the story "Tiger by the Tail" by James Hadley Chase (cited by van Dijk, 1980):

A tall slim blond in a white summer frock walking just ahead of him, caught Ken Holland's eye. He studied her, watching her gentle undulations as she walked. He quickly shifted his eyes. He hadn't looked at a woman like this since he had first met Ann. What's the matter with me? he asked himself. I'm getting as bad as Parker. (p. 52)

Readers can extract two macropropositions from this text: (1) Ken Holland is looking at a beautiful girl in the street; (2) he feels guilty about it because he is married (van Dijk, 1980, p. 56). These macropropositions provide a good summary of this section of the story. In general, the macrostructure provides an account of what has happened at a gist level. Readers are able to extract macropropositions, and build macrostructures, by fitting the facts of the story to the types of structure in memory (scripts and schemata) we discussed earlier.

Situation models. To reason about a text, readers must often go beyond propositions or macropropositions and create a *situation model* or *mental model* (Garnham, 1981; Johnson-Laird, 1980, 1983; Perrig & Kintsch, 1985; van Dijk & Kintsch, 1983). The situation model (the term we will use) is a unified representation of the content of the text. Imagine, for example, that the following series of statements was part of a narrative (Johnson-Laird, 1983):

[On the table] the spoon is to the left of the knife. The plate is to the right of the knife. The fork is in front of the spoon. The cup is in front of the knife. (p. 160)

A macroproposition describing this text might be *The table has been set.* That sort of representation would be rather inadequate if a reader were asked, as were the subjects in an experiment, to say whether the description is consistent with the following layout:

> spoon knife plate
> fork cup

Of more use would be a situation model representation corresponding directly to the layout. The reader could then simply compare the situation model to the display. A situation model also makes it possible to make global inferences. For example, with such a model in hand, it is relatively easy to verify that "The fork is to the left of the cup" is consistent with the earlier series of sentences; without a situation model, inferences of this kind are difficult to make (Mani & Johnson-Laird, 1982; see also Perrig & Kintsch, 1985). Situation models make it possible for readers to reason about texts at a level liberated from the actual words and sentences that have comprised the text.

Aspects of fictional worlds

In this section, we discuss some problems of text comprehension that arise particularly when people read fiction. First, we discuss the ways in which the differing knowledge states of readers and characters affect comprehension.

Second, we consider the difficulties readers may have in keeping information they acquire about fictional worlds from intruding on their real-world
knowledge.

What readers know and what characters know. The author of a work of fiction has almost total control over who − readers or characters − has what
information at what times in a text. Often, the power of fiction is enhanced
because authors create a dissociation between the knowledge states of the
readers and the characters. Consider, for example, Jay Cantor's novel, *The
Death of Che Guevera.* Simply by virtue of the title, the reader knows something that Che Guevera and the other characters do not, namely, that
Guevera will die during the limited time span described in the book. The
title adds drama for the reader that would be unperceived by the characters.

   The dissociation of knowledge states poses some interesting problems for
theorists of text comprehension. We will focus on issues relating to the interpretation of dialogue. Suppose, for example, the following utterances were
taken from works of fiction:

Shirley: It's raining. Close the windows.
Howard: The monster is coming. Run for your life.

Obviously we would not, as a consequence of reading these utterances, close
our own windows (Searle, 1975) or take flight from the monster (Walton,
1978). What this suggests is that we play a different role as comprehenders
of fictional dialogue than we do as comprehenders of everyday dialogue.
Rather than being participants in the conversation, we are overhearers −
but we are overhearers with a very privileged status.

   In everyday conversation, overhearers are generally greatly disadvantaged
with respect to real conversational participants (Clark & Carlson, 1982).
The problem for an overhearer is that the speakers are designing their utterances on the basis of *common ground* − the knowledge they know they
share with their addressees (Clark & Carlson, 1981; Clark & Murphy, 1982).
When overhearers do not possess the necessary common ground, they are
left uncomprehending. Suppose, for example, Karla makes the following
statement in a conversation with her friend Patty:

"I'm going to the movies with Superman tonight."

If Karla is being a cooperative conversationalist, she must have good reason
to believe that she and Patty share appropriate knowledge so that *Superman*
refers to some unique individual (Clark & Marshall, 1981; Grice, 1975).
However, Karla has no conversational responsibilities to anyone who might
overhear the statement. That is, she has no reason to produce an utterance
that will be comprehensible to anyone but Patty, and, in fact, she might
purposely select the term *Superman* to leave others, overhearers, in the dark.

   Characters in novels also design − that is, authors design for them −

utterances based on the knowledge they share with their addressees. Consider this utterance from Tony Morrison's novel *Tar Baby*:

"It's not important who this one loves and who this one hates and what bow-tie do or what machete-hair don't do . . . "

Here Gideon is speaking to Therese, with whom he shares the knowledge of which individuals the phrases *bow-tie* and *machete-hair* refer to. Fortunately, this information is also shared by the reader. Morrison provides another problematic referring phrase:

"What you want to know?" Gideon asked, drying his ears.
[Son answers,] "If she's there. If she's not, I need an address."

Who does Son mean by *she*? Under ordinary circumstances, we would expect to see a definite pronoun like *she* only if the immediately preceding text provided a referent. There is, however, no immediately prior textual referent for this *she*. The reference to *she* takes place at the beginning of the conversation. Gideon (and the readers) know who *she* is because there is only one female character in the book who is sufficiently salient in their common ground to be selected by this referring phrase (Gerrig, 1986). Although the knowledge is gained from different perspectives − that of conversational participant versus that of overhearer − both the characters and the readers must resort to common ground to interpret this unusual *she*.

Thus, as an overhearer of conversations, readers must bring whatever knowledge they share to bear on the interpretation of the characters' utterances. If, in the service of literary goals, the author is being purposely obscure, readers sometimes suffer the fate of everyday overhearers and are left uncomprehending. Usually, however, they know more than the characters − because the author has given them more information − which enables them to comprehend utterances in a different way than the characters. Fiction, for example, provides the ideal circumstances for achieving irony. According to one theory, irony requires two audiences that are differentiated by the knowledge they possess (Clark & Gerrig, 1984; Fowler, 1965). One audience comprises an inner circle that possesses the information necessary to perceive ironic intent. The second audience does not have such information. Consider this utterance:

Seth: Joel is a daredevil driver.

This would be perceived as ironic only by the circle of individuals who share the common ground that Joel is actually a timid driver. Other people would not appreciate Seth's ironic intent.

In fiction, an author can bring about the perception of irony by giving the readers information the characters do not have. Let us return to *The Death of Che Guevera*. Throughout the novel, Guevera makes pronouncements about the state of affairs "after the revolution." Because the title (and our knowledge of history) makes us privy to knowledge unknown to Guevera or the other characters, the perception of tragic irony is strong throughout the book. Thus, the author's manipulation of relative knowledge states has added another layer of understanding to our ordinary text comprehension.

The status of fictional information. One great difficulty facing a reader of fiction is the need to ignore fictional information that appears to be relevant to everyday life. Consider, for example, this excerpt from Thomas Pynchon's novel, *Gravity's Rainbow:*

Gustav is a composer. For months he has been carrying on a raging debate with Saure over who is better, Beethoven, or Rossini. . . . "I'm not so much for Beethoven qua Beethoven," Gustav argues, "but as he represents the German dialectic, the incorporation of more and more notes into the scale, culminating with dodecaphonic democracy, where all notes get an equal hearing. . . . While Rossini was retiring at the age of 36, womanizing and getting fat, Beethoven was living a life filled with tragedy and grandeur."

"So?" is Saure's customary answer. . . . "Which would you rather do? The point is, . . . a person feels *good* listening to Rossini. All you feel like listening to Beethoven is going out and invading Poland. Ode to Joy indeed . . . "

How seriously ought we to take these opinions about Beethoven and Rossini? A moment's thought suggests that we should discount them entirely because they are spoken by fictional characters: We have no reason to believe that any nonfictional person (even the author) would harbor these attitudes. Logically, therefore, we ought to enjoy the prose but ignore the opinions. We ought not to let fictional statements meld with nonfictional ones in our memories, nor in this case should we allow our attitudes toward Beethoven and Rossini to be manipulated by fictional statements. At issue, however, is whether psychologically we are able to avoid these situations.

The limited amount of relevant experimentation suggests that we may have some difficulty isolating what we read in fiction from what we know from the real world. In one study, participants were asked to commit to memory a number of *fantasy facts* about historical characters, for example, "George Washington wrote *Tom Sawyer*" and "Napoleon Bonaparte is a liberal senator" (Lewis & Anderson, 1976). Once they had learned these artificial facts, the participants were asked to identify as true or false a number of real pieces of information, for example, "George Washington crossed the Delaware." The study showed that people took more time to verify a nonfictional true statement about a historical figure − something they had known before they entered the laboratory − after they had learned the fictional facts. Longer verification times imply the need to search a larger memory structure. Thus, this result suggests that, rather than keeping fact and fiction distinct, participants had merged the fictional statements with their preexisting memory representations. Because the participants were required to memorize the fictional facts, the conditions of this study were different from ordinary circumstances of reading. Nonetheless, the experiment suggests that we do not maintain strict separation of fact and fiction in memory.

Expository and persuasive texts

We turn now to expository and persuasive texts. We distinguish these texts from narratives primarily in terms of the writer's goals and the reader's goals. It is often difficult to differentiate types of text simply by examining the prose itself: The same passage could entertain us, inform us, or persuade us at different times. The topics we address in this section arise when writers intend their text to inform or persuade and we intend as readers to let them do so. When that is the case, we can ask two questions: What features of the texts themselves affect our ability to be informed or persuaded; what features of *ourselves* affect the ability of texts to inform or persuade us?

Features of texts

Expository prose. Expository texts are most often useful to people who are trying to acquire information. Research on these texts, therefore, has often concerned itself with the ways in which texts should be constructed to facilitate learning. One difficulty most readers face with respect to much expository prose is that they have very little knowledge in memory relevant to the text domain. As described earlier for narratives, we have a number of knowledge structures related to the *content* of texts, for example, scripts and plan and goal schemata. This content information allows us to generate expectations about the details of a story, given an opening scenario. Unfortunately, we have few such content schemata for domains covered by expository prose (Kieras, 1985). Consider this passage from a biochemistry text (cited by Kieras, 1985):

Pancreatic RNase is a highly specific endonuclease which splits the bond between the phosphate residue at C-3' in a pyrimidine nucleotide to C'-5 in the next nucleotide in sequence. The basic feature of its actions is an intramolecular attack on the phosphodiester bond using the 2'-OH group to form an obligatory 2' : 3' cyclic phosphate intermediate, which is then hydrolysed by the enzyme to give pyrimidine 3'-phosphates either as free nucleotides or as a terminal nucleotide residue in an oligonucleotide. (p. 90)

We cannot use memory structures related to content to help us understand this passage. Instead, theorists have suggested, we use memory structures related to the typical presentation of information in expository texts. That is, we have abstract knowledge about the conventional organization of texts, and we use that knowledge to guide our processing of expository prose (Kieras, 1985; Meyer, 1977, 1984, 1985). For example, in the biochemistry passage we are first told that pancreatic RNase accomplishes some function and then we are told how it does so. Our comprehension of this text is facilitated if, given the first "function" sentence, we generate the expectation, based on our experience with a wide range of expository texts, that a second "mechanism" sentence will follow.

Because readers are using organizational expectations to drive processing of expository prose, writers' divergences from canonical arrangements of information can have a dramatic impact on comprehension. For example, instructors generally admonish would-be writers to devote the initial sentence of a paragraph to a statement of its topic. Research suggests that this is an expectation we have institutionalized as part of our prose processing. When paragraphs do not have an initial statement of the main idea we are at a great disadvantage. In general, it will take us longer to read such a passage (compared with a topic-first paragraph) and our recall of the material will be poorer (Kieras, 1978). We can easily see why that might be. When a topic sentence comes first, we can interpret the rest of the paragraph as information about that topic. We are able to generate expectations about the way subsequent information will be related to the general theme of the passage. If no main theme appears in the initial sentence, we must try to find one as we read, which causes grave difficulties: Our guess may be incorrect, and we may have to revise our idea of what the paragraph is about several times; we may discover that we have misjudged what information in the paragraph is critical to the argument and what is unimportant (Kieras, 1985). The uncertainty engendered by a missing initial topic sentence leads to poorer comprehension. As writers, we must heed our instructors' advice or knowingly hamper the comprehension of our texts.

Research also suggests that texts can be optimally structured to enable students to move beyond the information given. For example, many scientific texts are intended to enable the student to solve problems beyond the small number presented in the text. This goal is best accomplished when texts are made to highlight *explanative information*: prose that provides explanations of mechanisms underlying scientific ideas (Mayer, 1982, 1985). For example, suppose we wanted to teach someone how to calculate the probabilities of getting specific numbers of "heads" and "tails" when flipping a coin. One method would be simply to present the appropriate formula and then some examples of its use. A second method would be to start with the concepts that underlie the formula — trials, outcomes, and so on — and offer the formula itself only after the student had mastered the concepts that explain it. The efficacy of these two methods can be compared. When faced with problems similar to the examples, students trained by the first method perform with greater success than those trained by the second. However, as soon as the problems begin to diverge noticeably from the examples, students who have been trained with explanative information excel (Mayer, 1982). The latter outcome is highly valued in educational settings. The lesson for writers is that they should structure their texts to highlight explanative information (Mayer, 1985).

Persuasive prose. Extensive research has been undertaken to relate the structure of arguments to their capacity to persuade (see McGuire, 1985, for a review). A number of issues arise: Should the argument be stated at the beginning or at the end of a passage? Should opposition arguments be refuted before or after one's own position is defended? How should one's own arguments be ordered with respect to strength (i.e., should one put the best arguments first or last)? The pursuit of answers to questions like these has revealed complicated interactions between the cognitive factors that have dominated the discussion in this chapter and the social factors that arise when we try to influence other people.

Consider, for example, the issue of whether the target position should come first or last (imagine a passage in which an idea, e.g., "Colleges should not charge tuition," is stated and then evidence is given versus a passage in which the idea is stated last, as a logical consequence of the evidence). We learned when considering expository prose that the "idea-first" arrangement greatly facilitates comprehension. Thus, on the basis of cognitive considerations, we would recommend that writers use that structure. However, one difficulty associated with persuasion is getting disinclined individuals to listen to our arguments. If we are arguing against a position that some individuals hold, and announce that fact by putting the idea first, we may never get them to read our prose. Even if they do read on, the trumpeting of a foreign position may cause them to proceed with wariness. Thus, given social considerations, we might recommend that a statement of the target position not be made until the end (McGuire, 1985). What this brief analysis suggests is that considerations of optimal text processing cannot always prevail when the text must serve some real-world function.

Features of readers

Throughout this chapter, we have considered all readers to be equal with respect to the knowledge and skills they bring to text-processing situations. In this section, we relax this idealization to examine briefly some ways in which individual differences can affect the comprehension of a text. First, we consider how the goals that readers bring to text comprehension influence what they recall. Second, we discuss the effect of individual differences in readers' knowledge about subject areas on the comprehension of texts in those areas.

The goals of reading. Often, our processing of a text depends on our goals – what we want to get from the text. Differing goals do not affect processing word by word so much as they affect our choice of information to focus on in a passage. For example, if we are assigned the task of reporting the main theme of a text, our reading will differ markedly, in terms of where we devote our attention, from our reading of a passage without this goal (Kieras, 1978). Often, goals are assigned to us, particularly in educational settings. For example, we frequently read texts knowing that we will later be tested on the material. Our expectations about the type of test – recall, multiple-choice, and so on – will influence our selection of information to concentrate on while reading. Faced with a test that is different from the one we expected, we perform poorly (d'Ydewalle & Roselle, 1978). Similarly, as in the case of text structure, if our goal in reading a scientific text is to be able to solve problems that go beyond the material presented, we should adopt a reading strategy that requires us to reflect on the material and remember explanations (Mayer, 1985). Thus, the information that individuals will be able to remember from texts, and the uses to which they can put the information, depend on the goals that they brought to the reading situation.

Reader knowledge. Different readers approach a text with differing background knowledge about the topic. Recall, for example, the cryptic paragraph that was entitled "Christopher Columbus Discovering America." Someone who knew little or nothing about Columbus would benefit little by being informed of this title. In general, people differ in what they know about a domain, so we can ask how text comprehension differs as a function of expertise.

One important difference between experts and nonexperts is the structures they have in memory. When we discussed schemata, we suggested that these knowledge structures were abstracted over time from repeated exposure to a domain. Schemata encode generalizations, so the more experiences we have in forming them, the more accurately they will guide our comprehension. Consider, for example, the game of baseball. With more experience in watching the game, we will better understand the plans and goals that underlie particular actions, such as sacrifice hits and intentional walks. In an experiment, subjects with greater or lesser knowledge about baseball were asked to listen to an acount of a half-inning of a fictitious baseball game. The two groups of subjects were then asked to recall the text and to answer questions about it (Spilich, Vesonder, Chiesi, & Voss, 1979). The results of the experiment gave evidence of the better instantiated goal schemata of the "high-knowledge" subjects. First, they recalled more information overall, which suggested that they had more useful memory structures for recording information than did the "low-knowledge" subjects. Second, the details they remembered, such as which batters got on base and how runners advanced, were relevant to the outcome of the game. Low-knowledge individuals did better only on unimportant details like the names of the players. Thus, expertise in a domain enables us to distinguish what is important from what is trivial and to commit to memory more easily the information that is important.

Conclusions

We are all experts at text comprehension. An important goal of this chapter has been to enable its readers to examine their own intuitions about the processes that underlie understanding. As we read texts — narrative, expository, persuasive, or other types of prose — it is important that we reflect on the skills we muster to facilitate comprehension. The insights we gain can provide the catalyst for future research.

References

Abelson, R. P. (1981). Psychological status of the script concept. *American Psychologist, 36,* 715–29.

Abbott, V., Black, J. B., & Smith, E. E. (1985). The representation of scripts in memory. *Journal of Memory and Language, 24,* 179–99.

Alba, J. W., & Hasher, L. (1983). Is memory schematic? *Psychological Bulletin, 93,* 203–31.

Anderson, R. C., & Pichert, J. W. (1978). Recall of previously unrecallable information following a shift in perspective. *Journal of Verbal Learning and Verbal Behavior, 17,* 1–12.

Bartlett, F. C. (1932). *Remembering.* Cambridge University Press.

Black, J. B., & Bower, G. H. (1980). Story understanding as problem-solving. *Poetics, 9,* 223–50.

Black, J. B., & Wilensky, R. (1979). An evaluation of story grammars. *Cognitive Science, 3,* 213–30.

Bower, G. H. (1982). Plans and goals in understanding episodes. In A. Flammer & W. Kintsch (Eds.), *Discourse processing* (pp. 2–15). Amsterdam: North-Holland.

Bower, G. H., Black, J. B., & Turner, T. J. (1979). Scripts in memory for text. *Cognitive Psychology, 11,* 177–220.

Bransford, J. D., & Johnson, M. K. (1973). Considerations of some problems of comprehension. In W. G. Chase (Ed.), *Visual information processing* (pp. 383–438). New York: Academic Press.

Brewer, W. F., & Lichtenstein, E. H. (1982). Stories are to entertain: A structural-affect theory of stories. *Journal of Pragmatics, 6,* 473–86.

Brewer, W. F., & Nakamura, G. V. (1984). The nature and functions of schemas. In R. S. Wyer & T. K. Srull (Eds.), *Handbook of social cognition* (Vol. 1, pp. 119–60). Hillsdale, NJ: Erlbaum.

Brewer, W. F., & Treyens, J. C. (1981). Role of schemata in memory for places. *Cognitive Psychology, 13,* 207–30.

Clark, H. H., & Carlson, T. B. (1981). Context for comprehension. In J. Long & A. Baddeley (Eds.), *Attention and performance* (Vol. 9, pp. 313–30). Hillsdale, NJ: Erlbaum.

(1982). Hearers and speech acts. *Language, 58,* 332–73.

Clark, H. H., & Clark, E. V. (1977). *Psychology and language.* Orlando, FL: Harcourt Brace Jovanovich.

Clark, H. H., & Gerrig, R. J. (1984). On the pretense theory of irony. *Journal of Experimental Psychology: General, 113,* 121–6.

Clark, H. H., & Haviland, S. E. (1977). Comprehension and the given–new contract. In R. O. Freedle (Ed.), *Discourse production and comprehension* (Vol. 1, pp. 1–40). Norwood, NJ: Ablex.

Clark, H. H., & Marshall, C. R. (1981). Definite reference and mutual knowledge. In A. K. Joshi, B. Webber, & I. Sag (Eds.), *Elements of discourse understanding* (pp. 10–63). Cambridge University Press.

Clark, H. H., & Murphy, G. L. (1982). Audience design in meaning and reference. In J.-F. Le Ny & W. Kintch (Eds.), *Language and comprehension* (pp. 287–99). Amsterdam: North-Holland.

Coots, J. H. (Ed.). (1982). Stories [special issue]. *Journal of Pragmatics, 6*(5–6).

de Beaugrande, R. (1982). The story of grammars and the grammar of stories. *Journal of Pragmatics, 6,* 383–422.

Dooling, D. J., & Lachman, R. (1971). Effects of comprehension on retention of prose. *Journal of Experimental Psychology, 88,* 216–22.

d'Ydewalle, B., & Roselle, H. (1978). Test expectancies in text learning. In M. M. Gruneberg, P. E. Morris, & R. N. Skyes (Eds.), *Practical aspects of memory* (pp. 609–17). New York: Academic Press.

Fowler, H. (1965). *A dictionary of modern English usage* (2nd ed.). New York: Oxford University Press.

Galambos, J. A., & Rips, L. J. (1982). Memory for routines. *Journal of Verbal Learning and Verbal Behavior, 21,* 260–81.

Garnham, A. (1981). Mental models as representations of text. *Memory & Cognition, 9,* 560–5.

Gerrig, R. J. (1986). Process models and pragmatics. In N. E. Sharkey (Ed.), *Advances in cognitive science* (Vol. 1, pp. 23–42). Chichester, Eng.: Horwood.

Graesser, A. C. (1981). *Prose comprehension beyond the word.* New York: Springer-Verlag.

Graesser, A. C., Gordon, S. E., & Sawyer, J. D. (1979). Recognition memory for typical and atypical actions in scripted activities: Tests of a script pointer + tag hypothesis. *Journal of Verbal Learning and Verbal Behavior, 18,* 319–32.

Graesser, A. C., & Nakamura, G. V. (1982). The impact of a schema on comprehension and memory. In G. H. Bower (Ed.), *The psychology of learning and motivation* (Vol. 16, pp. 59–109). New York: Academic Press.

Grice, H. P. (1975). Logic and conversation. In P. Cole & J. L. Morgan (Eds.), *Syntax and semantics: Vol. 3. Speech acts* (pp. 41–58). New York: Academic Press.

Haviland, S. E., & Clark, H. H. (1974). What's new? Acquiring new information as a process in comprehension. *Journal of Verbal Learning and Verbal Behavior, 13,* 515–21.

Johnson, N. S., & Mandler, J. M. (1980). A tale of two structures: Underlying and surface forms in stories. *Poetics, 9,* 51–86.

Johnson-Laird, P. N. (1980). Mental models in cognitive science. *Cognitive Science, 4,* 71–115.
    (1983). *Mental models.* Cambridge, MA: Harvard University Press.

Kieras, D. E. (1978). Good and bad structure in simple paragraphs: Effects on apparent theme, reading time, and recall. *Journal of Verbal Learning and Verbal Behavior, 17,* 13–28.
    (1985). Thematic processes in the comprehension of technical prose. In B. K. Britton & J. B. Black (Eds.), *Understanding expository text* (pp. 89–107). Hillsdale, NJ: Erlbaum.

Kintsch, W. (1974). *The representation of meaning in memory.* Hillsdale, NJ: Erlbaum.
    (1978). Comprehension and memory of text. In W. K. Estes (Ed.), *Handbook of learning and cognitive processes: Vol. 6. Linguistic functions in cognitive theory* (pp. 57–86). Hillsdale, NJ: Erlbaum.

Kintsch, W., & van Dijk, T. A. (1978). Toward a model of text comprehension and production *Psychological Review, 85,* 363–94.

Lewis, C. H., & Anderson, J. R. (1976). Interference with real world knowledge. *Cognitive Psychology, 8,* 311–35.

Lichtenstein, E. H., & Brewer, W. F. (1980). Memory for goal-directed events. *Cognitive Psychology, 12,* 412–45.

Mandler, J. M. (1984). *Stories, scripts, and scenes: Aspects of schema theory.* Hillsdale, NJ: Erlbaum.

Mandler, J. M., & Goodman, M. S. (1982). On the psychological validity of story structure. *Journal of Verbal Learning and Verbal Behavior, 21,* 507–23.

Mandler, J. M., & Johnson, N. S. (1977). Remembrance of things parsed: Story structure and recall. *Cognitive Psychology, 9,* 111–51.

Mani, K., & Johnson-Laird, P. N. (1982). The mental representation of spatial descriptions. *Memory & Cognition, 10,* 181–7.

Mayer, R. E. (1982). Instructional variables in text processing. In A. Flammer & W. Kintsch (Eds.), *Discourse processing* (pp. 445–61). Amsterdam: North-Holland.
    (1985). Structural analysis of science prose: Can we increase problem-solving performance? In B. K. Britton & J. B. Black (Eds.), *Understanding expository text* (pp. 65–87). Hillsdale, NJ: Erlbaum.

McGuire, W. J. (1985). Attitudes and attitude change. In G. Lindzey & E. Aronson (Eds.), *Handbook of social psychology* (3rd ed., pp. 233–346). New York: Random House.

Meehan, J. R. (1982). Stories and cognition: Comments on Robert de Beaugrande's "The story of grammars and the grammar of stories." *Journal of Pragmatics, 6,* 455–62.

Meyer, B. J. F. (1977). The structure of prose: Effects on learning and memory and implications for educational practice. In R. C. Anderson, R. J. Spiro, & W. E. Montague (Eds.), *Schooling and the acquisition of knowledge* (pp. 179–200). Hillsdale, NJ: Erlbaum.

(1984). Text dimensions and cognitive processing. In H. Mandl, N. L. Stein, & T. Trabasso (Eds.), *Learning and comprehension of text* (pp. 3–51). Hillsdale, NJ: Erlbaum.

(1985). Prose analysis: Purposes, procedures, and problems. In B. K. Britton & J. B. Black (Eds.), *Understanding expository text* (pp. 11–64). Hillsdale, NJ: Erlbaum.

Minsky, M. (1975). A framework for representing knowledge. In P. H. Winston (Ed.), *The psychology of computer vision* (pp. 211–77). New York: McGraw-Hill.

Nakamura, G. V., Graesser, A. C., Zimmerman, J. A., & Riha, J. (1985). Script processing in a natural situation. *Memory & Cognition, 13,* 140–4.

Omanson, R. C. (1982). The relation between centrality and story category variation. *Journal of Verbal Learning and Verbal Behavior, 21,* 326–37.

Owens, J., Bower, G. H., & Black, J. B. (1979). The "soap opera" effect in story recall. *Memory & Cognition, 7,* 185–91.

Perrig, W., & Kintsch, W. (1985). Propositional and situational representations of text. *Journal of Memory and Language, 24,* 503–18.

Pichert, J. W., & Anderson, R. (1977). Taking different perspectives on a story. *Journal of Educational Psychology, 69,* 309–15.

Ratcliff, R., & McKoon, G. (1978). Priming in item recognition: Evidence for the propositional structure of sentences. *Journal of Verbal Learning and Verbal Behavior, 17,* 403–18.

Rieger, C. J. (1975). Conceptual memory and inference. In R. C. Schank (Ed.), *Conceptual information processing* (pp. 157–288). New York: Elsevier.

Rubin, D. C., & Kontis, T. C. (1983). A schema for common cents. *Memory & Cognition, 11,* 335–41.

Rumelhart, D. E. (1975). Notes on a schema for stories. In D. G. Bobrow & A. Collins (Eds.), *Representation and understanding: Studies in cognitive science* (pp. 211–36). New York: Academic Press.

(1977). Understanding and summarizing brief stories. In D. LaBerge & S. J. Samuels (Eds.), *Basic processes in reading: Perception and comprehension* (pp. 265–303). Hillsdale, NJ: Erlbaum.

(1980a). Schemata: The building blocks of cognition. In R. J. Spiro, B. C. Bruce, & W. F. Brewer (Eds.), *Theoretical issues in reading comprehension: Perspectives from cognitive psychology, linguistics, artificial intelligence, and education* (pp. 33–58). Hillsdale, NJ: Erlbaum.

(1980b). A reply to Black and Wilensky. *Cognitive Science, 4,* 313–16.

Rumelhart, D. E., & Ortony, A. (1977). The representation of knowledge in memory. In R. C. Anderson, R. J. Spiro, & W. E. Montague (Eds.), *Schooling and the acquisition of knowledge* (pp. 99–135). Hillsdale, NJ: Erlbaum.

Sanford, A. J., & Garrod, S. C. (1981). *Understanding written language.* New York: Wiley.

Schank, R. C. (1975). *Conceptual information processing.* New York: Elsevier.

(1982). *Dynamic memory.* Cambridge University Press.

Schank, R. C., & Abelson, R. P. (1977). *Scripts, plans, goals, and understanding.* Hillsdale, NJ: Erlbaum.

Schmandt-Besserat, D. (1978). The earliest precursor to writing. *Scientific American, 238,* 50–9.

Searle, J. R. (1975). The logical status of fictional discourse. *New Literary History, 6,* 319–32.

Seifert, C. M., Robertson, S. P., & Black, J. B. (1985). Types of inferences generated during reading. *Journal of Memory and Language, 24,* 405–22.

Sharkey, N. E., & Mitchell, D. C. (1985). Word recognition in a functional context: The use of scripts in reading. *Journal of Memory and Language, 24,* 253–70.

Spilich, G. J., Vesonder, G. T., Chiesi, H. L., & Voss, J. F. (1979). Text processing of domain-related information for individuals with high and low domain knowledge. *Journal of Verbal Learning and Verbal Behavior, 18,* 275–90.

Spiro, R. J. (1980). Accommodative reconstruction in prose recall. *Journal of Verbal Learning and Verbal Behavior, 19,* 84–95.

Stein, N. L., & Glenn, C. G. (1979). An analysis of story comprehension in elementary school children. In R. O. Freedle (Ed.), *New directions in discourse processing* (pp. 53–120). Norwood, NJ: Ablex.

Stein, N. L., & Trabasso, T. (1982). What's in a story: An approach to comprehension and instruction. In R. Glaser (Ed.), *Advances in instructional psychology* (Vol. 2, pp. 213–67). Hillsdale, NJ: Erlbaum.

Thorndyke, P. W. (1977). Cognitive structures in comprehension and memory of narrative discourse. *Cognitive Psychology, 9,* 77–110.

Trabasso, T., & van den Broek, P. (1985). Causal thinking and the representation of narrative events. *Journal of Memory and Language, 24,* 612–30.

Trabasso, T., Secco, T., & den van Broek, P. (1984). Causal cohesion and story coherence. In H. Mandl, N. L. Stein, & T. Trabasso (Eds.), *Learning and comprehension of text* (pp. 83–111). Hillsdale, NJ: Erlbaum.

Trabasso, T., & Sperry, L. L. (1985). Causal relatedness and importance of story events. *Journal of Memory and Language, 24,* 595–611.

Trabasso, T., Stein, N. L., & Johnson, L. R. (1981). Children's knowledge of events: A causal analysis of story structure. In G. H. Bower (Ed.), *The psychology of learning and motivation* (Vol. 15, pp. 237–82). New York: Academic Press.

van Dijk, T. A. (1977). Semantic macro-structures and knowledge frames in discourse comprehension. In M. A. Just & P. A. Carpenter (Eds.), *Cognitive processes in comprehension* (pp. 3–32). Hillsdale, NJ: Erlbaum.

   (1980). *Macrostructures.* Hillsdale, NJ: Erlbaum.

van Dijk, T. A., & Kintsch, W. (1983). *Strategies of discourse comprehension.* New York: Academic Press.

Walker, C. H., & Yekovich, F. R. (1984). Script-based inferences: Effects of text and knowledge variables on recognition memory. *Journal of Verbal Learning and Verbal Behavior, 23,* 357–70.

Walton, K. L. (1978). Fearing fictions. *Journal of Philosophy, 75,* 5–27.

Wilensky, R. (1982). Points: A theory of the structure of stories in memory. In W. G. Lehnert & M. H. Ringle (Eds.), *Strategies for natural language processing* (pp. 345–74). Hillsdale, NJ: Erlbaum.

10   Intelligence

Robert J. Sternberg

During most of the twentieth century, the dominant approach to theory, research, and practice in the field of human intelligence has been psychometric. Investigators taking this approach have examined patterns of individual differences in scores on mental tests, such as vocabulary, number facility, figure analogies, and mental rotation of geometric objects. Whereas psychometric theories deal primarily with the structural aspects of intelligence, cognitive theories deal primarily with its processing aspects. This chapter concentrates on these cognitive theories and, in general, the cognitive approach to understanding human intelligence.

The nature of information-processing components

The fundamental unit of analysis in most cognitive theories is the information-processing component. A component is an elementary information process that operates on the internal representation of objects or symbols (Newell & Simon, 1972; Sternberg, 1977). Components may translate a sensory input into a conceptual representation, transform one conceptual representation into another, or translate a conceptual representation into a motor output.

The organization of components of human intelligence

In this section we consider three theories of the organization of the information-processing components of intelligence.

Carroll's theory

According to Carroll (1976, 1981), performance on mental tests can be understood in terms of a relatively small number of basic information-processing components. Carroll has investigated the major tests used in both psychometric and cognitive research. On the basis of a "logical and partly intuitive analysis of the task" (Carroll, 1981, p. 14), Carroll has identified a tentative list of 10 types of cognitive components.

1. *Monitor.* This process is a cognitive set or "determining tendency" that drives the operation of other processes during the course of task performance.

267

2. *Attention.* This process evolves from an individual's expectations regarding the type and number of stimuli that are to be presented in the course of task performance.
3. *Apprehension.* This process is used in the registering of a stimulus in a sensory buffer.
4. *Perceptual integration.* This process is used in the perception of the stimulus or the attainment of perceptual closure of a stimulus and its matching with any previously formed memory representation.
5. *Encoding.* This process is used in forming a mental representation of the stimulus and in its interpretation in terms of its attributes, associations, or meaning, depending on the requirements of a particular task.
6. *Comparison.* This process is used to determine whether two stimuli are the same or at least of the same class.
7. *Corepresentation-formation.* This process is used to establish a new representation in memory in association with a representation that is already there.
8. *Corepresentation-retrieval.* This process is used to find in memory a particular representation in association with another representation on the basis of some rule or other basis for the association.
9. *Transformation.* This process is used to transform or change a mental representation on some prespecified basis.
10. *Response-execution.* This process is used to operate on some mental representation in such a way as to produce either an overt or a covert response.

Carroll (1981) emphasizes that this list may not cover all of the processes that might eventually be identified in the analysis of elementary cognitive tasks; however, it does include all of the processes that he has been able to identify so far. Although he is not certain that all of the processes are mutually distinct, they seem to be different enough to serve as the basis for an information-processing analysis of intelligent task performance.

In his 1981 article, Carroll analyzes a choice reaction-time task in terms of this set of processes. An individual is presented with two or more stimuli, for example, bulbs that can be lit. The subject's task is to make one of several responses as a function of what happens to a given stimulus. For example, there might be two light bulbs, one on the left and one on the right. The subject's task might be to press a button with his or her left hand if the bulb on the left lights up and to press a button with his or her right hand if the bulb on the right lights up (see also Jensen, 1980). Carroll's task analysis shows that the successful execution of even as simple a task as this requires a long and complicated set of information-processing components.

Brown's theory

Brown (1978; Brown & Campione, 1978; Campione & Brown, 1978) has divided processes of cognition into two kinds: metacognitive processes, which are executive skills used to control one's information processing, and cognitive processes, which are nonexecutive skills used to implement task strategies. An essentially identical distinction has been proposed by a number of other investigators, for example, Butterfield and Belmont (1977), Flavell (1981), Markman (1981), and Reitman (1965). In Brown's version of this process dichotomy, five metacognitive processes are of particular importance: (a) *planning* one's next move in executing a strategy, (b) *monitoring* the effectiveness of individual steps in a strategy, (c) *testing* one's strategy as one performs it, (d) *revising* one's strategy as the need arises, and (e) *evaluating* one's strategy in order to determine its effectiveness. Metacognitive processes such as these are used to decide which cognitive processes are appropriate for completing a task. For example, these processes might be used to decide that, in a learning task, the cognitive processes involved in rehearsal of material provide an appropriate way of memorizing a list of words.

Sternberg's theory

Sternberg (1980b, 1985) distinguishes among three kinds of information-processing components.

Metacomponents are higher order control processes used for executive planning, monitoring, and evaluation of one's performance in a task. Metacomponents are comparable to what Brown refers to as metacognitive processes. Collectively, these processes are sometimes referred to by psychologists as the *executive* or the *homunculus*. The eight metacomponents believed to be most important in intelligent functioning are (a) recognizing that a problem exists, (b) recognizing the nature of the problem, (c) selecting a set of lower order nonexecutive components for performance of a task, (d) selecting a strategy for task performance into which to combine the lower order components, (e) selecting one or more mental representations for information, (f) deciding how to allocate attentional resources, (g) monitoring or keeping track of one's place in task performance and of what has been done and has to be done, and (h) understanding internal and external feedback about the quality of task performance.

Performance components are lower order processes used to execute various strategies in task performance. Three examples are (a) *encoding* the nature of a stimulus, (b) *inferring* the relations between two stimulus terms that are similar in some ways and different in others, and (c) *applying* a previously inferred relation to a new situation.

Knowledge-acquisition components are processes involved in learning new information and storing it in memory. The three knowledge-acquisition components believed to be most important in intelligent functioning are (a) *selective encoding,* by which new information relevant to the process of learning is sifted out from irrelevant new information; (b) *selective combination,* by which the selectively encoded information is combined to maximize its internal coherence, or connectedness; and (c) *selective comparison,* by which the selectively encoded and combined information is related to information already stored in memory so as to maximize the connectedness of the newly formed knowledge structure to previously formed knowledge structures.

One applies these three kinds of components in task performance in order to reach a solution or attain some other goal. Components vary widely in the range of tasks to which they apply. Some components, especially meta-components, appear to be applicable over a wide range of tasks. Other components apply to a smaller range of tasks, and some apply to only a narrow range. The last-named components are of little theoretical interest and generally are of little practical interest.

Understanding human abilities from a cognitive point of view

In this section, some of the major sources of variation in performance on intelligence tests are considered with an eye toward understanding the information-processing bases of these abilities. The abilities considered here are verbal ability, quantitative ability, inductive and deductive reasoning abilities, learning and memory abilities, and spatial ability.

Verbal ability

Verbal ability is sometimes divided into two separate kinds of skills: verbal comprehension and verbal fluency (Thurstone, 1938). *Verbal comprehension* refers to a person's ability to understand linguistic material such as newspapers, magazines, textbooks, and lectures. *Verbal fluency* refers to a person's ability to generate words and strings of words easily and rapidly. Verbal comprehension is typically measured by tests such as reading comprehension and vocabulary. Verbal fluency is typically measured by tests such as word generation. For example, an individual might be asked to think of as many words as possible beginning with the letter *b* in, say, five minutes. In this section, only verbal comprehension will be considered, because it has received much more attention in psychological research than has verbal fluency.

Verbal comprehension abilities have been recognized as an integral part of intelligence in both psychometric theories (e.g., Guilford, 1967; Thurstone, 1938; Vernon, 1971) and information-processing theories (e.g., Carroll, 1976; Heim, 1970; Sternberg, 1980b) and have, under a variety of aliases, been a major topic of research in differential and experimental psychology for many years.

Three major information-processing approaches to understanding the nature of verbal comprehension are a knowledge-based approach, a bottom-up approach, and a top-down approach. The knowledge-based approach deals with the role of prior information in the acquisition of new information. The bottom-up approach deals with the speed of execution of certain very basic mechanistic cognitive processes. The top-down approach deals with the higher order utilization of cues in understanding complex verbal material. The three approaches are complementary rather than contradictory.

The knowledge-based approach. The knowledge-based approach assigns a central role to old knowledge in the acquisition of new knowledge. Although *knowledge* is often referred to in the sense of domain-specific knowledge, the knowledge-based approach can also encompass research focusing on general world knowledge, knowledge of structures or classes of text (as in story grammars), and knowledge about strategies for knowledge acquisition and application (see, e.g., Bisanz & Voss, 1981). Proponents of this approach differ in the respective roles they assign to knowledge and process in the acquisition of new knowledge.

Those who advocate this approach usually cite instances of differences between expert and novice performance − in verbal and other domains − that seem to derive more from knowledge differences than from processing differences. For example, Keil (1984) suggests that development in the use of metaphor and in the use of defining features of words is due more to differential knowledge states than to differential use of processes or speed of process execution. Chi (1978) has shown that whether children's recall performance is better than adults' depends on the knowledge domain in which the recall takes place and, particularly, the relative expertise of the children and the adults in the respective domains. Finally, Chase and Simon (1973) found that differences between expert and novice performance in chess seemed largely due to differential knowledge structures rather than processes.

The bottom-up approach. Bottom-up research has emerged from the tradition of investigation initiated by Earl Hunt (e.g., Hunt, 1978; Hunt, Lunneborg, & Lewis, 1975) and followed up by a number of other investigators (e.g., Jackson & McClelland, 1979; Keating & Bobbitt, 1978; see also Perfetti & Lesgold, 1977, for a related approach). According to Hunt (1978), two types of processes underlie verbal comprehension ability: knowledge-based processes and mechanistic (information-free) processes. Hunt's approach has emphasized the latter. Hunt et al. (1975) studied three aspects of what they called *current information processing,* which they believed to be key determinants of individual differences in developed verbal ability:

(a) sensitivity of overlearned codes to arousal by incoming stimulus information, (b) the accuracy with which temporal tags can be assigned, and hence order information can be processed, and (c) the speed with which the internal representations in STM and intermediate term memory (ITM, memory for events occurring over minutes) can be created and altered. (p. 197)

Their basic hypothesis was that individuals varying in verbal ability differ even in these low-level mechanistic skills − skills that are free from any contribution of disparate knowledge or experience. Intelligence tests are hypothesized to measure indirectly these basic information-processing skills by measuring directly the products of these skills, both in terms of their past contribution to the acquisition and storage of knowledge (such as vocabulary) and in terms of their present contribution to the current processing of information.

For example, in a typical experiment, subjects are presented with the Posner and Mitchell (1967) letter-matching task. The task comprises two experimental conditions: a physical-match condition and a name-match condition. In the physical-match condition, subjects are presented with pairs of letters that either are or are not physical matches (e.g., *AA* or *bb* versus *Aa* or *Ba*). In the name-match condition, subjects are presented with pairs of letters that either are or are not name matches (e.g., *Aa, BB,* or *bB* versus *Ab, ba,* or *bA*). Subjects must identify the letter pair either as a physical match (or mismatch) or as a name match (or mismatch) as rapidly as possible. The typical finding of these experiments is that the difference between mean name-match and physical-match times for each of a group of subjects is correlated about −.3 with scores on tests of verbal ability. The theoretical interpretation of this finding is that speed of lexical access, as measured by name-match minus physical-match time, is in some sense causal of acquired level of verbal ability.

The top-down approach. Top-down processing refers to expectation- or inference-driven processing, or to knowledge-based processing, to use Hunt's (1978) terminology. Top-down processing has been an extremely popular focus of research in the past decade: many researchers have attempted to identify and predict the sorts of inferences a person is likely to draw from a text and the effect of these inferences (or lack of inferences) on text comprehension (see, e.g., Kintsch & van Dijk, 1978; Rieger, 1975; Rumelhart, 1980; Schank & Abelson, 1977; Thorndyke, 1976). Usually, top-down researchers examine the way in which people combine information present in the text with their own store of world knowledge to create a new whole representing the meaning of the text (e.g., Bransford, Barclay, & Franks, 1972). To our knowledge, however, the top-down approach, although often used in models of text processing in general, has been only minimally applied to understanding individual differences in verbal ability or to understanding vocabulary acquisition as a special subset of knowledge acquisition.

The first of a handful of investigators who looked at the use of inference in the acquisition of word meanings from context were Werner and Kaplan (1952), who proposed that a child acquires the meanings of words principally in two ways. One is by explicit reference, either verbal or objective; the child learns to understand verbal symbols through the adult's direct naming of objects or through verbal definition. The second way is implicit or contextual reference. The meaning of a word is grasped in the course of conversation; that is, it is inferred from the cues of the verbal context (p. 3).

Werner and Kaplan (1952) were especially interested in the second way of acquiring word meanings – the inference of meaning from context. They devised a task in which subjects were presented with an imaginary word followed by six sentences containing that word. The subjects' task was to guess the meaning of the word on the basis of the contextual cues they were given. An example of the 12 imaginary words used is *contavish,* which Werner and Kaplan intended to mean *hole.* They presented the children with six sentences (p. 4):

1. You can't fill anything with a contavish.
2. The more you take out of a contavish the larger it gets.
3. Before the house is finished the walls must have contavishes.
4. You can't feel or touch a contavish.
5. A bottle has only one contavish.
6. John fell into a contavish in the road.

Children ranging in age from 8 to 13 years were tested on their ability to acquire new words presented in this way. Developmental patterns were analyzed in a number of ways. Werner and Kaplan (1952) found that (a) performance improves gradually with age, although the processes that underlie performance do not necessarily change gradually; (b) there is an early and abrupt decline in signs of immaturity that are related to inadequate orientation toward the task; (c) the processes of signification for words undergo a rather decisive shift between approximately 10 and 11 years of age; and (d) language behavior shows different organization at different ages.

Daalen-Kapteijns and Elshout-Mohr (1981) pursued the Werner–Kaplan approach by asking subjects to think aloud while solving Werner–Kaplan type of problems. They proposed an ideal strategy for learning from context with which subjects could form a model (provisional representation) of the meaning of a new word. According to this strategy, (a) the sentence is reformulated so that it can be brought to bear directly on the neologism (e.g., in Sentence 1 above, the strategy might yield the statement that "a contavish is not a substance that can be used to fill anything") and (b) the reformulated information is transformed into an aspect of the meaning of the neologism (e.g., "a contavish may be some kind of absence of substance").

Using ingenious protocol-analysis techniques, the investigators found that (a) word acquisition is guided by models, an initial model being chosen on the basis of the interpretation of the new word's meaning in the first sentence and subsequent processing being guided by this model; (b) the processing of each new word presentation in context can lead to the filling of slots in the model, to the adjustment of these slots, or to the formation of a new model altogether; (c) if the model is not sufficiently well articulated to permit active search and evaluation of possibly relevant information, as tends to be the case for low-verbal subjects, model-guided search can be replaced by the subsequent use of step (b) of this strategy; and (d) high- and low-verbal subjects learn word meanings differently, high-verbal subjects generally using both steps of the ideal strategy and low-verbal subjects generally using only the first step (sentence-based processing).

Whereas Daalen-Kapteijns and Elshout-Mohr (1981) specified strategies for word acquisition in some detail but the mental representation (what they referred to as the model) of information about the word in only minimal detail, Keil (1981) specified representation in considerable detail but strategy in only minimal detail. Keil presented children in kindergarten and grades 2 and 4 with simple stories in which an unfamiliar word was described by a single paragraph. The following is an example of such a story: "*Throstles* are great except when they have to be fixed. And they have to be fixed very often. But it's usually very easy to fix throstles." Subjects were asked what else they knew about the new word and what sorts of things the new word described. Keil found that even the youngest children could make sensible inferences about the general categories denoted by new terms and about the properties the terms might reasonably have. Errors were systematic and in accordance with Keil's (1979, 1981) theory of the structure of ontological knowledge. This theory provides a powerful basis for inferring a possible structure for storing (at least ontological) information about the meaning of a new word and for inferring the possible predicates of the word.

Jensen (1980) suggested that vocabulary is such a good measure of intelligence "because the acquisition of word meanings is highly dependent on the *eduction* of meaning from the contexts in which the words are encountered" (p. 146). Marshalek (1981) tested this hypothesis by using a faceted vocabulary test, although he did not directly measure learning from context. The vocabulary test was administered with a battery of standard reasoning and other tests. Marshalek found that (a) subjects sometimes gave correct examples of the way a given word is used in sentences, despite having inferred incorrect defining features of the word; (b) subjects with low reasoning ability had major difficulties in inferring word meanings; and (c) reasoning was related to vocabulary measures at the lower end of the vocabulary difficulty distribution but not at the higher end. Together, these findings suggested that a certain level of reasoning ability may be a prerequisite for the extraction of word meanings. Above this level, the importance of reasoning begins to decrease rapidly.

It has been assumed so far that the ability to learn from external context leads to a higher vocabulary level. It should be pointed out, however, that the relationship between learning from context and level of vocabulary is probably bidirectional (Anderson & Freebody, 1979; Sternberg, 1980b): Learning from context can facilitate an increase in vocabulary level at the same time that a higher vocabulary level can facilitate learning from context.

Sternberg and Powell (1983) presented a theory of verbal comprehension ability based on learning from context. The theory has three parts: contextual cues, mediating variables, and component processes of verbal learning.

Contextual cues are hints contained in a passage that facilitate (or, in theory and sometimes in practice, impede) the deciphering of the meaning of an unknown word. Consider the sentence "At dawn, the *blen* arose on the horizon and shone brightly." This sentence contains several external contextual cues that could facilitate one's inferring that *blen* means "sun." "At dawn" provides a temporal cue, describing when the blen arose; "arose" provides a functional descriptive cue, describing an action that a blen could perform; "on the horizon" provides a spatial cue, describing where the blen arose; "shone" provides another functional descriptive cue, describing a second action a blen could perform; finally, "brightly" provides a stative descriptive cue, describing a property (brightness) of the shining of the blen. With all of these cues, most people would find it very easy to figure out that the neologism *blen* is a synonym for the familiar word *sun*.

Whereas contextual cues provide information that might be used to infer the meaning of a word from a given verbal context, not all cues are applicable to a given concept, nor do all cues enable one to weed out irrelevant information or integrate the information gleaned into a coherent model of the word's meaning. For this reason, there is a set of mediating variables that specify relations between a previously unknown word and the passage in which it occurs and that mediate the usefulness of the contextual cues. Thus, whereas the contextual cues specify the information that an individual might use to figure out the meaning of an unfamiliar word, mediating variables specify those textual elements that can affect, either positively or negatively, the application of the contextual cues present in a given situation.

Consider, for example, how the variable "variability of contexts in which multiple occurrences of the unknown word appear" can mediate the utilization of contextual cues. Different contexts − for example, different kinds of subject matter or different writing styles, and even different contexts of a given type, such as two different illustrations in a given text of the use of a word − are likely to supply different types of information about the unknown word. Variability of contexts increases the likelihood that a wide range of cues will be supplied about a given word and thus increases the probability that a reader will get a full picture of a given word's meaning. In contrast, mere repetition of an unknown word in essentially the same context as that in which it previously appeared is unlikely to be as helpful as a variable-context repetition because it provides few or no new cues regarding the word's meaning. Variability can also present a problem in some situations and for some individuals: If the information is presented in a way that makes it difficult to integrate its parts, or if a given individual finds it difficult to make such an integration, then variable repetition may actually obfuscate rather than clarify the word's meaning. In some situations and for some individuals, variable contexts may cause a stimulus overload to occur, resulting in reduced rather than increased understanding. The other mediating variables for external context can similarly facilitate or inhibit the acquisition of a word's meaning from a given text.

Three components of knowledge acquisition are critical for the acquisition of word meanings and of verbal concepts in general: (a) selective encoding, (b) selective combination, and (c) selective comparison. Selective encoding involves sifting out relevant information from irrelevant information. When new information is presented in natural contexts, information that is relevant to one's purposes is embedded in a large amount of irrelevant information. A critical task facing the individual is that of sifting the wheat from the chaff: recognizing what information is relevant for his or her purposes. Selective combination involves combining selectively encoded information in such a way as to form an integrated, plausible whole. Simply sifting out relevant from irrelevant information is not enough to generate a new knowledge structure; one must know how to combine the pieces of information into an internally connected whole (see Mayer & Greeno, 1972). Selective comparison involves relating newly acquired information to information acquired in the past. Deciding what information to encode and how to combine it does not occur in a vacuum; rather, it is guided by the retrieval of old information. New information is all but useless if one cannot relate it to old knowledge in order to form an externally connected whole (Mayer & Greeno, 1972).

We initially tested the theory of decontextualization by asking 123 high school students to read 32 passages that were roughly 125 words in length and contained from one to four extremely low-frequency words (Sternberg & Powell, 1983). Thirty-seven such words (all nouns) were used in the passages; each target word could appear from one to four times, resulting in a total of 71 presentations. Passages were equally divided among four different writing styles: literary, newspaper, scientific, and historical. An additional sample passage was written in the literary style.

The students' task was to define as best they could each of the low-frequency words in each passage. (If a word appeared more than once in a given passage, only a single definition was required.) Students were not permitted to look back to earlier passages and definitions in making their current responses. Experienced raters evaluated the quality of the students' definitions. The correlations between predicted and observed goodness ratings were .92 for literary passages, .74 for newspaper passages, .85 for science passages, and .77 for history passages. All of these values were statistically significant. In an external-validation procedure, subjects' scores (mean rated goodness of all written definitions) on the learning-from-context task were correlated with scores on the psychometric tests. Correlations for the various passage types combined were .62 with IQ, .56 with vocabulary, and

.65 with reading comprehension. Correlations with the psychometric test scores were similar for learning-from-context scores computed for the individual passage types.

To conclude, three major approaches to the study of verbal comprehension have been proposed: knowledge-based, bottom-up, and top-down. Each deals with a somewhat different aspect of verbal comprehension. Ultimately, a complete theory will integrate aspects of all three theories.

Quantitative ability

Whereas models of verbal comprehension have been cast in the role of general models of the whole verbal comprehension domain, models of quantitative ability are generally models of more limited subdomains of knowledge and information processing. It is not clear whether the models of verbal ability actually are more general; it seems as likely that the major difference in generality with respect to models of quantitative ability lies in the generality of claims rather than that of coverage. In this section, I deal with two domains: computational and problem-solving abilities.

Computational abilities. The most salient ability of children in the primary grades is probably computational. At the very least, primary school children must demonstrate facility in addition and subtraction. The component skills involved in addition and subtraction have been studied by cognitive psychologists.

Groen and Parkman (1972) proposed three alternative models of the way children (as well as adults) add pairs of numbers. These models are predicated upon the assumption that addition processes can be understood as a set of discrete, serial operations. A *counter* is set to some initial value. Subsequently, an iterative process is executed whereby the value of the counter is incremented until it reaches the sum of two numbers. In order to illustrate how the three models differ from one another, I will show how they apply to the simple addition problem $4 + 2 = 6$.

In one model, Model A, the counter is initially set to zero. Then, it is incremented by the value of the first of the two addends. Finally, it is incremented by the value of the second addend. The final value of the counter is the sum of the two numbers. In the example, the counter is initially set to 0; then it is incremented by 4, the value of the first addend; finally, it is incremented by 2, the value of the second addend. The sum is thus found to be 6. Note that, in this model, the counter is incremented six times. In more general terms, if M is the first addend and N the second, the counter is incremented $M + N$ times. The number of increments made to the counter is important for predicting the reaction time for the computation of sums. The model predicts that reaction time will vary linearly as a function of $M + N$.

In Model B, the counter is initialized not as 0, but as a value corresponding to the first addend. After this initialization, the counter is incremented by a number of times corresponding to the value of the second addend. In the example, the counter is initially set at 4. It is then incremented by 2, so that the final value of the sum is 6. Note that, in this model, it is necessary to increment the counter only two, rather than six, times. In general, the number of times the counter must be incremented is equal to N, where N is the value of the second addend. Note that the predictions this model makes about reaction time are quite different from those made by model A. Whereas in Model A, reaction time is a linear function of $M + N$, in Model B, reaction time is a linear function simply of N.

In Model C, the counter is initially set to the value of whichever of the two addends is greater. The incrementing procedure is then applied to the other of the two addends. In the example, the counter would initially be set to 4 and then incremented by 2. Thus, for this problem, the predictions of Models B and C are identical. However, for $2 + 4 = 6$, the predictions of the models would be different. In Model B, the counter would initially be set to 2 and then incremented by 4; in Model C, the counter would initially be set to 4 and then incremented by 2. In Model C, therefore, reaction time is a linear function of either M or N, depending on which of these values is smaller.

Groen conducted a number of experiments to compare the fits of these three alternative models to reaction-time data for subjects solving addition problems. One study (Groen & Parkman, 1972) compared the capacities of the models to account for the reaction times of first graders. Groen and Parkman found that virtually all of the first-grade children used Model C, the most sophisticated of the three models. It thus appears that even young children are able to employ a relatively sophisticated strategy in solving simple addition problems. It should be noted that the model seems not to apply to problems in which both of the addends have the same value, for example, $3 + 3 = 6$ or $4 + 4 = 8$. Such problems are solved more rapidly than would be predicted by the model. This result suggests that the sums of addition problems in which both addends have the same value may be prestored in long-term memory. Some of these sums need not be computed when children are presented with such problems.

Woods, Resnick, and Groen (1975) extended this kind of information-processing modeling to subtraction, with good results. But the linear-modeling approach that characterizes the research described above is not the only approach to the understanding of arithmetic computation. Brown and Burton (1978) and Ginsburg (1977) have sought to understand the sources of error in children's computational algorithms. They even developed a computer program, BUGGY, that analyzes students' algorithms for three-column subtraction. The program analyzes students' answers to a large number of three-column subtractions, for example, $436 - 281 = 155$. If a student answers all items correctly, BUGGY categorizes the student as having used the correct algorithm for subtraction. If there are errors, however, BUGGY attempts to find the "bug" or "bugs" that best account for the source of the errors. Some examples of bugs are (a) not knowing how to borrow from zero, (b) not knowing how to subtract a larger digit from a smaller digit, and (c) not knowing how to subtract a digit from zero. It is interesting that, although the BUGGY program was able to identify hundreds of bugs or combinations of bugs in students' performance, it did not by any means diagnose all of the sources of students' errors. In fact, the program was able to find algorithms that either totally or partially produced the answers given by only 43% of the students. The remaining errors were either random or were at least in part inconsistent in the kinds of bugs involved. Thus, although the approach of Brown and Burton enables one to identify quite precisely the kinds of knowledge about computation students lack, it does so only for some problems and for some people.

To conclude, at least two approaches have yielded some success in understanding the way people solve arithmetic computation problems. One is based on information-processing modeling of the components individuals use in solving problems such as addition and subtraction. The idea is to predict *reaction time* in solving computation problems. The second approach involves the prediction of errors in solving computation problems. A computer program analyzes the kinds of errors students make in order to reveal what facts about computation they lack. Clearly, the two approaches are complementary rather than mutually exclusive. It would be useful to combine them in order to understand both the speed and accuracy with which people solve arithmetic computation problems.

Problem-solving ability. Mathematical problem solving is often broken down into two basic steps (Bobrow, 1968; Hayes, 1981; Mayer, 1983): problem representation and problem solution. In problem representation, a problem is converted from a series of words and numbers into an internal mental representation of the relevant terms. In problem solution, operations are performed so as to deduce a solution to the problem from the internal mental representation. Each of these stages is a source of differences among individuals' overall problem-solving abilities.

A striking example of the potential difficulty of problem representation, even for college students, was provided by Soloway, Lochhead, and Clement (1982). These investigators asked college students to represent statements such as "There are six times as many students as professors at this university" in terms of an equation. Roughly one-third of the students represented problems such as this one incorrectly. In this example, they represented the problem by the incorrect equation $6S = P$, where S refers to student and P to professor. An interesting sideline to this experiment showed the powerful effect of mental representation on students' ability to represent problems correctly. Consider the following problem: "At the last company cocktail party, for every 6 people who drank hard liquor, there were 11 people who drank beer." Some students were asked to translate this statement into a mathematical equation; other students were asked to translate the statement into a short program in the BASIC computer language. The error rate for students translating the problem into an equation was 55%, whereas the error rate for students translating the problem into the computer language was only 31%.

Mayer (1982) has also studied the ability of college students to represent mathematical problems. Two sets of data analyses are of particular interest in this research. In order to illustrate these analyses, I will consider the following algebra problem: "A river steamer travels 36 miles downstream in the same time that it travels 24 miles upstream. The steamer's engine drives in still water at a rate of 12 miles per hour more than the rate of the current. Find the rate of the current." The students were asked to recall problems such as these as well as they could.

In the first set of data analyses, Mayer focused on the kinds of content students tended most to forget. He divided problem content into three kinds: *assignments,* which assigned a value to a variable, for example, "A river steamer travels 36 miles downstream"; *relations*, which express a quantitative relation between two variables, for example, "The steamer's engines drive in still water at a rate of 12 miles per hour more than the rate of the current"; and *questions,* which ask for a solution to the problem, for example, "Find the rate of the current." Mayer found that students made about three times as many errors in recalling relational propositions (error rate, 29%) as in recalling assignment propositions (error rate, 9%). This result is consistent with that of Soloway et al. and others in suggesting that students have the greatest difficulty in representing relational information about mathematical problems.

In the second set of data analyses, Mayer examined the kinds of errors students make in recalling propositions: *omission errors,* in which the proposition is not recalled; *specification errors,* in which a variable in the original proposition is somehow changed to a different variable in recall (e.g., "A river steamer travels 36 miles downstream" is recalled as "A boat travels 36 mph downstream"); and *conversion errors,* in which the form of the proposition is changed from an assignment to a relation, or vice versa (e.g., "The steamer's engine drives in still water at 12 miles per hour more than the rate of the current" is translated into "The steamer's engine drives in still water at 12 miles per hour"). By far the largest proportion of errors was in errors of omission. The smallest number of errors was in errors of conversion. This pattern held true for assignment relations and questions. It is interesting that there was a systematic bias in the form taken by conversion errors. Of 21 cases of conversion, 20 involved changing a relation into an assignment, whereas only 1 involved changing an assignment into a relation. Thus, one can begin to see that students' greatest difficulty appears to lie in their represention of relational information.

Davidson and Sternberg (1984) compared the abilities of gifted and nongifted students to solve quantitative insight problems. An example of such a problem is as follows: "A man has black socks and blue socks in a drawer mixed in a ratio of 4 to 5. It is dark, and so the man cannot see the colors of the socks he removes from the drawer. How many socks need the man remove from the drawer in order to be assured of having a pair of socks of the same color?" The correct answer to the problem is 3. Davidson and Sternberg tested the hypothesis that the poorer performance of the nongifted students could be traced in part to their failure to generate spontaneously three kinds of insights: (a) *selective encoding,* in which information relevant to problem solution is distinguished from irrelevant information; (b) *selective combination*, in which relevant information is combined in such a way that the problem can be solved; and (c) *selective comparison,* in which new information in the problem is related to old information stored in long-term memory. In order to test this hypothesis, problems such as the socks problem were presented in either of two ways. In the standard presentation, the students read the problem and had to solve it. In the second presentation, the students were given one of the three kinds of insight in order to facilitate their problem solution. For example, a selective-encoding insight was provided in each problem by the underlining of only information that was relevant to the solution. In the socks problem, for instance, the ratio information is irrelevant to the solution; yet many students attempt to use it in order to solve the problem. Davidson and Sternberg found that providing insights of each of the three kinds significantly facilitated the performance of only the nongifted students. The gifted students seemed to generate the insights on their own.

The steps involved in representing and solving mathematical problems can become complicated, and some investigators have sought to do justice to this degree of complication by constructing computer simulations of students' problem-solving processes. For example, Greeno (1978) wrote a computer program, PERDIX, that simulates the performance of high school students in solving geometry problems. In fact, Greeno formulated the project on the basis of a fairly extensive study of students' thinking-aloud protocols as provided in the course of their actual solution of geometry problems. Two important features of this program are its use of a generate-and-test strategy and its use of subgoals. The generate-and-test strategy is used when one knows what kind of information is needed at a given point during problem solution but does not know which information given in the problem is of this kind. According to this strategy, one scans the list of items that may provide the information needed and tests each one to see if it fits the context of the problem. Resnick and Ford (1981) provide a good example of the generate-and-test strategy. Suppose one is asked to find the list of all prime numbers (i.e., numbers whose only factors are themselves and 1) in the range from 1 to 50. Usually, one tests each number between 1 and 50 to determine whether it has any factors other than itself and 1.

Plane-geometry theorem proving is usually too complicated for the use of a single goal. In order to construct a proof, students usually set up a series of subgoals that they must meet as they make their way toward the final solution of the proof.

In conclusion, mathematical abilities involve a number of information-processing skills. At least some of these skills are hierarchically related. For example, computational skills presuppose counting skills, and problem-solving skills presuppose at least some computational skills. Information-processing analyses of ability can tend to obscure the overall picture of quantitative abilities. Although quantitative abilities can be decomposed into a large number of component information processes, the abilities to use these processes are certainly correlated. Thus, some people seem to have greater quantitative ability, overall, than other people. There is a need for theories that combine the best aspects of psychometric and information-processing analysis. Psychometric analysis gives one a good sense of quantitative ability as comprising one factor or, at most, a small number of factors. It does not, however, specify the processing components involved. Information-processing analysis can specify processing components, but it is often hard to see how they fit together into an overall ability structure. Thus, there is a need for a theory that specifies the information-processing components of quantitative abilities but that also specifies how these components fit together into a higher order ability that distinguishes more quantitatively capable people from less quantitatively capable ones.

Learning ability

The relation between learning ability and intelligence is a perplexing one. Intuitively, learning ability would seem to be closely related to, perhaps central to, intelligence. This intuition is captured by many definitions of intelligence in terms of learning. For example, in a 1921 symposium on the nature of intelligence, Buckingham defined intelligence as the ability to learn, and similarly Dearborn defined intelligence as a capacity to learn and profit by experience. Investigators such as these not only believed that learning is the central ingredient of intelligence, but proposed that measures of learning would form the most suitable measures of intelligence. For example, Thorndike (1924) argued that measures of learning could well form a single basis for evaluating intelligence.

Between the 1920s and 1940s, a considerable amount of research was done on the relation between learning ability and intelligence as measured by standard intelligence tests. To the surprise of many investigators, the results were largely negative: Learning performance did not seem to be very highly related to intelligence. Indeed, most of the studies found no relation at all. (For a review of this literature, see Estes, 1982.) By 1946, Woodrow, as much a learning theorist as Thorndike, claimed that "intelligence, far from being identical with the amount of improvement shown by practice, has practically nothing to do with the matter" (p. 151). It is no surprise that Woodrow came to this conclusion. His own work had yielded some of the most disappointing findings of all. In one study, Woodrow (1917) found no differences in the learning performance of normal and mentally retarded children. In another study, Woodrow (1938) found no relation between level of intelligence of college students and their learning ability.

Why did the studies of Woodrow and many others fail to reveal a link between learning performance and intelligence? There seem to be at least five reasons. First, these investigators may have been focusing on the wrong aspects of learning, at least to the extent that the purpose was to relate learning to intelligence. Consider some recent work that suggests that differences can be found in the learning performance of normal and retarded subjects if one investigates the right phenomena of learning.

A frequent observation in the memory literature is the serial-position curve, whereby items presented near the beginning and near the end of a list tend to be recalled more easily than items near the middle of the list. The superior recall of the earlier items (the primacy effect) is usually attributed to the effects of long-term memory, whereas the superior recall of the later items (the recency effect) is usually attributed to the effects of short-term memory (Crowder, 1976). Several investigators have found that manipulating the rate at which items are presented has an effect on normal subjects' recall of earlier items; specifically, faster presentation reduces recall of words near the beginning of the list (Glanzer & Cunitz, 1966). Glanzer and Cunitz suggested that slow presentation permits more rehearsal than does fast presentation and that increased rehearsal of earlier items leads to greater recall of these items.

Retarded subjects do not show a reduction in primacy with faster presentation. This interaction between the performance of the normal and the retarded led Ellis (1970) to conclude that mentally retarded performers simply do not rehearse (or minimally rehearse) items, even under conditions of slow presentation. It seems unlikely that the deficit of the retarded results from their inability to rehearse items. Presumably, almost anyone is capable of repeating presented words subvocally. Rather, it seems more likely that retarded performers simply do not choose to rehearse. Belmont and Butterfield (1971) conducted an experiment to test this hypothesis. They concluded that, indeed, the deficiency of retarded performers in the recall of early items is due in large part to their failure to rehearse but that this failure stems from their failure to generate an appropriate strategy for learning the items. When the retarded subjects were told to rehearse, they made significant gains in primacy recall. Thus, the difficulty of retarded subjects lies not in learning processes, but in the executive processes by which a strategy for learning is generated. Early investigators, however, studied learning per se rather than the executive processes that contribute to learning.

Another example of research with a more analytic focus is that of Zeaman and House (1963). These investigators had subjects perform a concept-learning task that involved learning to attend to a relevant dimension in concept learning and choosing the correct value along that dimension. In a typical experiment, subjects saw two objects in each of a series of trials. The objects differed along a number of dimensions, such as color, shape, size, and number. The subjects' task was to choose the "correct" object. What made a specific object correct was its having a particular value along a particular dimension. For example, the experimenter might define in advance the color red as the basis for a correct answer. In this case, an object would be correct if it were red, and incorrect otherwise. The subject would thus have to learn to attend to the dimension of color and the value of red in the concept-learning task. Zeaman and House used an elegant mathematical-modeling technique to find the locus of the difference between retarded and normal subjects in performing this concept-learning task. They found that the major source of differences between the two groups was attentional. The normal subjects were more likely to attend to the relevant dimension early during the learning trial. Note that in this work, as in the work of Belmont and Butterfield, the study of learning per se would not have been enough: Whereas the Belmont and Butterfield research showed the locus of differences between retarded and normal subjects to lie in executive processes, the Zeaman and House work showed the differences between retarded and normal subjects in concept learning to lie in attentional processes.

A second reason for the generally poor correlation between scores on simple learning tasks and scores on intelligence tests may be the nature of the tasks. Typical memory tasks involve such exercises as learning and remembering a list of words in the exact order that the words were presented (serial recall); learning pairs of words such that later, when only the first word of the pair is presented, the examinee can recall the second word in the pair (paired-associate recall); and learning a list of words that can later be recalled in any order (free recall). These so-called episodic memory tasks are notable for their simplicity and relative lack of meaningful content. For example, the words in a list are usually either unrelated to one another or related in only the most casual ways.

More recent research has focused on learning of meaningful materials.

For example, it was noted earlier that performance on the Sternberg—Powell (1983) learning-from-context task is correlated at a level of approximately .6 with scores on standard IQ tests. The ability to recall final words of successive sentences is correlated at about the same level with tests of verbal intelligence (Daneman & Carpenter, 1980). Brown and Smiley (1977, 1978) studied the ability of grade 3 through grade 12 students to identify essential organizing features and crucial elements of meaningful texts. These texts had previously been rated by college students as involving material varying in importance for learning the content of the text. Third graders made no reliable distinctions between levels of importance in their attempts to rate such levels. Fifth graders could distinguish only the highest level of importance from the other levels. Seventh graders did not differentiate the two intermediate levels of importance, but they were able to distinguish the least important and the most important elements in the text. Twelfth graders were able to distinguish all four levels of importance in the text. Brown and Smiley also found that, when children were given extra time for studying, their tendency to use active strategies for learning, such as note taking or underlining, increased with age. The youngest students tended to favor a passive strategy involving nothing more than rereading of the text, whereas the older children tended to favor the more active strategies. Subsequent recall of material was greater for strategy users than for those who failed to use an active strategy.

The third reason for the failure of early studies to find a relation between learning and intelligence is, ironically, the completeness and clarity of the directions for carrying out the tasks. A number of investigators, including Resnick and Glaser (1976) and Campione, Brown, and Bryant (1984), have suggested that intelligence may involve in large part the ability to learn from incomplete instructions. Rohwer (1973) investigated the use of elaborative processes in facilitating paired-associate learning. An example of an elaborative process would be learning a paired associate by the mental creation of a sentence linking the two words. For example, if the paired associate to be learned were lion—potato, the subject might form a sentence such as "The lion mashed the potato." Alternatively, the subject might form an interactive visual image of a physical relation between the two items in the paired associate. For example, the subject might imagine a scene in which a lion is chomping on a large potato. Rohwer provided a variety of cues to facilitate subjects' use of elaborative strategies. Some of these cues were more explicit than others. Rohwer found that the younger or less intelligent the subjects, the more they needed a more explicit cue in order to make use of an elaborative strategy and to improve performance.

The fourth reason that early studies found no relation between learning and intelligence was their concentration on the immediate results of learning rather than on the extent to which learning transfers. In much of our lives, the real function of learning is the transfer of what is learned in old situations to new situations. If we are unable to carry over knowledge to new situations, the knowledge is essentially useless to us. Ferrara (1982) studied the possibility that a major distinction between students of average mental ability and those of above-average mental ability lies in their levels of transfer of learning. She taught students rules for solving series completion problems, which require inductive reasoning. A typical series completion of the kind Ferrara used is A B A C A D __ __. The subject's task is to fill in the blanks.

Ferrara had all subjects learn how to solve these problems to a uniform criterion. She then investigated three kinds of learning via new series completion items. *Maintenance* items were new examples of the same problem types that the subjects had been taught. *Near-transfer* items involved the same kinds of relations that the subjects had been taught, but with new combinations of letters. *Far-transfer* items included new relations as well as other potential new features. Ferrara found that above-average children learned more quickly than did average children, although all children were able to learn the original material to criterion. The more interesting results concerned transfer. On the maintenance items, the performance of both the average and above-average subjects was almost perfect. Similarly, both groups of subjects did quite well on the near-transfer problems. On the far-transfer problems, however, large group differences emerged. The above-average subjects performed at a distinctly higher level than did the average subjects. Thus, the above-average subjects showed greater ability to transfer learning, even though their original learning was to the same criterion as that set for the average subjects.

The fifth reason for the low correlation in early studies between scores on learning tasks and intelligence is that, whereas the early studies used impoverished content with minimal semantic relatedness to test the relation between learning and intelligence, it may be precisely the opposite kind of material that most shows the relation. A number of investigators have now demonstrated the strong effect of prior knowledge on new learning, and because more intelligent individuals can be expected, on the average, to have a richer knowledge base than lower ability individuals, the more intelligent, higher knowledge individuals may learn more quickly.

What has become the classic study of the effect of knowledge on learning and recall was performed by Chase and Simon (1973). These investigators had individuals at various levels of expertise in chess learn and later recall patterns of chess pieces on a chessboard. The critical finding was that the better chess players were no better than the worse chess players at recalling the board configurations when the configurations were random (i.e., the pieces were placed on the board in a way that bore no correspondence to the way in which they would appear in a normal chess game). However, when the pieces were placed in sensible configurations, the chess experts' recall of the pieces was much better than the recall of the lesser players. A developmental twist to this finding was demonstrated by Chi (1978). Chi showed that, when child chess experts were pitted against adult chess novices in recall, the adults performed better on a standard task of memory span (serial recall of digits), but the children performed better in recalling configurations of pieces on a chessboard. In other words, the children's greater knowledge of chess enabled them to outperform the adults on the chess-recall task, even though their memory of less meaningful materials was inferior. In a related study, Chi and Koeske (1983) studied a child's recall of names of dinosaurs. These investigators had previously determined that some of the names of dinosaurs on the list to be learned were more well known than others. They found that recall of dinosaur names was largely a function of prior knowledge about the dinosaurs. In other words, the more familiar the dinosaur was to the subject before the experiment began, the more likely it was that the subject would recall the name of the dinosaur when it was presented in a list of words. Results similar to those reported by Chase and Simon and by Chi have been reported in other domains, such as the learning of baseball information (Chiesi, Spilich, & Voss, 1979).

An intriguing notion about the relation between learning and intelligence has been proposed by Vygotsky (1978) and expanded by Feuerstein (1979). This notion is the so-called zone of potential development. The idea is that a person's latent, or unexpressed, ability can be measured by the extent to which the person profits from guided instruction in performing a task. In other words, one would measure a person's zone of potential development by comparing the person's performance on a task without guided instruction to the person's performance with guided and graded instruction. Vygotsky and Feuerstein have claimed that individuals who profit from such sequenced instruction have latent ability that may not be measured by standard tests of intelligence. Brown and Ferrara (1985) have provided some evidence that this may be the case, but at present the zone of potential development remains an interesting but unverified construct.

To conclude, there definitely appears to be a relation between learning and intelligence, but this relation tended not to be expressed in early correlational studies involving simple learning tasks. There has been a tendency, however, for more recent studies emphasizing the role of fairly complex information processing to demonstrate the relation. It now appears that learning is central to intelligence, rather than peripheral or unrelated to it. But the learning that is related to intelligence is the kind that occurs in our everyday interactions with the environment, rather than the very simple kinds that have often been studied in the laboratories of experimental psychologists. Psychologists are often implored to make their research "ecologically valid," that is, relevant to performance in the real world. The results of the research on the relation between learning and intelligence show that the quest for ecological validity is not merely well intentioned yet inconsequential. To the contrary, ecologically valid research can yield results that are quite different from those that are not as relevant to the real world.

Inductive-reasoning ability

Inductive-reasoning problems are characterized by the absence of a single, logically certain response. Although an inductive-reasoning problem may have one solution that seems better than alternative solutions, this solution is a consensually agreed-upon one rather than a logically necessary one. Consider, for example, a prototypical inductive-reasoning problem: the series completion. One might see in an inductive-reasoning test the series completion 1, 2, 3, 4, ___. One's task would be to complete the series. Most people would have no hesitation in completing the series with the number 5, and, indeed, if this problem appeared in an intelligence test for children, it is virtually certain that 5 would be viewed as the correct answer. However, 5 is not the only possible answer: An equation can be generated that will yield as a correct answer any rational number at all (Skyrms, 1975). In the typical interpretation of this problem, the generating equation is $K + 1$, where K takes on the value of each successive number in the series. An alternative equation, however, is $(K - 1)(K - 2)(K - 3)(K - 4) + K$. This equation generates 29 as the fifth value in the series. Other equations would generate other completions. One might argue that some completions are simpler, more elegant, or more natural than others. That is precisely the point: In inductive-reasoning problems, some completions may seem better than others, but there is no logically defined, uniquely correct response.

Inductive-reasoning performance has long been considered a keystone of intelligence. One of the first theorists of general intelligence, Spearman (1923), used analogies as prototypes for intelligent performance. Spearman exemplified three basic principles of cognition through the use of the analogy. The ability to perceive second-order relations, or relations between relations, serves as the marker of the transition between concrete and formal operations in Piaget's (1972) theory of intelligence; and analogies, because they require the ability to perceive relations between relations for their solution, can serve as a useful measure for distinguishing concrete-operational from formal-operational children (Sternberg & Rifkin, 1979). Certain forms of series completion and classification problems also require the ability to perceive second-order relations. Finally, induction problems, and especially analogies, have played a major role in information-processing theories of intelligence. Reitman (1965) and Sternberg (1977) have used analogies as cornerstones for information-processing theories of intelligence, and other investigators also consider analogies as well as other kinds of induction problems to be fundamental to information-processing notions of intelligence (e.g., Pellegrino & Glaser, 1980; Whitely, 1977). Thus, induction problems have played a central part in differential, Piagetian, and information-processing theories of intelligence.

Whereas in some areas of the study of intelligence, the disagreements among theorists are more salient than the agreements, in the study of inductive reasoning, the agreements among investigators regarding the way in which induction problems are solved are much more striking than the disagreements.

Sternberg (1977, 1979; Sternberg & Gardner, 1983; Sternberg & Nigro, 1980) has proposed a theory of inductive reasoning that he has applied to analogies, series completions, classifications, and metaphorical understanding. (For a complete review of this theory and the research it has generated, see Sternberg, 1985.) The theory of information processing specifies the processing components alleged to be involved in inductive reasoning. Consider what these components are in a simple analogy: *lawyer : client : : doctor :* (a) *medicine,* (b) *sick person.* The seven components are (a) *encoding,* by which the individual recognizes the terms of the problem and accesses attributes of the analogy terms that are stored in semantic memory and that might be relevant to task solutions: (b) *inference,* by which the individual figures out the relation between the first two terms of the analogy (e.g., that a lawyer renders professional consulting services to a client): (c) *mapping,* by which the individual figures out the higher order relation between the two halves of the analogy (e.g., that both a lawyer and a doctor render professional services), (d) *application,* by which the individual takes the relation inferred between the terms in the first half of the analogy as mapped to the third term in the second half of the analogy and uses this relation to generate an "ideal" completion to the analogy (e.g., the individual might generate *patient* as an ideal completion); (e) *comparison,* by which the individual compares each of the given answer options (in multiple-choice analogies) to the ideal and decides which is better (in the sense of more closely resembling the ideal) (e.g., the individual will compare each of *medicine* and *sick person* to *patient*); (f) *justification,* in which the individual decides whether the preferred answer option is close enough to the ideal option to warrant its selection, or whether the possibility ought to be entertained, and perhaps acted upon, that an error has been made in earlier information processing (e.g., the individual might decide that *sick person,* although not an ideal response, is at or above some criterion for a minimally acceptable response); and (g) *response,* by which the individual communicates his or her choice of answer (e.g., the individual might circle an answer or press a button indicating his or her choice of *sick person*).

As already noted, the theory can be applied to other kinds of induction problems. Consider, for example, the series completion 2, 5, 8, 11, (a) 14,

(b) 15. In this series completion, the individual must *encode* the terms of the problem, *infer* the relation between each successive pair of given digits, *apply* this relation so as to generate the next digit in the series, *compare* each of the two answer options to the generated option, possibly *justify* the chosen option if it does not correspond exactly to one of the given options, and respond. Note that mapping is not required in this series completion because the problem does not require any recognition of higher order relations between relations. The series completion problem thus requires only a subset of the component processes required by the analogy.

This theory was originally tested in a set of experiments involving Stanford undergraduates (Sternberg, 1977). In these experiments, the subjects solved schematic-picture, verbal, and geometric analogies and were timed while they did so. The reaction-time data provided strong support for the theory. In a later set of experiments, the theory was extended to series completions and classifications presented to adult subjects. Again, there were three contents (schematic pictures, words, and geometric figures) (Sternberg & Gardner, 1983). This research showed that the theory could be successfully extended to the other kinds of induction problems. In both sets of experiments, individuals' scores on each component of inductive reasoning were correlated with scores on standard psychometric tests of inductive-reasoning abilities and perceptual-speed abilities. The idea was to show that the components of reasoning did correlate strongly with inductive reasoning but did not correlate strongly with perceptual speed. The results of the first set of studies were somewhat ambiguous, but the results of the second set of studies, which entailed far more reliable observations than did the first, were not. The three components of inductive reasoning alleged to be most critical for reasoning – inference, mapping, and application – were shown to be strongly correlated with psychometric tests of inductive-reasoning ability but not at all correlated with psychometric tests of perceptual-speed ability. The comparison component also correlated significantly and substantially with psychometrically measured reasoning abilities. The encoding and justification parameters showed mixed patterns of correlation (some statistically significant, but others not). The response parameter did not correlate significantly with reasoning in any studies in the second set, although it did show significant correlations in the first set.

In further experiments, the theory was tested developmentally (Sternberg & Nigro, 1980; Sternberg & Rifkin, 1979). In the Sternberg–Nigro study, verbal items were used, and the investigators looked at the use of word association as well as reasoning in the solution of the items. For example, in the analogy *tree : animate :: pencil :* (a) *inanimate,* (b) *paper,* the word *pencil* has the greater associative relation to *paper,* even though the correct answer to the analogy is *inanimate.* Children ranging in educational levels from grade 2 to college received either one of two kinds of schematic-picture analogies (Sternberg–Rifkin) or verbal analogies (Sternberg–Nigro). In these experiments, the most interesting data proved to be qualitative data illustrating the functioning of metacomponents rather than quantitative data illustrating the functioning of performance components. With regard to the latter, the main result was that the theory of analogical reasoning was supported for both kinds of contents and at all grade levels.

In sum, Sternberg's theory of inductive reasoning contains two parts: a theory of information processing and a theory of response choice. The theory of information processing specifies the processing components used by individuals when they solve an induction problem. It includes processing components such as inferring relations, applying relations, and mapping relations. The theory of response choice, based on a theory proposed by Rumelhart and Abrahamson (1973), seeks to predict individuals' response choices in inductive reasoning. It uses a representation of a multidimensional psychological space in order to make predictions. Both theories have been tested on a number of empirically collected data sets and have been found to predict both reaction time and response-choice data with high accuracy.

Pellegrino and Glaser have proposed a theory of inductive reasoning (Mulholland, Pellegrino, & Glaser, 1980; Pellegrino & Glaser, 1980, 1982) that differs from Sternberg's theory in two major respects. First, a second inference component is substituted for the application component; second, mapping (which these investigators call *comparison*) occurs near the end of analogy solution rather than in the middle and is slightly different from mapping in Sternberg's theory.

Motivated by the Pellegrino–Glaser theory, Goldman, Pellegrino, Parseghian, and Sallis (1982) studied developmental differences in verbal analogical reasoning. Goldman and her colleagues conducted two experiments with 8- and 10-year-olds. Although this work was partly motivated by the Pellegrino–Glaser theory, it did not directly test it. Rather, it focused explicitly on developmental changes in solution processes and strategies for solving verbal analogies. Goldman et al. (1982) found evidence for both quantitative and qualitative changes in children's solutions to analogies. Older children were more accurate than younger children in inference and application processes, and they were also more likely to recognize the correct response in a set of alternatives when either their inference or application had been incorrect. (Note that, although the Pellegrino and Glaser theory did not include an application process, Goldman et al. did make use of such a process, following Sternberg's theory.) In addition, older children were less likely to be distracted than younger children by associative choices in the alternative set. These are choices in which one of the options is highly related to the third term in the analogy stem but is nevertheless an incorrect analogical completion. Consider, for example, the analogy *lemon : sour :: apple :* (a) *fruit,* (b) *sweet.* Although *fruit* is more highly associated with *apple* than is *sweet,* the word *sweet* is the correct answer to the analogy.

In both of Goldman et al.'s experiments, children were also asked to explain their choice of answer. Their responses were classified into three major categories: parallel relations, nonparallel relations, and no relation. Statements indicating comprehension that the $A : B$ and $C : D$ relations of an analogy must match were classified in the parallel-relation category. Statements that violated the property of matching relations were classified in the nonparallel category. Statements that did not relate the subject's response to anything else were classified in the no-relation category. Goldman and her colleagues found that 10-year-olds had significantly more statements in the parallel-relations category than did 8-year-olds. The investigators interpreted these results as indicating that younger children understand that they are supposed to use parallel relations when they solve analogy problems but do not, in fact, always use these relations when solving the analogies. When they do choose the correct answer to an analogy problem, they are just as likely as the older children to verbalize the appropriate reason. But they choose inappropriate answers more often than do older children, and when they do so, they come up with rationalizations for their answers that show little cognizance of the relational properties of the four analogy terms (see Pellegrino, 1984). The developmental trends observed by Goldman and her colleagues have also been observed in older students. Heller (1979) studied the performance of vocational high school and college students in verbal analogical reasoning. She found that the college students used analogical solutions 99% of the time. However, the most capable (upper 25% in verbal ability) of the high school students used analogical solutions 71% of the time, whereas the least capable (lower 25% of verbal ability) used analogical solutions only 34% of the time.

In collaboration with Holzman (Holzman, Glaser, & Pellegrino, 1976; Holzman, Pellegrino, & Glaser, 1983), Pellegrino and Glaser have examined the processes, strategies, and knowledge involved in the solution of series completion problems. However, the empirical work has not been based primarily on the Pellegrino and Glaser theory of analogical reasoning. Rather, the Holzman et al. (1976) work derives from a model of series completions formulated by Simon and Kotovsky (1963), whereas the Holzman et al. (1983) study emphasizes the role of knowledge in series completions rather than the processes of the Simon and Kotovsky theory.

In the Simon and Kotovsky (1963) theory (see also Kotovsky & Simon, 1973), there are three basic components of solution of series completions. The theory applies most clearly to letter series and can be applied as well to number series. It does not apply in as straightforward a manner to other kinds of series problems, such as verbal or geometric series.

The first component is the detection of relations. This component requires an individual to scan the terms of a series and to hypothesize how each element of a series is related to another. Thus, this component is similar to inference in Sternberg's theory. In letter-series problems, only three relations need be considered: identity (which is adjacent repetitions of a given letter), next (which is transition from a given letter of the alphabet to the next letter of the alphabet, as in AB), and backward next (which is transition from one letter to another in reverse alphabetical order, as in BA). In number-series problems, a much greater variety of relations is possible. For example, number series can involve relations of addition, subtraction, multiplication, division, exponentiation, and so on.

The second component of solution is the discovery of periodicity. The period of a series is the number of elements that constitutes one complete cycle of the pattern that makes up the series. For example, in the series problem 1, 5, 2, 6, 3, 7, 4, . . . , a period consists of just two relations, +4 and -3. A longer period would be possible in a more complex series problem. Individuals can use either of two principal methods for discovering the periodicity of a series (see Pellegrino, 1984). In an "adjacent" approach, one discovers periodicity by noting regularly occurring breaks in relations between adjacent elements. To take a simple example, in the series 1, 2, 5, 6, 1, 2, 5, 6, 1, 2, . . . , there is a break separating the 1, 2 sequence from the 5, 6 sequence. In the "nonadjacent" approach, one discovers period length by noting regular intervals at which a given relation repeats itself. For example, if one noticed that the relation +4, -3 repeats itself again and again, one would have used a nonadjacent approach to discovering the periodicity of the series.

The third component of series-completion solution is the completion of the pattern description, whereby the individual extrapolates the rule that he or she has discovered in order to generate the next term or terms of the series problem. Extrapolation involves identifying the position in the period in which the answer should occur, discovering that part of the rule that governs the answer position, and using that part of the rule to find the correct solution. Whereas Simon and Kotovsky (1963) tested this theory by computer simulation, comparing the computer's performance with the performance of human subjects, Kotovsky and Simon (1973) tested the theory primarily by examining data of human subjects. With series problems, Holzman and his colleagues tested the theory by means of three training experiments. The results of all three studies supported the theory.

In conclusion, a variety of theories have been proposed to account for information processing in inductive reasoning. There seems to be a consensus that the components of information processing are the same, or at least highly overlapping, across a variety of induction tasks (Greeno, 1978; Pellegrino & Glaser, 1980; Simon, 1976; Sternberg & Gardner, 1983; Whitely, 1980). If this contention is correct, and the data described in this section suggest that it is, we may have at least one basis for understanding why tests of general intelligence tend to be highly intercorrelated and to yield a general (g) factor. Tests of general intelligence almost always involve at least some induction items. The Raven Progressive Matrices (Raven, 1938, 1960) and the Cattell Culture-Fair Test of g (Cattell & Cattell, 1963), for example, involve induction items exclusively. The general factor may arise as a function of common information-processing components that are relevant to problem solving across induction items and other items as well.

Deductive reasoning

In deductive reasoning, the information contained in the premises of a problem is logically (although not necessarily psychologically) sufficient to reach a valid conclusion. Several kinds of deductive-reasoning problems have been studied. For example, mathematical word problems, propositional reasoning, and syllogistic reasoning all involve primarily deductive inference. Because mathematical word problems were considered in an earlier section and studies of propositional reasoning have not tended to intersect with the human abilities domain, the focus of this section is on the study of syllogistic reasoning.

The three most commonly studied syllogisms are categorical syllogisms, conditional syllogisms, and linear syllogisms. A categorical syllogism usually contains three statements: a major premise, a minor premise, and a conclusion. The individual's task may be to decide whether a given conclusion is logically valid or to decide which of several conclusions is logically valid or best serves as a conclusion to the syllogism. The following is an example of a categorical syllogism: "All Danians are Eleuseans. Some Richters are Danians. Can one conclude that all Richters are Eleuseans?" Premises of categorical syllogisms can be presented in either affirmative or negative form (e.g., "All Etruscans are ancients" versus "No Etruscans are ancients"). Furthermore, the premises can be presented in either universal or particular form (e.g., "All Etruscans are ancients" versus "Some Etruscans are ancients"). By combining polarity (affirmative versus negative) with quantification (universal versus particular), it is possible to obtain four basic kinds of syllogistic statements: universal affirmatives ("All X are Y"), universal negatives ("No X are Y"), particular affirmatives ("Some X are Y"), and particular negatives ("Some X are not Y"). Some of the major theories of categorical syllogistic reasoning that have been proposed are the atmosphere theory of Woodworth and Sells (1935), the conversion theory of Chapman and Chapman (1959), the complete- and random-combination theories of Erickson (1974, 1978), the analogical theory of Johnson-Laird and Steedman (1978), and the transitive-chain theory of Guyote and Sternberg (1981).

Conditional syllogisms also involve a major premise, a minor premise, and a conclusion. However, these problems are rather different in form from categorical syllogisms. The following is an example of a conditional syllogism: "If Conrad the Clown performs, people laugh. Conrad the .Clown performs. Can one conclude that people laugh?" As is the case with categorical syllogisms, premises may be negated (e.g., "If Conrad the Clown performs, people do not laugh," or "Conrad the Clown does not perform"). There appears to be a great deal of similarity between the way people solve categorical and conditional syllogisms, although the commonalities in these two forms of deductive reasoning have received less theoretical and empirical attention than have the commonalities in inductive reasoning (but see Guyote & Sternberg, 1981).

In linear syllogisms, two relations are presented between each of two pairs of items. One item of each pair overlaps between the two pairs. The individual's task is to figure out the relation between the nonoverlapping terms in the two linear-syllogistic premises. The following is an example of a linear syllogism: "John is taller than Pete. Pete is taller than Bill. Who is tallest?" In these problems, a logically valid conclusion is implied by the premises only if it is assumed that the relations linking the terms are transitive. For example, the relation *taller than* would satisfy transitivity, whereas the relation *plays better tennis than* might not. Of the three kinds of syllogisms, linear syllogisms have received the greatest attention in the literature on human intelligence, and therefore the remainder of this section is devoted to a review of theories and research pertinent to such syllogisms.

The linear syllogism has played an important part in theorizing about intelligence. In Piaget's (1928, 1955) developmental theory of intelligence, the ability to perform transitive inferences, as required by linear syllogisms, is alleged to differentiate preoperational from concrete-operational children. In a more psychometric vein, Burt (1919) used linear syllogisms as a problem for measuring the intelligence of school children, and the problem has been used on subsequent tests as well. In more recent work, to be described below, performance on linear syllogisms has been found to be highly correlated with performance on tests of verbal, spatial, and abstract reasoning ability (Shaver, Pierson, & Lang, 1974; Sternberg, 1980a; Sternberg & Weil, 1980). Correlations with such tests generally fall in the range from .30 to .60.

Although theorists of intelligence and cognitive processes agree that capacity for linear syllogistic reasoning is an important ingredient of intelligence, they disagree about the process by which linear syllogisms are solved. The major disagreement regards the way in which information encoded in the linear syllogism is mentally represented. The three major classes of theories are spatial theories, linguistic theories, and spatial—linguistic mixture theories. We shall consider each of these in turn.

Spatial theorists such as DeSoto, London, and Handel (1965), Huttenlocher (1968), and Huttenlocher and Higgins (1971) have argued that information from linear syllogisms is represented in the form of a spatial array that functions as an internal analog of a physically realized or realizable array.

Linguistic theorists argue that information is represented in the form of linguistic, deep-structural propositions of the type originally proposed by Chomsky (1965). For example, the sentence "John is taller than Pete" might be represented by (John is tall +; Pete is tall).

Mixture theories are of two basic kinds. One kind postulates that individuals solve linear syllogisms via different forms of mental representation at different points during practice. Thus, Shaver, Pierson, and Lang (1974) proposed that, during the course of practice with linear syllogisms, individuals use a linguistic representation for information during initial trials but later switch to a spatial representation for information. Johnson-Laird (1972) has made the opposite proposal, namely, that individuals use a spatial representation early during practice and later switch to a linguistic representation (see also Wood, Shotter, & Godden, 1974). Thus, both theories postulate that individuals switch formats of mental representation during the course of practice with linear syllogisms. However, the theories differ in terms of the direction the switch takes.

Sternberg (1980a) has proposed a different sort of mixture model in which individuals use both spatial and linguistic representations of information in the course of solving a single linear syllogism. In other words, the mixture of representations occurs within problems rather than between problems, as in the other two theories. Sternberg (1980a) offered two major classes of evidence to support this claim.

First, he performed *internal validation* of a mixture theory of linear syllogistic reasoning. In a series of experiments with college students, Sternberg quantified alternative information-processing models of task performance and assessed their capacity to fit reaction-time data. Regardless of experimental manipulations (e.g., whether the question came after or before the two premises), adjective pair, or session of practice, the mixture theory provided a better fit to the group reaction-time data than did either of the spatial or linguistic theories. Moreover, there was no evidence of an interaction between quantitative fit and amount of practice. The squared correlation (R^2) between predicted and observed reaction time was generally in the range of .8 to .9 across experiments. Additional evidence for the mixture theory is the fact that parameter estimates (mathematically estimated latencies for particular component operations) were highly similar across experiments in which the mixture theory was tested. This fact, combined with the good fit between the mixture theory and the data, suggests that the component processes specified by the mixture theory give a good account of individuals' processing of linear syllogisms.

Although the mixture theory was better able to account for latency data than either the spatial theory or the linguistic theory, there are differences in the way individuals process these problems. When the latency data of individual subjects is modeled mathematically, it turns out that, although most individuals use a strategy for solving the linear syllogisms that is specified by the mixture theory, a nontrivial proportion of individuals use either a spatial strategy or a linguistic strategy. In other words, the fit of the model to the group basically reflects the process that the majority of subjects follow. However, when data are modeled individually, individual differences can, and in fact do, show up (Sternberg, 1980a; Sternberg & Weil, 1980).

External-validation procedures also generally support the mixture theory over the alternative theories. Sternberg (1980a) found that latencies for solving linear syllogisms tend to be significantly correlated with scores on both verbal and spatial ability tests. Moreover, when individuals' scores on particular components of information processing are correlated with the psychometric tests, the information-processing components that are theorized to be linguistic tend to show higher correlations with verbal ability tests and lower correlations with spatial ability tests; conversely, when information-processing components theorized to be spatial are correlated with the psychometric ability tests, these components show high correlations with spatial tests and relatively lower correlations with verbal tests. In other words, the correlations of component latencies with the verbal and spatial ability tests show the pattern of convergent-discriminant validation predicted by the mixture theory. Again, it should be kept in mind that there are differences in the strategies that individuals use. For individuals who use a basically spatial strategy, significant correlations are obtained with spatial but not with verbal tests. Conversely, for subjects who use a basically linguistic strategy, significant correlations are obtained with verbal but not with spatial tests (Sternberg & Weil, 1980). None of the quantitative fits of theory to data were consistent with the notion of strategy change across time. In other words, the theories of Shaver et al. (1974) and of Johnson-Laird (1972) received no support from the data.

To conclude, the mixture theory appears to give the best general account of performance in the solution of linear syllogisms. There are, however, differences in the strategies subjects employ. In general, however, individuals appear to use both spatial and linguistic mental representation in solving linear syllogisms. Solutions to other kinds of syllogisms, such as categorical and conditional syllogisms, appear to rely even more heavily on the use of spatial representations than do linear syllogisms (Guyote & Sternberg, 1981). One's working memory capacity plays an important part in one's ability to solve any of these syllogisms. This is especially true in the case of categorical syllogisms, where the working-memory requirements can be simply overwhelming.

Spatial ability

Although many tests of intelligence include items measuring spatial ability, the construct of spatial ability remains somewhat ill defined. All such items require some kind of mental manipulation of objects that simulates a manipulation that could occur physically as well.

The classic experiment that essentially initiated information-processing research on spatial ability was performed by Shepard and Metzler (1971). In that experiment, the subjects were asked to determine whether pairs of perspective drawings of three-dimensional geometric forms were identical to each other in shape or, instead, were mirror images. The complexity introduced into the task was that the objects could differ from each other in angle of orientation either in the picture plane or about an axis of depth. For example, a subject might see on the left a picture of a given geometric form and on the right a picture of that same form rotated 45 degrees. In this case, the subject would have to indicate that the two forms were the same. Had the 45-degree-rotated object been a mirror image of the original object, the subject would have had to indicate that the two forms were different. The most striking result of the study was that the time subjects needed to make the same–different discrimination increased linearly as a function of the difference in the portrayed orientations of the two objects in each (same-shaped) pair. Shepard and Metzler interpreted these results as suggesting that the subject performs the mental rotation task by imagining one of the two objects mentally rotated into a congruent orientation with the other object. Once the two objects are in the same orientation, the subject then determines whether their shapes match or do not match. The investigators interpreted the slope of the reaction-time function as indicating the rate at which mental rotation takes place. An interesting subsidiary finding was that rate of rotation was not a function of whether the rotation was in the picture plane or in a third dimension that cut across the picture plane.

In more recent work, Cooper and Shepard (1973) demonstrated that when familiar visual stimuli, such as letters of the alphabet, are shown individually in nonstandard orientations, the time required to determine whether the stimuli are in their normal form or in a reflected form increases approximately linearly as a function of the extent of the stimuli's departure from the standard, upright position. In other words, the most difficult position would be a 90-degree departure from the upright position of, say, a letter. Linear reaction-time functions for a mental rotation task have also been demonstrated for random polygons (Cooper, 1975). Cooper and Podgorny (1976) showed that the rate of mental rotation for such random polygons is unaffected by the complexity of the polygon. The linear reaction-time function found in the mental rotation task can be found in other spatial tasks as well. For example, Shepard and Feng (1972) found that reaction times for a mental paper-folding task, in which subjects have to fold shapes mentally, increase approximately linearly with the number of foldings to be performed.

Although Cooper and Podgorny found that the complexity of a figure had no effect on mental rotation time, it would seem that at some point, variations in figures would affect the time required to rotate these figures mentally. Pellegrino, Mumaw, Kail, and Carter (1979) investigated this hypothesis. Ninety-nine adults were engaged in mental rotation tasks involving either alphanumeric characters or two-dimensional geometric forms of the kind found on the spatial subtest of the Primary Mental Abilities Test. The rate of mental rotation of the more familiar figures, the alphanumeric ones, was significantly higher than that of the other forms. Moreover, the time required to encode the alphanumerics, as measured by the intercept of the reaction-time function, was less than the time required to encode the geometric forms.

There now appears to be substantial evidence for the existence of sex differences in scores on psychometric measures of spatial ability. According to Maccoby and Jacklin (1974), reliable sex differences do not appear until early adolescence, but once they appear, they are maintained throughout adulthood. Information-processing studies of spatial ability help isolate the locus of the difference between males and females. Metzler and Shepard (1974) found a nonsignificant tendency for women to have steeper slopes (i.e., slower rates of mental rotation) and also greater intercepts (i.e., slower rates of figural encoding) than men. Tapley and Bryden (1977) performed some experiments related to those of Metzler and Shepard. In experiments with concrete rather than abstract three-dimensional stimuli, women had nonsignificantly larger intercepts than men. In an experiment with abstract stimuli, women had significantly steeper slopes than men and nonsignificantly greater intercepts. Kail, Carter, and Pellegrino (1979) undertook a more definitive study than these in order to test for sex differences. They found that men rotated stimuli significantly faster than did women, both with familiar alphanumeric characters and with unfamiliar geometric characters of the kind found on the Primary Mental Abilities Test. These authors argued that the main locus of the difference between men and women in spatial information processing is the rate of mental rotation.

All of the studies described here have been conducted with adults. However, work has been conducted with children as well. Kail, Pellegrino, and Carter (1980) tested 8-, 9-, 11-, and 19-year-olds on a mental rotation task, again using both alphanumeric stimuli and geometric characters of a form found on the Primary Mental Abilities Test. Error rates were low (under 10%) at each grade level, indicating that even children as young as 8 can perform the mental rotation task with little difficulty. Moreover, the reaction-time data at each age level were well fit by a linear function, again implicating an analog mental rotation process. The main developmental findings were these: First, rates of mental rotation decreased approximately monotonically with grade level. Thus, older children performed mental rotation at a higher rate than the younger children. Second, the unfamiliar geometric stimuli were rotated more quickly than the familiar alphanumerics by all groups except the 8-year-olds: interpretation of the results in the latter case proved to be problematic owing to the reduced fit of the model to the data. Third, intercepts (i.e., encoding and response time) also declined monotonically with age. Children improved in all aspects of performance with increasing age.

The data described so far suggest that there are systematic differences in rates of mental rotation both among subjects of different ages and even within subjects of the same age. These differences might be viewed as "quantitative" ones, in that they portray differences in amounts of spatial ability but not differences in strategies in spatial ability. One might ask whether the ways in which subjects process spatial information also differ "qualitatively." Data collected by Cooper (1980) suggest that there do exist at least some qualitative differences in the strategies by which individuals solve spatial problems. In her research, Cooper shows subjects two randomly constructed geometric forms in various degrees of angular orientation with respect to each other. The subjects' task is to determine whether the two forms are identical to or different from each other. Forms that are different may differ in variable amounts. In other words, different forms may be either quite close to or quite different from each other in appearance. Cooper discovered two kinds of subjects in her research. For one kind, the speed of deciding whether the two forms were the same or different was a monotonically decreasing function of the difference between the two stimuli. In other words, the greater the difference between the two geometric forms, the easier it was for these subjects to tell the geometric forms apart. For the other kind of subjects, however, the degree of difference between the two forms had no effect on reaction time. Reaction time exhibited a flat function no matter what the degree of difference between the two forms.

Cooper (1980, 1982) has suggested that individuals can be characterized as either analytic or holistic spatial information processors. Analytic information processors compare the two spatial forms feature by feature and hence take longer to differentiate stimuli that exhibit greater similarity to each other than do other spatial forms. The idea here is that the response of subjects in Cooper's experiments would be "different" as soon as they found a difference between two stimuli, but it would take longer to find such a difference with similar stimuli than it would with stimuli that differed to a greater extent. For holistic processors, the degree of difference between the two geometric figures has no effect on reaction time because the two figures are compared holistically only. If they are not identical, they are characterized as "different," regardless of the degree of difference between the two figures.

The results described above indicate that information-processing analyses of spatial aptitude can be useful in pinpointing the sources of differences on spatial ability tests. However, they do not provide a comprehensive information-processing theory of spatial ability. Such a theory has been provided by Kosslyn (1980, 1981). The theory specifies both the mental structures and the mental processes that comprise spatial abilities. I shall describe here only the four classes of processes specified by the theory: image generation, image inspection, image transformation, and image utilization.

Image generation occurs when one forms a visual image on the basis of information stored in long-term memory. *Image inspection* occurs when one surveys a mental image in order to answer a question about it. For example, if one is asked, "Which is larger, a mouse or a beaver?" one might picture a mouse and picture a beaver and then compare their sizes. The process of inspecting the images in order to determine their sizes is the critical process here. *Image transformation* occurs when one changes the appearance of an image. For example, one might be imagining a gray elephant in one context and then, upon hearing the term *white elephant,* change the image so that the elephant now appears white. *Image utilization* occurs when an image is used in some other mental operation, such as fact retrieval. For example, suppose one is asked whether a kangaroo has a tail. If one does not remember spontaneously the answer to this question, one might generate a mental image of a kangaroo and search for a tail. If one's mental image has a tail, one responds affirmatively to the question; otherwise, one responds negatively.

Kosslyn's (1980, 1981) theory assumes that mental images are represented in an analog fashion. In other words, associated with the mental images are some of the spatial properties that actual physical objects demonstrate. Indeed, Kosslyn defines mental processes such as *scan, zoom,* and *rotate,* which sound like operations that could be performed as well on physical objects as they could be on mental objects. The other investigators whose work is cited in this section also assume spatial analog representations. It should be noted, however, that not all theorists share this assumption. For example, Pylyshyn (1973, 1979) has disputed whether such analog representations actually exist in the head. He has claimed instead that all mental representations are fundamentally propositional. Moreover, he has attempted to show how propositional representations of information might generate the empirical results that Kosslyn, Shepard, Cooper, and others have obtained. Anderson and Bower (1973) took a similar position, although Anderson (1978) believes that there is probably no conclusive way of distinguishing between propositional and analog representational theories. At the present time, the debate among theorists continues, some arguing for analog representations of spatial information, some for propositional representation, and still others arguing that the debate will not be a fruitful one. Whatever the underlying representation, however, the work on information processing suggests that it is possible to understand at least some of the sources of individual differences in psychometric test and factor scores in terms of differences in rates and strategies of spatial information processing.

Conclusions

In this chapter, I have reviewed a small subset of the work that has been done on the relations between cognition and intelligence. Research along these lines has been actively pursued in the past decade and shows no sign of abatement. Several conclusions follow from the results of these investigations. First, identification of the components of information processing does not in itself give an adequate account of the nature of intelligent performance. One must also identify the strategies into which the components are combined and the mental representations on which both the components and the strategies act. It has been customary in much psychometric and cognitive research to pursue a *nomothetic* approach to understanding individual differences. Those who take this approach assume that all individuals have essentially the same abilities, whether these abilities are measured by factors or components. Thus, the factors and components of mental abilities would be the same across subjects, and only their values would differ qualitatively. It now appears, however, that individuals differ qualitatively as well as quantitatively so that, as a result, a more *idiographic* approach is necessary for the study of human abilities. Several investigators have found that individuals sometimes differ widely in the strategies they bring to bear on information-processing tasks measuring intelligent performance. Averaging over these strategies yields a composite that may mean little or nothing in individual cases. Thus, it is necessary to understand data at the individual as well as the group level. In practice, cognitive techniques probably lend themselves more readily to this kind of analysis than do psychometric techniques, although it is possible, in theory, to perform factor analysis on data of individual subjects obtained over multiple trials.

Second, in order to understand intelligent behavior, we must move beyond the fairly restrictive tasks that have been used both in experimental laboratories and in psychometric tests of intelligence. The work on learning, in particular, shows that very different patterns of results can be obtained as a function of the ecological validity of the learning task. In more general terms, the abilities one applies to laboratory tasks or intelligence tests may not transfer to one's performance in everyday life, or, conversely, the abilities one exercises in everyday life may not express themselves in laboratory tasks or intelligence tests. Thus, there is a pressing need to investigate the components of intelligence as they operate in everyday life as well as in fairly artificial laboratory settings.

Third, there is a need to integrate theory and research on various aspects of intellectual performance. At the present time, research on such topics as verbal comprehension, learning, inductive reasoning, deductive reasoning, and spatial relations is quite distinct. It is usually a simple matter to classify a given theory or research project into a single domain. But mental abilities cross-cut the domains that we so readily assign to them, and there is a need to understand how this cross-cutting takes place. The appearance of general and major group factors in intelligence tests argues strongly for the generality of at least some abilities. Clearly, not all abilities are domain-general. In fact, the current *Zeitgeist* in cognitive psychology is toward emphasis on domain-specific abilities. It appears, however, that at least some abilities, such as those represented by metacomponents or executive processes, are quite general, and their application in various domains of endeavor must be more fully understood.

Finally, there is a need to bring developments in cognitive research into the arenas of current technology. The technologies of testing and training of intellectual skills are still dominated largely by psychometric perspectives. Although this in itself is not bad, it appears certain that the cognitive perspective could have a great deal to offer to technologies of testing (Sternberg, 1981) and training (Sternberg, 1983). A cognitive perspective could not by itself facilitate efforts in these domains, but it might well contribute to the improvement of the outcome of these efforts.

In sum, the cognitive approach to understanding intelligence has provided a new and exciting perspective on the nature and function of intelligence. It has provided much more detail regarding the nature of mental abilities than have any of the other approaches used to date. No one approach to the study of intelligence is apt to be complete, and thus the cognitive approach, like any other, must be supplemented by other approaches. A continuing challenge for the future will be the integration of results from various paradigms of research so that our understanding of intelligence will be transparadigmatic. Regardless of the theoretical or methodological approach one prefers, one should not lose sight of the fact that our ultimate goal is to understand the psychological phenomenon of *intelligence* and that our understanding of this mental construct must transcend any one paradigm.

References

Anderson, J. R. (1978). Arguments concerning representations for mental imagery. *Psychological Review, 85,* 249–77.

Anderson, J. R., & Bower, G. H. (1973). *Human associative memory.* New York: Wiley.

Anderson, R. C., & Freebody, P. (1979). *Vocabulary knowledge* (Tech. Rep. No. 136). Champaign: University of Illinois, Center for the Study of Reading.

Belmont, J. M., & Butterfield, E. C. (1971). Learning strategies as determinants of memory deficiencies. *Cognitive Psychology, 2,* 411–20.

Bisanz, G. L., & Voss, J. F. (1981). Sources of knowledge in reading comprehension. In A. Lesgold & C. A. Perfetti (Eds.), *Interactive processes in reading* (pp. 215–39). Hillsdale, NJ: Erlbaum.

Bobrow, D. G. (1968). Natural language input for a computer problem solving system. In M. Minsky (Ed.), *Semantic information processing* (pp. 146–227). Cambridge, MA: MIT Press.

Bransford, J. D., Barclay, J. R., & Franks, J. J. (1972). Sentence memory: A constructive versus interpretive approach. *Cognitive Psychology, 3,* 193−209.

Brown, A. L. (1978). Knowing when, where, and how to remember: A problem of metacognition. In R. Glaser (Ed.), *Advances in instructional psychology* (Vol. 1, pp. 77−165). Hillsdale, NJ: Erlbaum.

Brown, A. L., & Campione, J. C. (1978). Permissible inferences from cognitive training studies in developmental research. *Quarterly Newsletter of the Institute for Comparative Human Behavior, 2,* 46−53.

Brown, A. L., & Ferrara, R. A. (1985). Diagnosing zones of proximal development. In J. Wertsch (Ed.), *Culture, communication, and cognition: Vygotskian perspectives* (pp. 273−305). Cambridge University Press.

Brown, A. L., & Smiley, S. S. (1977). Rating the importance of structural units of prose passages: A problem of metacognitive development. *Child Development, 48,* 1−8.

(1978). The development of strategies for studying texts. *Child Development, 49,* 1076−88.

Brown, J. S., & Burton, R. R. (1978). Diagnostic models for procedural bugs in basic mathematical skills. *Cognitive Science, 2,* 155−92.

Buckingham, B. R. (1921). Intelligence and its measurement: A symposium. *Journal of Educational Psychology, 12,* 271−5.

Burt, C. (1919). The development of reasoning in school children. *Journal of Experimental Pedagogy, 5,* 68−77.

Butterfield, E. C., & Belmont, J. M. (1977). Assessing and improving the executive cognitive functions of mentally retarded people. In I. Bialer & M. Sternlicht (Eds.), *The psychology of mental retardation: Issues and approaches* (pp. 277−318). New York: Psychological Dimensions.

Campione, J. C., & Brown, A. L. (1978). Toward a theory of intelligence: Contributions from research with retarded children. *Intelligence, 2,* 279−304.

Campione, J. C., Brown, A. L., & Bryant, N. R. (1984). Individual differences in learning and memory. In R. J. Sternberg (Ed.), *Human abilities: An information processing approach* (pp. 103−26). New York: Freeman.

Carroll, J. B. (1976). Psychometric tests as cognitive tasks: A new "structure of intellect." In L. B. Resnick (Ed.), *The nature of intelligence* (pp. 27−56). Hillsdale, NJ: Erlbaum.

(1981). Ability and task difficulty in cognitive psychology. *Educational Researcher, 10,* 11−21.

Cattell, R. B., & Cattell, A. K. (1963). *Test of g: Culture Fair, Scale 3.* Champaign, IL: Institute for Personality and Ability Testing.

Chapman, L. J., & Chapman, A. P. (1959). Atmosphere effect re-examined. *Journal of Experimental Psychology, 58,* 220−6.

Chase, W. G., & Simon, H. A. (1973). The mind's eye in chess. In W. G. Chase (Ed.), *Visual information processing* (pp. 215−82). New York: Academic Press.

Chi, M. T. H. (1978). Knowledge structures and memory development. In R. S. Siegler (Ed.), *Children's thinking: What develops?* (pp. 73−176). Hillsdale, NJ: Erlbaum.

Chi, M. T. H., & Koeske, R. D. (1983). Network representations of a child's dinosaur knowledge. *Developmental Psychology, 19,* 29−39.

Chiesi, H. L., Spilich, G. J., & Voss, J. F. (1979). Acquisition of domain-related information in relation to high and low domain knowledge. *Journal of Verbal Learning and Verbal Behavior, 18,* 257−74.

Chomsky, N. (1965). *Aspects of the theory of syntax.* Cambridge, MA: MIT Press.

Cooper, L. A. (1975). Mental rotation of random two-dimensional shapes. *Cognitive Psychology, 7,* 20−43.

(1980). Spatial information processing: Strategies for research. In R. Snow, P. A. Federico, & W. E. Montague (Eds.), *Aptitude, learning, and instruction: Cognitive process analyses* (pp. 149−76). Hillsdale, NJ: Erlbaum.

(1982). Strategies for visual comparison and representation: Individual differences. In R. J. Sternberg (Ed.), *Advances in the psychology of human intelligence* (Vol. 1, pp. 77−124). Hillsdale, NJ: Erlbaum.

Cooper, L. A., & Podgorny, P. (1976). Mental transformations and visual comparison processes: Effects of complexity and similarity. *Journal of Experimental Psychology: Human Perception and Performance, 2,* 503–14.

Cooper, L. A., & Shepard, R. N. (1973). Chronometric studies of the rotation of mental images. In W. C. Chase (Ed.), *Visual information processing* (pp. 75–176). New York: Academic Press.

Crowder, R. G. (1976). *Principles of learning and memory.* Hillsdale, NJ: Erlbaum.

Daalen-Kapteijns, M. M. van, & Elshout-Mohr, M. (1981). The acquisition of word meanings as a cognitive learning process. *Journal of Verbal Learning and Verbal Behavior, 20,* 386–99.

Daneman, M., & Carpenter, P. A. (1980). Individual differences in working memory and reading. *Journal of Verbal Learning and Verbal Behavior, 19,* 450–66.

Davidson, J. E., & Sternberg, R. J. (1984). The role of insight in intellectual giftedness. *Gifted Child Quarterly, 28,* 58–64.

Dearborn, W. G. (1921). Intelligence and its measurement: A symposium. *Journal of Educational Psychology, 12,* 210–2.

DeSoto, C. B., London, M., & Handel, S. (1965). Social reasoning and spatial paralogic. *Journal of Personality and Social Psychology, 2,* 513–21.

Ellis, N. R. (1970). Memory processes in retardates and normals. In N. R. Ellis (Ed.), *International review of research in mental retardation* (Vol. 4, pp. 1–32). New York: Academic Press.

Erickson, J. R. (1974). A set analysis theory of behavior in formal syllogistic reasoning tasks. In R. L. Solso (Ed.), *Theories of cognitive psychology: The Loyola Symposium* (pp. 305–30). Hillsdale, NJ: Erlbaum.

   (1978). Research on syllogistic reasoning. In R. Revlin & R. E. Mayer (Eds.), *Human reasoning.* New York: Wiley.

Estes, W. K. (1982). Learning, memory, and intelligence. In R. J. Sternberg (Ed.), *Handbook of human intelligence* (pp. 170–224). Cambridge University Press.

Ferrara, R. A. (1982). *Children's learning and transfer of inductive reasoning rules: A study of proximal development.* Unpublished master's thesis, University of Illinois, Champaign.

Feuerstein, R. (1979). *The dynamic assessment of retarded performers: The learning potential assessment device, theory, instruments, and techniques.* Baltimore, MD: University Park Press.

Flavell, J. H. (1981). Cognitive monitoring. In W. P. Dickson (Ed.), *Children's oral communication skills* (pp. 35–60). New York: Academic Press.

Ginsburg, H. (1977). *Children's arithmetic.* New York: Nostrand.

Glanzer, M., & Cunitz, A. R. (1966). Two storage mechanisms in free recall. *Journal of Verbal Learning and Verbal Behavior, 5,* 351–60.

Goldman, S. R., Pellegrino, J. W., Parseghian, P. E., & Sallis, R. (1982). Developmental and individual differences in verbal analogical reasoning by children. *Child Development, 53,* 550–9.

Greeno, J. G. (1978). A study of problem solving. In R. Glaser (Ed.), *Advances in instructional psychology* (pp. 13–76). Hillsdale, NJ: Erlbaum.

Groen, G. J., & Parkman, J. M. (1972). A chronometric analysis of simple addition. *Psychological Review, 79,* 329–43.

Guilford, J. P. (1967). *The nature of human intelligence.* New York: McGraw-Hill.

Guyote, M. J., & Sternberg, R. J. (1981). A transitive-chain theory of syllogistic reasoning. *Cognitive Psychology, 13,* 461–525.

Hayes, J. R. (1981). *The complete problem solver.* Philadelphia: Franklin Institute Press.

Heim, A. (1970). *Intelligence and personality: Their assessment and relationship.* Harmondsworth: Penguin Books.

Heller, J. I. (1979). *Cognitive processing in verbal analogy solution.* Unpublished doctoral dissertation, University of Pittsburgh.

Holzman, T. G., Glaser, R., & Pellegrino, J. W. (1976). Process training derived from a computer simulation theory. *Memory and Cognition, 4,* 349–56.

Holzman, T. G., Pellegrino, J. W., & Glaser, R. (1983). Cognitive variables in series completion. *Journal of Educational Psychology, 75,* 602–17.

Hunt, E. B. (1978). Mechanics of verbal ability. *Psychological Review, 85,* 109–30.

Hunt, E. B., Lunneborg, C., & Lewis, J. (1975). What does it mean to be high verbal? *Cognitive Psychology, 7,* 194–227.

Huttenlocher, J. (1968). Constructing spatial images: A strategy in reasoning. *Psychological Review, 75,* 550–60.

Huttenlocher, J., & Higgins, E. T. (1971). Adjectives, comparatives, and syllogisms. *Psychological Review, 78,* 487–504.

Jackson, M. D., & McClelland, J. L. (1979). Processing determinants of reading speed. *Journal of Experimental Psychology: General, 108,* 151–81.

Jensen, A. R. (1980). *Bias in mental testing.* New York: Free Press.

Johnson-Laird, P. N. (1972). The three-term series problem. *Cognition, 1,* 57–82.

Johnson-Laird, P. N., & Steedman, M. (1978). The psychology of syllogisms. *Cognitive Psychology, 10,* 64–99.

Kail, R. V., Carter, P., & Pellegrino, J. W. (1979). The locus of sex differences in spatial ability. *Perception and Psychophysics, 26,* 182–6.

Kail, R. V., Pellegrino, J. W., & Carter, P. (1980). Developmental changes in mental rotation. *Journal of Experimental Child Psychology, 29,* 102–16.

Keating, D. P., & Bobbitt, B. L. (1978). Individual and developmental differences in cognitive processing components of mental ability. *Child Development, 49,* 155–67.

Keil, F. C. (1979). *Semantic and conceptual development.* Cambridge, MA: Harvard University Press.

  (1981). Constraints on knowledge and cognitive development. *Psychological Review, 88,* 197–227.

  (1984). Transition mechanisms in cognitive development and the structure of knowledge. In R. J. Sternberg (Ed.), *Mechanisms of cognitive development* (pp. 81–99). New York: Freeman.

Kintsch, W., & van Dijk, T. A. (1978). Toward a model of text comprehension and production. *Psychological Review, 85,* 363–94.

Kosslyn, S. M. (1980). *Image and mind.* Cambridge, MA: Harvard University Press.

  (1981). The medium and the message in mental imagery. *Psychological Review, 88,* 46–66.

Kotovsky, K., & Simon, H. A. (1973). Empirical tests of a theory of human acquisition of concepts for sequential events. *Cognitive Psychology, 4,* 399–424.

Maccoby, E. E., & Jacklin, C. N. (1974). *The psychology of sex differences.* Stanford, CA: Stanford University Press.

Markman, E. M. (1981). Comprehension monitoring. In W. P. Dickson (Ed.), *Children's oral communication skills* (pp. 61–84). New York: Academic Press.

Marshalek, B. (1981). *Trait and process aspects of vocabulary knowledge and verbal ability* (NR154-376 ONR Tech. Rep. No. 15). Stanford, CA: Stanford University, School of Education.

Mayer, R. E. (1982). Memory for algebra story problems. *Journal of Educational Psychology, 74,* 199–216.

  (1983). *Thinking, problem solving, and cognition.* New York: Freeman.

Mayer, R. E., & Greeno, J. G. (1972). Structural differences between learning outcomes produced by different instructional methods. *Journal of Educational Psychology, 63,* 165–73.

Metzler, J., & Shepard, R. N. (1974). Transformational studies of internal representations of three-dimensional objects. In R. Solso (Ed.), *Theories in cognitive psychology: The Loyola Symposium* (pp. 147–202). Hillsdale, NJ: Erlbaum.

Mulholland, T. M., Pellegrino, J. W., & Glaser, R. (1980). Components of geometric analogy solution. *Cognitive Psychology, 12,* 252–84.

Newell, A., & Simon, H. A. (1972). *Human problem solving.* Englewood Cliffs, NJ: Prentice-Hall.

Pellegrino, J. W. (1984). Inductive reasoning ability. In R. J. Sternberg (Ed.), *Human abilities: An information-processing approach* (pp. 195–225). New York: Freeman.

Pellegrino, J. W., & Glaser, R. (1980). Components of inductive reasoning. In R. E. Snow, P. A. Federico, & W. Montague (Eds.), *Aptitude, learning, and instruction: Vol. 1. Cognitive process analyses of aptitude* (pp. 177–217). Hillsdale, NJ: Erlbaum.

(1982). Analyzing aptitudes for learning: Inductive reasoning. In R. Glaser (Ed.), *Advances in instructional psychology* (Vol. 2, pp. 269–345). Hillsdale, NJ: Erlbaum.

Pellegrino, J. W., Mumaw, R. J., Kail, R. V., & Carter, P. (1979). *Different slopes for different folks: Analyses of spatial ability.* Paper presented at the annual meeting of the Psychonomic Society, Phoenix, AZ.

Perfetti, C. A., & Lesgold, A. M. (1977). Discourse comprehension and individual differences. In P. Carpenter & M. Just (Eds.), *Cognitive processes in comprehension: The 12th Annual Carnegie Symposium on Cognition* (pp. 141–83). Hillsdale, NJ: Erlbaum.

Piaget, J. (1928). *Judgment and reasoning in the child.* London: Routledge & Kegan Paul.

(1955). *The language and thought of the child.* New York: Meridian.

(1972). *The psychology of intelligence.* Totowa, NJ: Littlefield, Adams.

Posner, M. I., & Mitchell, R. F. (1967). Chronometric analysis of classification. *Psychological Review, 74,* 392–409.

Pylyshyn, Z. W. (1973). What the mind's eye tells the mind's brain: A critique of mental imagery. *Psychological Bulletin, 80,* 1–24.

(1979). Validating computational models: A critique of Anderson's indeterminacy of representation claim. *Psychological Review, 86,* 383–94.

Raven, J. C. (1938). *Progressive matrices: A perceptual test of intelligence.* London: Lewis.

(1960). *Guide to the standard progressive matrices.* London: Lewis.

Reitman, W. (1965). *Cognition and thought.* New York: Wiley.

Resnick, L. B., & Ford, W. W. (1981). *The psychology of mathematics for instruction.* Hillsdale, NJ: Erlbaum.

Resnick, L. B., & Glaser, R. (1976). Problem solving and intelligence. In L. B. Resnick (Ed.), *The nature of intelligence* (pp. 205–30). Hillsdale, NJ: Erlbaum.

Rieger, C. (1975). Conceptual memory. In R. C. Schank (Ed.), *Conceptual information processing* (pp. 157–288). Amsterdam: North-Holland.

Rohwer, W. D., Jr. (1973). Elaboration and learning in childhood and adolescence. In H. W. Reese (Ed.), *Advances in child development and behavior* (Vol. 8, pp. 1–57). New York: Academic Press.

Rumelhart, D. E. (1980). Schemata: The building blocks of cognition. In R. J. Spiro, B. C. Bruce, & W. F. Brewer (Eds.), *Theoretical issues in reading comprehension: Perspectives from cognitive psychology, linguistics, artificial intelligence and education* (pp. 33–58). Hillsdale, NJ: Erlbaum.

Rumelhart, D. E., & Abrahamson, A. A. (1973). A model for analogical reasoning. *Cognitive Psychology, 5,* 1–28.

Schank, R., & Abelson, R. (1977). *Scripts, plans, goals, and understanding.* Hillsdale, NJ: Erlbaum.

Shaver, P., Pierson, L., & Lang, S. (1974). Converging evidence for the functional significance of imagery in problem solving. *Cognition, 3,* 359–75.

Shepard, R. N., & Feng, C. (1972). A chronometric study of mental paper folding. *Cognitive Psychology, 3,* 228–43.

Shepard, R. N. & Metzler, J. (1971). Mental rotation of three-dimensional objects. *Science, 171,* 701–3.

Simon, H. A. (1976). Identifying basic abilities underlying intelligent performance of complex tasks. In L. B. Resnick (Ed.), *The nature of intelligence* (pp. 65–98). Hillsdale, NJ: Erlbaum.

Simon, H. A., & Kotovsky, K. (1963). Human acquisition of concepts for sequential patterns. *Psychological Review, 70,* 534–46.

Skyrms, B. (1975). *Choice and chance* (2nd ed.). Encino, CA: Dickenson.

Soloway, E., Lochhead, J., & Clement, J. (1982). Does computer programming enhance problem solving ability? Some positive evidence on algebra word problems. In R. J. Seidel, R.

E. Anderson, & B. Hunter (Eds.), *Computer literacy* (pp. 171–86). New York: Academic Press.

Spearman, C. (1923). *The nature of intelligence and the principles of cognition.* New York: Macmillan.

Sternberg, R. J. (1977). *Intelligence, information processing, and analogical reasoning: The componential analysis of human abilities.* Hillsdale, NJ: Erlbaum.

    (1979). The nature of mental abilities. *American Psychologist, 34,* 214–30.

    (1980a). Representation and process in linear syllogistic reasoning. *Journal of Experimental Psychology: General, 109,* 119–59.

    (1980b). Sketch of a componential subtheory of human intelligence. *Behavioral and Brain Sciences, 3,* 573–84.

    (1981). Testing and cognitive psychology. *American Psychologist, 36,* 1181–9.

    (1983). Criteria for intellectual skills training. *Educational Researcher, 12,* 6–12, 26.

    (1985). *Beyond IQ: A triarchic theory of human intelligence.* Cambridge University Press.

Sternberg, R. J., & Gardner, M. K. (1983). Unities in inductive reasoning. *Journal of Experimental Psychology: General, 112,* 80–116.

Sternberg, R. J., & Nigro, G. (1980). Developmental patterns in the solution of verbal analogies. *Child Development, 51,* 27–38.

Sternberg, R. J., & Powell, J. S. (1983). Comprehending verbal comprehension. *American Psychologist, 38,* 878–93.

Sternberg, R. J., & Rifkin, B. (1979). The development of analogical reasoning processes. *Journal of Experimental Child Psychology, 27,* 195–232.

Sternberg, R. J., & Weil, E. M. (1980). An aptitude–strategy interaction in linear syllogistic reasoning. *Journal of Educational Psychology, 72,* 226–34.

Tapley, S. M., & Bryden, M. P. (1977). An investigation of sex differences in spatial ability: Mental rotation of three-dimensional objects. *Canadian Journal of Psychology, 31,* 122–30.

Thorndike, E. L. (1924). The measurement of intelligence: Present status. *Psychological Review, 31,* 219–52.

Thorndyke, P. W. (1976). The role of inferences in discourse comprehension. *Journal of Verbal Learning and Verbal Behavior, 15,* 437–46.

Thurstone, L. L. (1938). *Primary mental abilities.* University of Chicago Press.

Vernon, P. E. (1971). *The structure of human abilities.* London: Methuen.

Vygotsky, L. S. (1978). *Mind in society: The development of higher psychological processes.* Cambridge, MA: Harvard University Press.

Werner, H., & Kaplan, E. (1952). The acquisition of word meanings: A developmental study. *Monographs of the Society for Research in Child Development* (Vol. 15, Serial No. 51).

Whitely, S. E. (1977). Information-processing on intelligence test items: Some response components. *Applied Psychological Measurement, 1,* 465–76.

    (1980). Latent trait models in the study of intelligence. *Intelligence, 4,* 97–132.

Wood, D., Shotter, J., & Godden, D. (1974). An investigation of the relationships between problem solving strategies, repesentation, and memory. *Quarterly Journal of Experimental Psychology, 26,* 252–7.

Woodrow, H. A. (1917). Practice and transference in normal and feeble-minded children. 1. Practice. *Journal of Educational Psychology, 8,* 85–96.

    (1938). The effect of practice on groups of different initial ability. *Journal of Educational Psychology, 29,* 268–78.

    (1946). The ability to learn. *Psychological Review, 53,* 147–58.

Woods, S. S., Resnick, L. B., & Groen, G. J. (1975). An experimental test of five process models for subtraction. *Journal of Educational Psychology, 67,* 17–21.

Woodworth, R. S., & Sells, S. B. (1935). An atmosphere effect in formal syllogistic reasoning. *Journal of Experimental Psychology, 18,* 451–60.

Zeaman, P., & House, B. J. (1963). The role of attention in retardate discrimination learning. In N. R. Ellis (Ed.), *Handbook of mental deficiency* (pp. 159–223). New York: McGraw-Hill.

11 Creativity and the quest for mechanism

D. N. Perkins

Beethoven opens the final movement of his Ninth Symphony with several passages that together could be taken as a symbol of creative thinking. First come motifs from the earlier movements, each sounded for a moment and set aside. Interspersed are episodes of recitative in the cellos, a kind of searching rumination: None of these old themes will do, it seems. Then a few measures of the "Ode to Joy" sound briefly in the treble, immediately dismissed by more recitative that actually overwrites the last bars of the theme. Will this be the idea that lingers and grows? Yes, for back it comes after a firm cadence, a single soft unharmonized melodic line in the cellos, still far from its triumphant orchestral and choral tutti.

Creativity could be like that. The creator harks back to old ideas, wanders among them, picks them up and fits them together this way and that, tries a new one. Perhaps the new one holds promise. The maker explores it tentatively. Yes, it might do. Creativity could be this sort of sensitive searching and trying out until something shows potential. In more psychological terms, it could be primarily a process of search and selection, success being dependent on the adequate "targeting" of the search process and the sensitivity of selection. But, of course, creativity might more often take other paths altogether. When we ask what path creativity characteristically takes − and why some people routinely take that path whereas others do not − we are asking about the mechanism of creativity.

The episode of search, conception, and acceptance that begins the last movement of the Ninth Symphony is no real evidence of the nature of the creative mechanism. The same passages could no doubt be interpreted in social, political, or even agricultural terms by someone with a different ax to grind. Chances are that Beethoven was simply constructing a bridge between the prior movements and the innovative choral finale (Thayer, 1921, p. 149). Moreover, even if we take his foyer to the Ninth as an emblem of the process of invention, it is, after all, Beethoven's contrivance. What *his* processes were is quite a different question from what processes he chose to represent.

As it happens, however, the image of invention one can read from, or at least read into, Beethoven's opening does not fall so far from what we know about Beethoven's composing practices. If anything, in its brief gropings it understates the highly exploratory way in which Beethoven searched out motifs, reworked them, and developed them toward complete compositions. In Beethoven's notebooks are pages of scratchings and scratching out in which he evolved, among other motifs, the "Ode to Joy" theme (Thayer, 1921, p. 148). From such evidence, we gain a little more insight into the mechanism of Beethoven's thinking.

What is this quest for mechanism and why might we want to make it? Broadly speaking, the quest for mechanism is a search for causal models of the phenomenon in question. In the case of creativity, a causal model might answer such questions as these: What happens in a person's mind that results in invention? What sorts of abilities, skills, values, and attitudes dispose a person to invention? The reasons for the quest seem much the same as those in any other domain – understanding and empowerment. We hunger after an understanding of mysterious things – black holes, quarks, and creativity. Also, understanding often empowers us. We find ways of applying our understanding to gain more of whatever it is we want. In the case of creativity, a better understanding of its mechanism might help us to be more creative and to educate for creativity, for example.

But the quest for a mechanism of creativity poses dilemmas that the quest for an understanding of black holes does not. Some believe that creativity is intrinsically inexplicable: How can one hope to explain a process that by definition breaks existing patterns? Some think that, although perhaps in principle explicable, creativity presents such a mysterious face that in practice little progress is likely. Still others argue that, whether or not one can, one *should not* probe the mechanism of creativity. Theorizing, even if correct, could yield a self-consciousness of the nature of the process that undermines the process itself. Some things work better when left alone.

Here we rush in where at least some angels fear to go. There follows an account of the mechanism of creativity that encompasses a good deal of what is now known about the phenomenon. Inevitably, that perspective reflects some personal ways of thinking about the nature of creativity, but at the same time it reflects a conscious effort to be reasonably evenhanded. I take a stronger position elsewhere (Perkins, 1981, 1985b). As to the problem of treading on inviolable ground, in my view the dangers of excessive self-consciousness are minor compared with the potential benefits of understanding and mining more deeply the natural resource of our creative capabilities.

Creativity as overt conduct

To understand Beethoven's or anyone else's creativity on the inside, we need to understand it on the outside. What is it that we are trying to explain, that is? Under what conditions do we call a person creative or identify instances of creative thinking? Unless we have an answer to these questions, we do not have in focus what it is we are trying to find a mechanism for.

A brief and somewhat simplistic sounding answer actually serves the purposes of inquiry rather well: (a) A creative result is a result both original and appropriate. (2) A creative person – a person with creativity – is a person who fairly routinely produces creative results. Both (a) and (b) call for a very broad interpretation of results – they could be paintings, poems, or theories but also jokes, styles of dress, gardens, car repairs, and so on.

What sense do these propositions make? They capture fairly well our actual practices in talking about creativity. We do not call something creative unless we classify it as both original and appropriate. If we do not see it as original, it may count as finely crafted but not as creative. If we do not see it as appropriate, its originality simply makes it bizarre. Likewise, we do not call a person creative unless the person regularly produces original, appropriate results of some sort.

There are a number of misgivings one might have about Definitions (a) and (b). Many people wince at the notion of defining creativity in terms of results. Creativity, they emphasize, is something inside a person, not outside. Actually, it is both. We call people creative because they produce creative results routinely; this is the outside view. We want to know what about their psychology yields such results; this is the quest for an inside view. If we want, we can say that the inside view is the "real" creativity, just as we say a baseball is "really" a swarm of atoms. At the same time, it is worth keeping in mind that both inner creativity and the swarm of atoms have pragmatic "outside" meanings in our everyday world and that this, in the last analysis, is what makes us interested in the inside.

A less easily resolved misgiving about Definitions (a) and (b) concerns their ambiguity. Is Beethoven's music creative? To be sure, we think so now. But though he had a commanding reputation during his lifetime, certain of his compositions were disdained by many. When a student discovers a theorem long known in mathematics, is it original or not? It is original to the student but not to the field.

These ambiguities actually challenge the clarity of our concept of creativity more than they challenge Definitions (a) and (b) per se. When, for instance, the student rediscovers a theorem, we ourselves feel a tension about whether to call this creative. We want to say something like, "Well, it depends what you mean by 'original' in this case." In general, originality and appropriateness are no *more* ambiguous than our use of the term *creative*. On the contrary, they help us to explain its ambiguity by helping us to isolate where the ambiguity lies in particular cases.

The ambiguity, however, seems to threaten the quest for mechanism from the outset. Seeking a mechanism requires identifying clear instances of what the mechanism is supposed to explain. This threat leads to a variety of tactical solutions that involve evading the problem. As to the dilemma of the student rediscovering a theorem, we have to remember that from the standpoint of psychological mechanism it makes no difference whether or not a discovery is a rediscovery. Another dilemma might be "How original is original enough?" But here we can focus on unimpeachable cases, such as Beethoven, or remind ourselves that we should be interested not only in the grand creative achievements of civilization but also in more modest and everyday creative achievements, in which we settle for less originality. As to the ambiguity of what is appropriate, we can again try to confine ourselves to clear-cut cases. In short, in the quest for mechanism we should dodge the problems of ambiguity in our concept of creativity rather than repair them. Why dodge rather than repair? Because the problems are not just confusions – they are intrinsic to the concept. But simply because a concept has a large fuzzy border, it does not necessarily lack a clear center. In the quest for mechanism we must address the center.

Creativity as ineffable

There are those who recommend that the quest for a mechanism of creativity be called off at once. However much we may strive to understand the workings of Beethoven's creative mind, the endeavor will fail – not just because minds are subtle things but because the quest itself contains a logical paradox that makes it impossible. The essence of the typical argument is something like this: (a) True creativity by definition breaks boundaries in unpredictable ways. (b) A model of something, creativity for instance, contains rules that predetermine the behavior of that something. But predetermination and unpredictability are inconsistent. Therefore, the very concept of a model of creativity contains an internal contradiction. Carl Hausman, for one, has advanced arguments of roughly this form (Hausman, 1976, 1985).

The challenge has a certain surface appeal: How can one capture the essence of something whose essence is freedom? However, much hangs on the kind of capturing one has in mind. Let us for the moment grant the first premise of the argument, that true creativity characteristically breaks boundaries in unpredictable ways. The second premise is that any true model of creativity would predetermine discoveries. But many a predictive scientific theory does not make *exact* predictions. The theory of gases, for instance, predicts global phenomena of pressure and temperature but not what molecule will be where at a given point in time. Quantum theory predicts the probability distribution of the position and momentum of an electron, not its exact position and momentum in a particular case. Analogously, a mechanism of creativity that predicted *that* certain people would be creative and *how* in broad terms the process worked, without predetermining exactly the discoveries to be made or even the boundaries to be broken, would be a model that met the standards of science.

Although this is perhaps the easiest counterargument, the first premise can be challenged too. To be sure, true creativity characteristically breaks boundaries in unpredictable ways – but unpredictable *in principle* or simply unpredictable *in normal practice?* If only the latter, the way is open for a model of creativity that does in fact predict particular creative discoveries. Such a model would go beyond what we now manage to predict, but this in itself should not surprise us. New scientific theories routinely enable us to predict what before we could not. Therefore, to maintain the argument, one has to take the premise to be that true creativity characteristically breaks boundaries in ways that are unpredictable not just in practice but in principle.

Now we can ask, what is the argument for this premise of unpredictability in principle? One possibility is an empirical argument. Perhaps we can tell from our experience of the world that discoveries we consider creative are unpredictable in principle. But the fact that such discoveries have not been predicted does not mean they cannot in principle be: The absence of something from our experience does not prove its impossibility, especially in an advancing field.

Then perhaps the unpredictability in principle of creative discoveries follows from the very meaning of creativity, much as being unmarried follows from the very meaning of being a bachelor. If so, however, another dilemma presents itself: How do we know that discoveries we have always considered creative – such as the theory of relativity – *are* creative by that standard; how do we know that they were in principle unpredictable? Perhaps the sorts of discoveries we normally consider creative are not in fact creative by this stringent rule. We do not want to fall into the trap of being so idealistic about the meaning of creativity that discoveries we normally consider to be creative do not meet the standard.

In summary, the argument that creativity is ineffable in principle does not hold. It depends on an unreasonably idealistic concept of what a model is – one much more stringent than normal practice – and an unreasonably idealistic concept of what creativity is – one that for all we can tell may exclude discoveries that we normally take to be creative. Beethoven may well slip through our net in the quest for mechanism; but he will not slip through because the quest is impossible in principle.

Creativity as computation

The origins of things commonly exert a special fascination and pose a special dilemma. Consider, for instance, the "big bang" with which the universe supposedly began. We would like to understand its mechanism, but the laws of physics governing the routine behavior of our universe break down under the extreme conditions that are thought to have prevailed during the first microseconds in which the universe was born. To probe the origin of the universe, we have either to remake radically or to build anew our physics.

Many believe that human invention poses a similar puzzle of origins. Whatever principles govern ordinary human thought do not account for that special kind of thinking that yields invention. One cannot understand invention in terms of such prosaic processes as reasoning, memory retrieval, rule following, and pattern recognition.

By this logic, computers could not create. They, after all, are ideal mechanisms of precise rule following, memory storage, and memory retrieval. If, on the contrary, computers can in some sense create, then we have to revise upward our estimate of the possibility of accounting for creativity in terms of prosaic processes of mind. Perhaps creativity is just computation, albeit computation of the right sort.

One claim for the computer's capacity for invention concerns a program called BACON. Named after Francis Bacon, BACON examines numerical data sets for systematic mathematical relations of various sorts. Using some relatively simple tactics, BACON has proved capable of rediscovering many important relatinships in physics and chemistry, such as Boyle's law. To be sure, these are only rediscoveries. But as noted earlier, from the standpoint of theorizing about the process a rediscovery may be as good as a discovery.

It is easy to argue that BACON captures only a very limited aspect of creativity. Why would a scientist be examining a particular data set in the first place? Why not some other data set? What paradigms or other patterns of expectation motivate a particular way of addressing nature (see Kuhn, 1962)? What drives the scientist to make the effort? What broad questions does the scientist formulate and where do they come from? At the same time, one can grant BACON its due. It does have a certain scientific "aesthetic" built in, one that values parsimony of a mathematical kind. It does search for and discover such relationships. To be sure, this *is* a part of what a creative scientist does.

Lenat (1983) developed a program called AM that perhaps captures something more of the nature of invention. AM "thinks about" elementary set and number theory, seeking to make and test interesting conjectures. Built into the processing of AM are a number of criteria for what makes a concept "interesting" and how to combine concepts in search of "interesting" ones. For instance, a relationship that sometimes, but only rarely, holds up gets points for being "interesting." By this measure, a prime number, divisible only by itself and 1, is interesting. Using its criteria for "interestingness" and its rules of combination, AM in fact generated the very concept of a prime number, along with a number of other concepts and principles familiar in elementary number theory.

Again one can complain that AM leaves out a great deal. AM is given its mission: what primitives to start with, what aesthetic to apply, what rules of combination to try. To be sure, AM goes far beyond those beginnings to discover some surprising things. However, human creators do not receive those beginnings on a platter. Naturally, a large part of the question of creativity concerns where the givens for AM come from. Again, however, in recognizing some of the limitations of AM one cannot dismiss it. AM is in no sense given the answers, but genuinely works toward interesting mathematical ideas in a quite divergent way.

The way BACON and AM achieve originality points to a broad limitation of both. Neither one breaks boundaries in its "thinking." Often, a human creator achieves originality in part by challenging rules or assumptions that have governed prior thinking. BACON and AM do nothing of the sort, but work entirely within the rules and assumptions they start with. To be sure, humans have made some significant original discoveries by applying old rules and assumptions. This is closer to what BACON and AM do. Broadly speaking, one might measure BACON and AM by Thomas Kuhn's concept of paradigms and paradigm change in science: The programs work within a paradigm but do not challenge the boundaries of paradigms as human invention often does (Kuhn, 1962). Of course, work within a paradigm can be creative.

How can we understand broadly the mechanism by which BACON and AM achieve their (limited) creativity? A general tactic is common to both. The programs are equipped with generative rules that allow the construction of candidate relationships. The rules are biased so that they tend to generate certain sorts of relationships considered "interesting" and likely to be valid. At the same time, both programs incorporate ways of evaluating the interestingness and validity of a relationship after it is generated. Interestingness gives the programs an aesthetic. Correctness of results comes from tests of validity: Does the relationship match the entire data set or hold up when checked against several numbers? In summary, a generate-and-select plan applied at various levels with well-chosen criteria of interestingness and validity driving both the generation and selection processes can yield what, coming from a human being, would certainly be considered discoveries. Furthermore, the generate-and-select plan is not at all alien to the human condition. People organize their behavior that way in problem-solving situations generally – as Beethoven's notebooks reveal that he did (see Newell & Simon, 1972; Perkins, 1981; Thayer, 1921).

The tactic of generation and selection even points to the way that descendants of BACON and AM might "think" in a more boundary breaking way. In principle, a computer program can work with representations of parts of itself, including representations of some of the rules it is following. One could imagine a program that, to some extent, generates and selects new rules for itself that displace old ones. Indeed, Lenat (1983) is extending the work on AM in just that direction. In other words, there is nothing intrinsically impossible about a computer program adding to and even discarding some of its own starting rules, although BACON and AM do not.

How does all this help the quest for mechanism? It shows that well-defined computational procedures can make significant bits of discovery. In principle, at least, those procedures can even be self-revising, allowing for a kind of boundary breaking. Broadly speaking, the computational procedures involved are not terribly exotic. They are procedures of generation and selection and associated functions of storage, retrieval, representation, and so on. Although research on such procedures comes no where near to capturing the breadth of creativity, it does encourage the idea that the building blocks of the mechanism of creativity might be more prosaic than one would at first think. Perhaps the processes that account for most of our thinking — processes such as reasoning, pattern recognition, memory retrieval, and evaluating — can, in the right combination, account for human creativity, without there being any need to resort to exotic explanations. This theme is revisited in later sections.

Levels of mechanism

Although experiments with computers can tell us something about the role of rules in invention, most of all we want to trace the sources of creativity in the human mind. What mechanisms there explain creativity? In examining that question, it is useful to focus on three broadly contrasted levels of explanation: potencies, plans, and values. Of course, we could discuss each of these in far more detail, highlighting a host of subdistinctions and interrelations, but for purposes of organizing this discussion, a relatively straightforward treatment will do.

Potencies. Here *potencies* refer to computational powers of the mind at or near the neurological level — mental muscle, so to speak. Perhaps creativity depends on a person's performing certain mental operations very efficiently or effectively, operations that do not lend themselves to a strategic approach. For example, one view of IQ holds that IQ in large part reflects basal neurological efficiency (Jensen, 1984). According to this account, IQ measures a potency. One can ask in what way potency is related to creativity. In the case of Beethoven, one can ask what general or even specifically musical potencies nourished his creativity — a powerful musical memory, the ability to "image" sounds, cognitive operations that tended to dissect and recompose conventional musical structures?

Plans. Here *plans* refer to the patterns by which a person's deployment of his or her potencies is organized. In terms of terminology well established in psychology, a plan is the same thing as a schema or frame. Although the meanings of *schema* and *frame* vary slightly from author to author, the general notion is sharp enough for present purposes. Note that plans need not be conscious. Creativity might reflect the persistent use of certain plans —

the plan of challenging assumptions for example. Beethoven's plan of exploring ideas in his notebooks is one example of a generic plan that many inventive, and not so inventive, people use: The plan of planning. His numerous revisions point to another plan mentioned earlier: generation and selection on criteria of interestingness and validity.

Values. Here *values* refer to the larger values that shape the direction of a person's endeavors. For instance, in the generate-and-select plan, the criteria that apply during the generation and screening processes reflect values. Whether, for instance, a person cherishes originality and tolerates ambiguity might influence considerably the person's tendency to engage in creative activities. Part of Beethoven's genius seems to have been his zest for going beyond the conventions of his day.

As the examples accompanying the comments on potencies, plans, and values suggest, all three potentially influence creativity. The question is, Can any generalizations be made about which is most influential and how? The question is especially tricky because potencies, plans, and values might foster creativity in quite different ways. For one contrast, it is important to distinguish between a characteristic (whether potency, plan, or value) *enabling* creativity and a characteristic *promoting* creativity. An enabling characteristic equips a person for creativity without particularly pressing the person to use his or her abilities in a creative way, much as being tall equips one to play better basketball without otherwise encouraging one to play basketball. A promoting characteristic, in contrast, yields such a press. It is also important to contrast characteristics that promote creativity *specifically* versus achievement *in general*. For example, desire for public notice might promote any of a range of aspirations, some of which would be creative and some not.

These distinctions have some importance because a very different picture of creativity emerges depending on the way a characteristic that fosters creativity does so. General intelligence, or *g*, makes a good case in point. At one extreme, someone might propose that a high *g* simply *enables* a person to be a good academic and hence perhaps a creative one. At the other extreme, someone might propose that a high *g* *specifically promotes* creativity in an academic. In the first case, *g* explains no more about academic creativity than having a hand explains writing; in the second, it explains much more.

Finally, note that for the sake of simplicity potencies, plans, values, enabling, and promoting have been treated rather categorically: One has a potency or not; it promotes creativity or it does not. Of course, all this, as with creativity itself, is a matter of degree. Even a plan or a value can be pursued more or less persistently.

Armed with the rough contrast between potencies, plans, and values and the distinctions between enabling, generally promoting, and specifically promoting creativity, we turn now to the findings of empirical work on the sources of creativity.

Creativity as potencies

The notion that creativity depends on one or more potencies has a natural appeal, because it amounts to a direct translation of an ability into a provision for that ability. To caricature the matter for clarity, perhaps creative people have a "creativity lobe" in their brains. This creativity lobe has the special purpose of performing those cognitive operations important for creativity — perhaps analogy making, assumption challenging, and so on. In the terms of the previous section, the creativity lobe promotes creativity specifically. To be sure, other parts of the brain play an enabling role, providing basic psychological functions without which a person could not do anything. But the creativity lobe is key.

Of course, no one since the phrenologists has proposed anything so simplistic as a creativity lobe, but the idea of mental functions that foster creativity remains an attractive one. Let us consider a number of candidates.

Intelligence

One of the broadest and most straightforward proposals about creativity is that creativity amounts simply to g, general intelligence. Whether this yields an interpretation of creativity as a matter of potency rather than of plans and values depends on one's theory of g. As mentioned earlier, Arthur Jensen (1984) views general intelligence as a reflection of the basal precision and efficiency of the nervous system, whereas Baron (1978) among others urges the importance of cognitive strategies and styles in g. Whatever the resolution, a reduction of creativity to intelligence forecasts a correlation between IQ and creative achievement. To the contrary, a number of investigations comparing performance within a discipline have failed to find much connection between intelligence and creative achievement or indeed postschool achievement of any sort (Baird, 1982; Barron, 1969; Wallach, 1976a,b).

The qualification "within a discipline" is crucial; there are substantial relations between various disciplines and intelligence. For example, one does not find professional physicists or mathematicians with IQs much lower than 120 or 130. Correlations between creative achievement and intelligence involving a general population are positive, if for no other reason than that disciplines in which creative work occurs typically require above-average IQs for the attainment of academic credentials and entrance into the disciplines. Torrance's (1972a,b, 1981) data offer such correlations, for instance. Moreover, there are grounds for concluding that creativity and intelligence are more highly correlated in the lower and midrange of intelligence than in its upper reaches (Crockenberg, 1972; Torrance, 1966; Yamamoto, 1965). The evidence depends not on biographical measures of creativity but rather on scores from the Torrance Tests of Creative Thinking (Torrance, 1966, 1974). However, the Torrance tests have some validity (Torrance, 1972a, 1980, 1981; Torrance & Wu, 1981), so the conclusion seems reasonable.

What does this pattern of results suggest about the relationship between general intelligence and creativity? Intelligence appears to enable creativity to some extent but not to promote it. The pattern of decreasing correlation with increasing intelligence signifies an enabling rather than a promoting relationship: The more intelligent one is, the more one *can* be, but still *may not* be, creative. Even if intelligence did promote creativity, intelligence in view of its definition and the ways it is tested would not appear to be specific to creativity. Finally, the absence of within-field relationships between intelligence and creativity argues that the enabling character of intelligence has more to do with entry into a field than subsequent success: If one is bright enough to become a professional in the field, how *creative* a professional one becomes is another matter. For a long time it has been argued that professional excellence in general (whether creative or just exceptionally competent) calls for much more than intelligence as classically construed. Sternberg (1985) has offered a broadened view of intelligence that makes room for the sorts of savvy that underlie such matters as managing one's professional life well.

Ideational fluency and flexibility

These terms refer to a person's ability to produce relatively quickly numerous relevant ideas on a topic, varied ideas in the case of flexibility (Guilford & Hoepfner, 1971; Wallach, 1970). As with intelligence, some psychologists might argue for viewing ideational fluency and flexibility as plans; the fluent person perhaps has strategies for idea production that the less fluent person lacks. However, by and large there is a tendency in the literature to treat ideational fluency and flexibility as atomic capacities that perhaps can be improved by practice. This has the character of a potency.

The matter of enabling versus promoting gains some clarity simply from the concepts of ideational fluency and flexibility. Ideational fluency yields a number of options but not necessarily options that range widely. By definition invoking varied types of ideas, ideational flexibility imparts a divergent cast to the options and hence makes a novel outcome more likely. Therefore, it makes most sense to say that ideational fluency would enable creativity whereas ideational flexibility would promote it specifically.

However, this question of a potency specifically promoting creativity is tricky, depending on a subtle issue about the organization of mind. Potency of flexibility would not in itself yield creative behavior. That potency must be brought into play by something, perhaps a value attached to variety in options or a plan of searching widely. In those cases, it is the value or plan that must get credit for promoting creativity; the ideational fluency simply enables the process. Perhaps, however, one's ideational fluency is "self-starting," coming into play whenever possible. In that case, it would specifically promote creativity. To pose the question more generally, do we function from the "top down," with particular value and plans recruiting exactly those potencies needed and so dominating the character of the results, or from the "bottom up," with potencies springing into action spontaneously whenever they can and so directly shaping the results? Such questions are notoriously difficult to resolve, and broadly speaking "some of both" often seems to be the most likely answer.

Fortunately, we can approach the question of ideational fluency and flexibility psychometrically, without having to resolve the matter of top-down versus bottom-up organization. The proposal that ideational fluency and flexibility contribute to creativity in any degree forecasts a positive correlation with measures of actual creative achievement. In fact, empirical research offers only scattered support for such a relation. In their review of testing for creativity in science and engineering, Mansfield and Busse (1981) examined five tests scored by idea counts and originality or other quality ratings of ideas. Each test was represented by several studies, all involving supervisor ratings or other real-world measures of creativity. No test showed a consistently positive relation to creativity, but most presented at least one positive result. Curiously, the best-known way of gauging ideational fluency and flexibility yielded the poorest results. An "unusual-uses" test requires that one list in a limited period as many unusual uses for an ordinary object such as a brick or a paper clip as one can. A number of assessments based on unusual-uses tests disclosed hardly any relation to creativity.

Further discouragement comes from research with the Wallach and Kogan Creativity Battery (Wallach & Kogan, 1965), which gauges number and uniqueness of responses on a variety of tasks. Wallach (1976b) himself argued against the criterion validity of this instrument after a considerable effort had been made to investigate its predictive powers. Other negative evidence comes from a process-tracing study of poets reported by Perkins (1981, chap. 5). The poets rated higher did not search longer for options in the course of creating, although perforce they thought of better options. Perkins (chap. 6) also discussed the general relationship between a poet's rate of work and reputation as a creator, noting that fluency varies widely among acknowledged masters and hacks alike, there being no obvious relation to quality.

The Torrance Tests of Creative Thinking offer findings that are more supportive of a relationship between fluency, flexibility, and creativity. Long-term studies have disclosed correlations of the order of .5 between Torrance test scores and creative achievement (Torrance, 1972a, 1980, 1981; Torrance & Wu, 1981). However, even here concerns arise. First of all, Torrance test scores appear somewhat related to IQ, so the results may reflect a relation to general intelligence in part. In one study (Torrance, 1972a), a measure of intelligence correlated with later creative achievement only slightly less than did Torrance scores, and in another (Torrance, 1972b) intelligence was sometimes a slightly better predictor. Torrance (1981) reported a much stronger relationship between Torrance scores and creative achievement than between intelligence and creative achievement, but the latter correlations were still statistically significant. Finally, one must ask what, exactly, the Torrance test measures. Plass, Michael, and Michael (1974) factor-analyzed a body of results from the Torrance test, with each subtest scored for fluency, flexibility, originality, and elaboration. They found that the emergent factors corresponded to the subtests themselves rather than the traits scored. So the Torrance tests may not measure fluency, flexibility, originality, and elaboration so much as they do performance on several tasks globally related to creativity.

In summary, efforts to demonstrate a relationship between ideational fluency and flexibility and creativity have yielded vexed results. Some instruments supposedly measuring the same trait have fared better than others. Considerable although not complete redundancy with general intelligence appears. When a test shows some criterion validity, it is not clearly attributable to the theoretical constructs of ideational fluency and flexibility. With such a pattern of findings, it seems too bold to conclude that ideational fluency and flexibility promote creativity, and perhaps they do not even enable it. One might say that tests in that style sometimes measure *something* that at least generally enables and promotes creativity, but what that something is and whether it is more a matter of potencies, plans, or values remains elusive.

Remote associative ability

Another well-known proposal for a creative potency is a *flat associative hierarchy*. Although in most people the close associations between concepts are strong and the more remote associates far weaker, in some people strength of association might taper off more slowly with remoteness of association. For such people, remote associates with their creative potentials would be more accessible. Mednick (1962), elaborating this viewpoint, developed the Remote Associates Test (RAT) to measure flatness of associative hierarchy. The RAT posed trios of terms such as *surprise, line,* and *birthday* and required that the test taker find the common remote associate of the three, in this case *party*. Such a potency would enable creativity specifically by making accessible options that otherwise would never be conceived.

Unfortunately, empirical work casts doubt on the relevance of the RAT and a flat associative hierarchy. First of all, findings on the correlation between real-world creative achievement and RAT scores have been inconsistent and unpersuasive (Blooberg, 1973; Mansfield & Busse, 1981; Mendelsohn, 1976). Moreover, people taking the RAT report going about it by forming hypotheses and testing them, an account that suggests a plan-driven process more than ripples of excitation spreading through an associative network. Several studies have measured directly subjects' ability to produce remote associates, sought correlations with RAT scores, and failed to find them (Mendelsohn, 1976). Apparently the RAT does not actually measure flatness of associative hierarchy, even though that was the intent.

Multiple intelligences

Conceptualizations of intelligence other than the traditional one deserve consideration here. One such has been proposed by Howard Gardner (1983), who posits the existence of seven aspects or dimensions of intelligence with distinct neurological bases: linguistic, musical, logical-mathematical, spatial, bodily-kinesthetic, intrapersonal, and interpersonal. Gardner holds that, under normal circumstances of social opportunity and instruction, exceptional achievement in any domain reflects a substantial initial endowment of the appropriate intelligences. (Most demanding activities call for special contributions from more than one intelligence.) However, Gardner notes that unusually effective instruction may help an individual with only ordinary talent to achieve far beyond the normal expectation, as with the Suzuki violin method.

How might one of Gardner's intelligences contribute to creativity? For example, high musical or mathematical intelligence would at least generally enable and promote creativity in music or mathematics. The greater intelligence would allow and encourage the individual to explore more options and choose sensitively among them. Nothing about Gardner's concept, however, suggests that high intelligence in a domain would enable or promote creativity specifically. One might have enormous talent in music or mathematics without much inclination toward creative expression. Whether or not the prediction of a generally enabling and promoting influence holds up calls for empirical inquiry that by and large has not been carried out.

One particular study illustrates the complexity of relating potency measures to creativity. Getzels and Csikszentmihalyi (1976) report that perceptual and, in fact, cognitive factors figured little in the relative success of male student artists enrolled in fine arts programs. It is as though sheer perceptual talent took a back seat to matters of personality and values, which substantially correlate with the criterion variables – grades, in which creativity seemed to figure and, a direct rating of originality and artistic potential. In contrast, female fine arts majors displayed a positive correlation between perceptual skills and the criterion variables but not between the values and personality measures and the criterion variables. Getzels and Csikszentmihalyi took this to mean that male and female art students were appraised on different grounds, males in terms of the personalities and values that would lead them to be creative and females in terms of competencies. Both male and female fine arts majors fell well above college norms in their perceptual abilities, suggesting that perceptual talent equipped them to function competently as artists. All in all, this study of student artists provides an interesting snapshot of the complex rather than straightforward role a particular talent may play in the development of creative abilities. Identifying creativity as such with talent clearly would be unwarranted.

Although other less familiar interpretations of creativity as a reflection of potencies could be considered (see Perkins, 1981), those reviewed here suffice to give the general picture. They make plain the pattern in efforts to account for creativity by way of potencies: Sometimes empirical evidence suggests that a potency enables creativity. There is no clear evidence that any potency promotes creativity, much less promotes it specifically in preference to other sorts of achievement. To put this another way, potencies equip a person for doing something well, but the person may or may not do that something creatively. The potencies do not *make* a person creative but simply *allow* the person to be creative if other factors encourage it. At least, that seems to be the trend of the results to date.

Creativity as plans

Any intricate course of thought will call on a host of mediating plans – what hue to mix, what cadence to use, what statistical test to apply, and so on, depending on the field involved. Such highly context specific plans hold no great interest in the quest for the general mechanism of creativity. Extremely broad plans such as the generate-and-select plan mentioned earlier help us to understand how a creative person can work toward a final result. But such plans plainly do not promote creativity specifically; they figure in nearly any sort of mindful endeavor, creative or not. What plans are candidates for the promotion of creativity specifically? First, consider some examples with a documented connection to inventive thinking.

Problem finding

Getzels and Csikszentmihalyi (1976) conducted a study of male student artists that involved examining their thinking processes in the studio, gathering assessments of their creativity, and checking their professional advancement a number of years later. The investigators identified a pattern of behavior they termed *problem finding*, which was exhibited by some students much more than others. Problem-finding behaviors included spending more time exploring approaches to a work before settling on one, remaining ready to change directions when a new approach suggested itself later, and not viewing a work as fixed, even when finished for the moment. Getzels and Csikszentmihalyi found strong correlations between degree of problem finding and both creativity ratings of the artists' student works and professional success several years later.

Basically, problem-finding behaviors fend off closure: Problem finders explore extensively before committing themselves to a direction, remain open to new directions, and resist viewing a work as finished. Problem finding promotes creativity specifically by downrating the weight of precedent and prior thought. The question remains whether problem-finding behavior can be considered a plan that one follows. Certainly we can phrase the conduct displayed by problem-finders as plans: "At the outset, spend time exploring alternative approaches," or "When a new approach suggests itself, entertain it seriously," for example. However, a critic might argue that problem-finding behavior simply follows automatically from certain potencies. Driven by the spontaneous activity of some potency generative of insight, a creative individual explores the problem before engaging it in ways that a less creative person would not.

This is a reasonable concern. Not only that, but it can be raised in rebuttal to the other plans discussed below just as well as to problem finding. But there is a flaw in the argument: What potency provokes the appearance of the plan in question? If that plan correlates with creativity, so should the potency. If one would count the plan as promoting creativity specifically, one should count the potency in that way too. However, as we concluded in the discussion of potencies in the previous section, none of the potencies put forth to date can be considered any more than enabling factors. The challenge that a potency rather than a plan accounts for the pattern of behavior in question suffers for lack of good candidate potencies.

A set-breaking set

The psychotherapist Albert Rothenberg has developed a view of creativity that highlights the tendency of creative people to think in negations, contraries, and opposites. As an icon for such thinking, Rothenberg adopts the Roman deity Janus, who, having two faces, looks two ways at once. Rothenberg (1979) makes an extensive case for "Janusian thinking" by examining a number of creations in the arts and the sciences.

A logical weakness impairs Rothenberg's historical evidence. Creativity, by definition involving originality, must always break boundaries in some way; hence, negations, contraries, or opposites in some sense have to figure. To speak of Janusian thinking is merely to say in different words what is implicit definitionally in creativity. Likewise, the statement that creativity somehow involves set breaking is merely circular.

But to demonstrate a disposition in creative people to break set even in trivial contexts is another matter. The supposed historical evidence aside, Rothenberg has performed experiments that offer more substantive support (Rothenberg, 1979, pp. 196–206). The experiments document a tendency for creative people to think in opposites even on simple word association tests, with appropriate controls for vocabulary. A plausible interpretation of such a trend holds that creative people maintain a contrary bias in their thinking as a plan. They harbor a set-breaking set, one might say. Such a plan would promote creativity specifically. It seems likely that there is some overlap between this tendency toward contrary thinking and problem finding, with its caution against committing oneself to a particular approach.

So far, two plans with a demonstrated relation to creativity have been discussed. Unfortunately, the literature offers empirical evidence of a connection between generic plans and creativity specifically in only a couple of instances. There are many other plans that might figure in the natural repertoire of creative individuals. It is worth discussing several.

Brainstorming

Brainstorming as a formal technique of group ideation was developed by Osborn (1953). The method involves banning criticism, deferring closure, stressing the fluent production of novel ideas, and encouraging add-ons and analogies to enrich the sample. The group method aside, the term *brainstorming* applies informally to any individual effort to generate a pool of ideas, deferring criticism and closure. It is a natural conjecture that many creative individuals brainstorm without ever having heard of the idea. They have discovered for themselves that deferred criticism and closure provides for a rich array of ideas from which to select. Certainly there is evidence in plenty of undersearching as a recurrent characteristic of ineffective natural problem solving (e.g., Bereiter & Scardamalia, 1985; Gettys, 1983; Gettys & Engelmann, 1983; Markman, 1977; Markman, 1979; Perkins, 1985a). However, I know of no empirical evidence one way or the other on whether creative people commonly brainstorm. If, indeed, such a process serves natural creative thinking, it would promote creativity specifically.

Analogical thinking

Numerous writers have emphasized on historical grounds the importance of analogical thinking in invention (e.g., Koestler, 1964; Schon, 1963). Like brainstorming, analogical thinking is a formal technique. Gordon (1961), in his book *Synectics*, presented a sequence of steps for group problem solving based on several types of analogies. Perhaps analogizing does not figure as frequently or powerfully in discovery as has sometimes been maintained; Perkins (1983) argued that novel remote analogies contribute less often to invention than is commonly supposed, both because more prosaic means lead to invention and because there may not be that many *powerful* analogies to be found. The caveat notwithstanding, one might hypothesize that at least some creative individuals discover for themselves or from others the powers of analogizing and maintain analogizing as one plan mediating ideation. If so, analogizing would seem to promote creativity specifically.

In addition to plans that might promote creativity, there are others that might be thought to do so but are better considered to be generally enabling.

Heuristics for mathematical problem solving

Considerable writing and research have addressed effective problem solving in mathematics while saying little about mathematical creativity as such (Polya, 1954, 1957; Schoenfeld, 1979a,b, 1980; Wickelgren, 1974). This work locates mathematical problem-solving ability in large part in a repertoire of problem-solving heuristics and self-management strategies possessed by the sophisticated mathematician. One experiment in particular makes a persuasive empirical case for the relevance of such a repertoire (Schoenfeld, 1982; Schoenfeld & Herrmann, 1982). The investigators taught students a number of heuristics and a self-management strategy, documented very substantial improvement in problem-solving performance, and demonstrated that the students came to classify problems to a greater extent, as did professional mathematicians, a sign that their patterns of encoding problems were becoming more expert (see Chase & Simon, 1973; Chi, Feltovich, & Glaser, 1981; Larkin, McDermott, Simon, & Simon, 1980).

How might these heuristics and management strategies contribute to creativity? In fact, little in the plans involves originality, nor are the characteristic values for mathematical proofs, such as elegance and parsimony, strongly represented. Moreover, no empirical results document a correlation with creativity as such. All in all, these plans are best considered enabling rather than promoting of creativity. They make a person a better mathematical problem solver but not necessarily a more creative mathematician.

Selective encoding, combination, and comparison

As part of his triarchic theory of intelligence, Robert Sternberg proposes a theory of insight, a process he places at the core of creative thinking (Sternberg, 1985, pp. 79–93). Sternberg maintains that an occasion of insight depends on one or more of three related but distinct psychological processes: selective encoding, selective combination, and selective comparison. *Selective encoding* refers to the encoding of available information with a selectivity appropriate to the context and task demands. *Selective combination* signifies synthesizing appropriate pieces of information into a relevant whole. *Selective comparison* denotes aptly relating new to previously acquired information. In all three cases, the term *selective* highlights the need for such processes to discriminate keenly between relevant and irrelevant information. (Their placement in the plans rather than potencies section reflects my judgment that the processes are commonly initiated as subgoals and pursued in a problem-solving fashion. This is in keeping with Sternberg's general view that the components in his theory are not primitive but can be broken down; see Sternberg, 1985, p. 98. In any case, the comments to follow do not depend on the way in which the three are categorized.)

Sternberg suggests that these processes are related specifically to insight and help to explain why psychologists have had so much difficulty in pinning down the nature of insight: Three processes are involved rather than one. Clearly, the three would at least generally enable creativity, but would they promote it, and promote creativity specifically rather than intellectual achievement in general? At least on the surface, the processes seem general to intelligent functioning, rather than specific to insight or creativity. Consider addressing a difficult math problem, for example. One would gain from good selective encoding discrimination of the crucial information among distractions: from good selective combination, synthesis of the information into a solution: and from good selective comparison, discernment of those previously solved problems that might inform one's approach to the present problem. In general, it seems plain that any challenging problem would tend to call upon the three processes, whether or not it had a creative cast.

Someone might object that solving any difficult problem requires insight. If, by *insight*, we mean the understanding that arises when things suddenly fall into place, this plainly does not hold: Many a difficult problem yields to intensive intelligent analysis without there being any one crucial breakthrough. If, by *insight*, we mean simply a good understanding of the problem achieved in the process of seeking a solution, then insight becomes confounded with understanding generally, losing its distinctive character, which was the very thing to be explained. Someone also might object that solving any difficult problem requires creativity. Such a demurral would suffer from the flaw just mentioned: Creativity is collapsed into intelligence generally, losing the distinctive phenomenon to be explained. In summary, selective encoding, combination, and comparison may be important components of intelligence that enable and even promote insightful and creative thinking, but they do not appear to be specifically associated with either one. This accords with Perkins's (1981) argument that the mental operations mediating creativity figure in all sorts of other activities.

In summary, this section samples several plans that have the potential to explain aspects of creativity. The discussion reveals a complete spectrum, from plans with a demonstrated relation to creativity, to plans that may well contribute directly to creativity but for which there is no empirical evidence, to plans that on logical grounds would appear simply to be enabling or perhaps generally promoting. Although the picture is not monolithic, one can find at least some plans that promote creativity specifically. This means that we can understand the character of creativity more fully in terms of the plans creative people deploy than in terms of the potencies they possess.

Creativity as values

What values might promote creativity? One answer concerns the contextually appropriate values for different disciplines. Cultivators of roses have their criteria, and cultivators of cabbage, theirs. Likewise, the mathematician would benefit from a love for rigor and elegance, the general an appreciation for the deceptive maneuver and the critical target. But of more concern here are broad standards and values that might figure in nearly any context and foster creativity generally.

Originality

One such value is originality, a component of the very concept of creativity, as explained earlier. Plentiful research argues that creative individuals cherish originality as such and seek it out. For example, personality studies of creative artists and scientists have documented a strong tendency toward autonomy and independence (Barron, 1969, 1972; Getzels & Csikszentmihalyi, 1976; Helson, 1971; MacKinnon, 1962, 1965; Mansfield & Busse, 1981). Biographical studies of scientists have disclosed that creative scientists self-consciously seek out what they take to be the "hot" areas inviting challenging original work (Mansfield & Busse, 1981; Roe, 1952a,b, 1963). A brief review of these sources can be found in Perkins (1981, chap. 9). It seems plain that such values promote creativity specifically, because they act as constraints guiding the search processes by which people generate and select options (on creative endeavor as a search process see Perkins, 1981, chap. 5).

Generic qualities

Appropriateness was the generic standard coupled with originality in explaining the concept of creativity. What can be said about general types of appropriateness and their contribution to creativity? Whereas many standards of appropriateness are context specific, some broadly stated standards are worth mentioning. In the sciences, for example, consistency, parsimony, generality, fundamentalness, and predictive power are widely accepted values. Biographical studies suggest that many creative scientists are quite conscious of such desiderata (Mansfield & Busse, 1981; Roe, 1952a,b). In studies of student artists, Getzels and Csikszentmihalyi (1976) found that the more creative artists displayed a concern for fundamental problems of, for instance, life and human nature in conceiving works, even when their products carried no obvious philosophical message. Encouraging the rejection of the narrow and mediocre and a search for the broad and fundamental as they do, such values certainly promote achievement generally.

Whether they promote creativity in particular depends on one's sense of promotion. The argument that they do not do so is as follows. Recalling the previous contrast of work within a paradigm versus work that challenges a paradigm, the values mentioned can be exercised fully within a paradigm. In that sense, they do not press a person to break boundaries as happens in the most dramatic examples of creativity. But it can also be argued that values do promote creativity. It was mentioned earlier that originality is not necessarily confined to the breaking of boundaries; it may consist, for instance, in the discovery of heretofore neglected opportunities. The press for fundamentalness, parsimony, and so on would tend to promote the discovery of such opportunities. Moreover, according to Kuhn (1962), paradigms are challenged seriously only when their flaws become perceptible. One could say, therefore, that it is the drive to rescue the parsimony, fundamentalness, and so on at risk of being lost that leads some thinkers to challenge the boundaries. In such a course of events, originality is not sought so much for its own sake but as a necessary path toward a new integration. In sum, the values mentioned promote creativity specifically in one sense but not in another. These complications in the meaning of *promote* are a reality that we do well simply to accept.

Critical tolerances

Another face of the matter of values concerns what a person does *not* attach a very negative value to, but comfortably tolerates. Creative work routinely involves confronting the uncertainties of new frontiers, for example. In keeping with this, Roe (1963) has noted the tolerance of creative scientists for ambiguity, along with their drive to resolve that ambiguity. Getzels and Csikszentmihalyi (1976) report an interesting result concerning panels of lay persons and professional critics assessing the creativity of works of art: Although both groups accurately discriminated the more from the less original, the lay panelists *disliked* the more original works. In general, intolerance for originality, ambiguity, and other characteristics of creative products or processes would inhibit creative endeavor. Accordingly, such tolerances specifically enable but do not specifically promote creativity: They free a person to search for more creative options but do not discourage the person from accepting less creative options.

In summary, creative people tend to share a certain broad aesthetic involving a positive affinity for the general, fundamental, elegant, and original, along with a tolerance for and even enjoyment of ambiguity and complexity. Such an aesthetic provides the individual with a strong intrinsic motivation to create. Amabile (1983) has presented extensive arguments and evidence regarding the importance of such intrinsic motivation in sustaining creative endeavor.

So far, the discussion of values by and large supports their promoting creativity specifically, perhaps even more so than plans. But someone could object that values merely reflect a person's potencies: Those who are well equipped for creative endeavor would find it easy and so fall into a creative pattern of values. According to such a reading, certain potencies would make up the essence of creativity, values being a side effect. This challenge has some merit: Certainly a person ill equipped cognitively for the demands of creative endeavor would tend to find such endeavor frustrating and so might form values antagonistic to creativity.

Common experience, however, offers counterexamples to viewing values merely as an echo of potencies. Many people aspire to creative success but are ill equipped for it; other individuals with great technical flair for, let us say, music or mathematics sometimes display no great inclination toward creativity. The same partial independence of values and potencies appears in other activities as well. Many who aspire to athletic excellence lack the talent, whereas some with natural strength and coordination show no great interest. Finally, we should remember again the lack of evidence that potencies promote creativity. With these counterarguments in mind, it seems most reasonable to view the value profile characteristic of creative individuals as something that directly promotes creativity, rather than as a side effect of potencies.

Creativity as expertise

So far little has been said directly about whether creativity is specific to a field or is general. After all, people function creatively in innumerable domains – gardening, physics, law, humor, architecture, and parenting to name a few. Is creativity the same thing across these varied contexts?

Contemporary psychology offers abundant evidence of the importance of particular knowledge for achievement in a field. Research has revealed that expertise depends on a sizable repertoire of schemata quite specific to the field in question. This seems generally true, since the sources of evidence include such domains as mathematics (Schoenfeld & Herrmann, 1982), physics (Chi et al., 1981; Larkin et al., 1980), computer programming (Schneiderman, 1976; Soloway & Ehrlich, 1984), music (Hayes, 1981; Slaboda, 1976), chess play (Chase & Simon, 1973; de Groot, 1965), and art (Gombrich, 1961, 1979). In terms of our framework, expertise means having and deploying fluently those potencies, plans, and values that are distinctive to a field. The expert acquires them through long-time involvement supported by initial values that motivate the effort, initial plans that organize the expert's learning, and initial potencies – natural talents – that help the expert to learn readily the requisite details, as suggested by Gardner (1983).

There can be little question that expertise in a field at least enables creativity. That is, without some expertise, one lacks the competency required for significant creative achievement. The question remains whether some field-specific aspects of expertise promote creativity specifically. For instance, recalling Beethoven, is creativity in music promoted in large part by certain specifically musical plans or perhaps specifically musical "metaplans" that have to do with the transformation of existing musical conventions? A strongly affirmative response for music and other fields would mean that not just expertise but creativity is a rather field-specific trait. A strongly negative answer would indicate that, although the components of expertise differ from field to field, the character of creativity per se remains much the same. The question is hard to answer because one would not expect individuals to display great creative achievement in two or more fields very often in any case. Even if their creativity were general, accumulating sufficient expertise for significant achievement would require too much time and commitment (Chase & Simon, 1973; Hayes, 1981). To test the question, one should look for a creative *approach* across domains rather than for significant creative achievement.

I have no hard evidence to offer here, but some arguments from analogy and experience point toward a provisional answer. First of all, the values and plans identified earlier as promoting creativity appear to have considerable generality. Cherishing originality, valuing one's autonomy, tolerating and even enjoying complexity, displaying a passion for the fundamental, problem finding, analogy making, a set to break set, and so on, are all characteristics that, in principle, apply across domains. These facts encourage the view that creativity per se is domain independent.

Someone might counterargue, however, that we are comparing apples and oranges here: A "passion for the fundamental" might amount to quite a different thing in physics and music, for instance. But at least a partial rebuttal presents itself. If what is "fundamental" varies from field to field, the restlessness with the status quo captured by the personality trait of autonomy involves no obvious domain specificity. Moreover, if "a passion for the fundamental" *might* mean something radically different in music versus physics, it seems to mean rather the same thing across many domains – a commitment to overarching principle. In general, although there may be reasons to doubt the complete field universality of creative characteristics, the default position need not be complete field specificity. Finally, personal experience suggests to me that creative people typically display a creative approach to matters outside their domains of expertise, even though they usually lack the competence required for achievement at the professional level.

In summary, the provisional arguments favor the view that creativity as such is a somewhat field independent trait. However, creative achievement at the professional level depends on finding a field for which one has an affinity, having some field-specific talent, and securing the opportunity to develop the expertise required for substantial achievement.

Why did Beethoven have better ideas?

At this point in our quest for mechanism, it makes sense to circle back to Beethoven. What have we learned about the mechanisms of creativity? Why, in particular, did Beethoven have better ideas than other composers?

Perhaps the first comment to make is that Beethoven did not just *have* brilliant ideas; he worked them up and worked them out, as his notebooks testify. In short, there were numerous cycles of generation and selection. These cycles reflect a very broad plan that enables (but does not promote) achievement in nearly any context. But why did Beethoven's results have a creative slant? One contribution surely came from his extensive exploration of the motifs around which to construct a whole work – a straightforward example of the plan of problem finding, which promotes creativity specifically. Another contribution surely came from his archetypically romantic values, which would bias toward originality and other standards his acts of generating ideas and selecting among them. To be sure, if you or I had the same plans and values we probably would not do anywhere near as well. But Beethoven's efforts were underwritten by remarkable potencies that did not in themselves promote creativity but enabled Beethoven to achieve fully what his plans and values disposed him to.

Much the same broad account applies to any creative individual. The general mechanism is something like this: potencies organized by plans and directed by values. In particular, we can itemize at least the following submechanisms. Although it is simpler to describe these mechanisms categorically, we do well to remember that enabling, promoting, and creativity itself are always matters of degree, not of all or nothing.

1. Potencies do not promote creative results. However, they enable creative results by enabling the execution of plans that may promote creative results.
2. Certain plans promote creative results specifically – problem finding or a set to break set, for example.

3. Certain plans simply promote sound results generally. "Divide a problem into parts" has no strongly creative bias, for example.
4. Still other plans need not but can promote creative results, when the plans make room for values with a creative bias. For example, the generate-and-select plan requires criteria that govern the generation and selection processes; originality and related criteria will lead to applications of the generate-and-select plan biased toward creative results.
5. Values promote creative results by biasing what plans are chosen and what criteria fill up plans that have "slots" for criteria, as mentioned above. Delight in originality, tolerance for ambiguity, and desire for the fundamental are relevant values, for example.
6. Values that cannot be satisfied by conventional means can promote creative results as a side effect. Circumstances press a person to challenge prior assumptions in order to solve the problem in question.

According to this perspective, creativity is an emergent phenomenon dependent on a complex conspiracy in which potencies, plans, and values interlock in certain patterns – those listed above and perhaps more. When this occurs once in an individual, creative results follow. When it occurs frequently, creative results follow frequently and we think of the person as creative or as "having creativity." What is this creativity? It consists of certain persisting values, plans, and potencies that supply the conspiracy. Taken together, these values, plans, and potencies *are* a person's creativity.

Sketches of mechanism like this sometimes provoke nontechnical reservations along the lines "But my experience of creativity isn't *like* that." Such concerns actually can mean a couple of things. One is that an account of mechanism does not "feel like" the experience of invention. The answer to this is that it is not supposed to. Einstein is reported to have said that the chemical analysis of a cup of soup should not be expected to taste like the soup. In other words, it is not the job of a mechanism of creativity to "feel like" the experience of creativity but simply to explain creativity.

The other interpretation is that, looking into one's own experience, one does not find these potencies, plans, and values. Actually, many people seem to be able to articulate their values easily, and potencies are more a matter for testing than for self-reports; pinning down plans presents a greater problem. The answer to those who deny that they use such plans is that people are not very good at investigating and reporting their own mental processes without special guidance (Nisbett & Wilson, 1977). Even notable creators in a field may be quite naïve about how they create; indeed, expertise tends to work *against* clear reporting because many plans have been automatized and are not fully accessible to consciousness (Ericsson & Simon, 1984). However, under proper conditions of observation, one can detect and even elicit reports of the sorts of plans discussed here (Ericsson & Simon, 1984; Getzels & Csikszentmihalyi, 1976; Perkins, 1981).

Therefore, if the mechanism uncovered so far falls short, it does so more in technical ways than in ways identified by casual reaction. And to be sure, this precis leaves a host of questions unanswered – some of which we shall list, lest we become self-satisfied with the current state of knowledge: Are the potencies that figure in high achievement generic, as Jensen (1984) would argue, or field specific, as Gardner (1983) would argue? What plans demonstrably foster creativity, considering that empirical evidence is available for only some of the plans discussed here? How do people acquire the kinds of values that foster creativity? To what extent is creativity really a cross-disciplinary phenomenon?

At the same time, the quest for mechanism has advanced in the past several years. Whereas at first creativity might seem utterly mysterious and beyond the pale of explanation by the tools available to psychology, one discovers that one can talk about it sensibly in terms of psychological factors such as potencies, plans, and values that also figure in explanations of other sorts of human behavior. One can even program computers to mimic some limited aspects of creative thinking. Morever, the research to date signals a shift in the character of explanation. For some time, a "potency" perspective was most popular; the mechanism of creativity was sought in potencies like ideational flexibility that specifically promoted creative thinking. The weight of logic and empirical inquiry now tends toward certain plans and values promoting creativity, whereas potencies simply enable it. Meanwhile, despite all this prying into the clockwork, the "Ode to Joy" survives, sounding just as joyous as ever.

References

Amabile, T. M. (1983). *The social psychology of creativity*. New York: Springer-Verlag.

Baird, L. L. (1982). *The role of academic ability in high-level accomplishment and general success* (College Board Rep. No. 82–6). New York: College Entrance Examination Board.

Baron, J. (1978). Intelligence and general strategies. In G. Underwood (Ed.), *Strategies in information processing* (pp. 403–50). New York: Academic Press.

Barron, F. (1969). *Creative person and creative process*. New York: Holt, Rinehart & Winston.

Barron, F. (1972). *Artists in the making*. New York: Seminar Press.

Bereiter, C., & Scardamalia, M. (1985). Cognitive coping strategies and problem of inert knowledge. In S. S. Chipman, J. W. Segal, & R. Glazer (Eds.), *Thinking and learning skills: Vol. 2. Current research and open questions* (pp. 65–80). Hillsdale, NJ: Erlbaum.

Blooberg, M. (1973). Introduction: Approaches to creativity. In M. Blooberg (Ed.), *Creativity: Theory and research*. New Haven, CT: College and University Press.

Chase, W. C., & Simon, H. A. (1973). Perception in chess. *Cognitive Psychology, 4,* 55–81.

Chi, M., Feltovich, P., & Glaser, R. (1981). Categorization and representation of physics problems by experts and novices. *Cognitive Science, 5,* 121–52.

Crockenberg, S. B. (1972). Creativity tests: A boon or boondoggle for education? *Review of Educational Research, 42*(1), 27–45.

de Groot, A. D. (1965). *Thought and choice in chess*. The Hague: Mouton.

Ericsson, K. A., & Simon, H. A. (1984). *Protocol analysis: Verbal reports as data*. Cambridge, MA: MIT Press.

Gardner, H. (1983). *Frames of mind*. New York: Basic.

Gettys, C. F. (1983). *Research and theory on predecision processes* (Tech. Rep.). Norman: University of Oklahoma, Decision Processes Laboratory.

Gettys, C. F., & Engelmann, P. D. (1983). *Ability and expertise in act generation* (Tech. Rep.). Norman: University of Oklahoma, Decision Processes Laboratory.

Getzels, J., & Csikszentmihalyi, M. (1976). *The creative vision: A longitudinal study of problem finding in art.* New York: Wiley.

Gombrich, E. H. (1961). *Art and illusion: A study in the psychology of pictorial representation.* Princeton, NJ: Princeton University Press.

(1979). *The sense of order: A study in the psychology of decorative art.* Ithaca, NY: Cornell University Press.

Gordon, W. J. (1961). *Synectics: The development of creative capacity.* New York: Harper & Row.

Guilford, J. P., & Hoepfner, R. (1971). *The analysis of intelligence.* New York: McGraw-Hill.

Hausman, C. R. (1976). Creativity and rationality. In A. Rothenberg & C. R. Hausman (Eds.), *The creativity question* (pp. 343–51). Durham, NC: Duke University Press.

(1985). Can computers create? *Interchange, 16*(1), 27–37.

Hayes, J. R. (1981). *The complete problem solver.* Hillsdale, NJ: Erlbaum.

Helson, R. (1971). Women mathematicians and the creative personality. *Journal of Consulting and Clinical Psychology, 36,* 210–20.

Jensen, A. R. (1984). Test validity: g versus the specificity doctrine. *Journal of Social and Biological Structures, 7,* 93–118.

Koestler, A. (1964). *The act of creation.* New York: Dell.

Kuhn, T. (1962). *The structure of scientific revolutions.* University of Chicago Press.

Larkin, J. H., McDermott, J., Simon, D. P., & Simon, H. A. (1980). Modes of competence in solving physics problems. *Cognitive Science, 4,* 317–45.

Lenat, D. B. (1983). Toward a theory of heuristics. In R. Groner, M. Groner, & W. Bischof (Eds.), *Methods of heuristics* (pp. 351–404). Hillsdale, NJ: Erlbaum.

MacKinnon, D. W. (1962). The nature and nurture of creative talent. *American Psychologist, 17,* 484–95.

(1965). Personality and the realization of creative potential. *American Psychologist, 20,* 273–81.

Mansfield, R. S., & Busse, T. V. (1981). *The psychology of creativity and discovery.* Chicago: Nelson-Hall.

Markman, E. M. (1979). Realizing that you don't understand: Elementary school children's awareness of inconsistencies. *Child Development, 50,* 643–55.

Mednick, S. A. (1962). The associative basis of the creative process. *Psychological Review, 69,* 220–32.

Mendelsohn, G. A. (1976). Associative and attentional processes in creative performance. *Journal of Personality, 44,* 341–69.

Newell, A., & Simon, H. (1972). *Human problem solving.* Englewood Cliffs, NJ: Prentice-Hall.

Nisbett, R., & Wilson, T. D. (1977). Telling more than we can know: Verbal reports on mental process. *Psychological Review, 84,* 231–59.

Osborn, A. (1953). *Applied imagination.* New York: Scribner.

Perkins, D. N. (1981). *The mind's best work.* Cambridge, MA: Harvard University Press.

(1983). Novel remote analogies seldom contribute to discovery. *Journal of Creative Behavior, 17,* 223–39.

(1985a). Postprimary education has little impact on informal reasoning. *Journal of Educational Psychology, 77*(5), 562–71.

Perkins, D. N. (1985b). What else but genius? Six Dimensions of the creative mind. In M. R. Raju, J. A. Phillips, & F. Harlow (Eds.), *Creativity in science* (pp. 15–27). Los Alamos, NM: Los Alamos National Laboratory.

Plass, H., Michael, J. J., & Michael, W. B. (1974). The factorial validity of the Torrance Tests of Creative Thinking for a sample of 111 sixth-grade children. *Educational and Psychological Measurement, 34,* 413–14.

Polya, G. (1954). *Mathematics and plausible reasoning* (2 vols.). Princeton, NJ: Princeton University Press.

(1957). *How to solve it: A new aspect of mathematical method* (2nd ed.). New York: Doubleday.

Roe, A. (1952a). A psychologist examines 64 eminent scientists. *Scientific American, 187*(5), 21–5.

(1952b). *The making of a scientist*. New York: Dodd, Mead.

(1963). Psychological approaches to creativity in science. In M. A. Coler & H. K. Hughes (Eds.), *Essays on creativity in the sciences*. New York: New York University Press.

Rothenberg, A. (1979). *The emerging goddess: The creative process in art, science, and other fields*. University of Chicago Press.

Schneiderman, B. (1976). Exploratory experiments in programmer behavior. *International Journal of Computer and Information Sciences, 5*, 123–43.

Schoenfeld, A. H. (1979a). Can heuristics be taught? In J. Lochhead & J. Clement (Eds.), *Cognitive process instruction* (315–38). Hillsdale, NJ: Erlbaum.

(1979b). Explicit heuristic training as a variable in problem solving performance. *Journal for Research in Mathematics Education, 10*(3), 173–87.

(1980). Teaching problem-solving skills. *American Mathematical Monthly, 87*, 794–805.

(1982). Measures of problem-solving performance and of problem-solving instruction. *Journal for Research in Mathematics Education, 13*(1), 31–49.

Schoenfeld, A. H., & Herrmann, D. J. (1982). Problem perception and knowledge structure in expert and novice mathematical problem solvers. *Journal of Experimental Psychology: Learning, Memory, and Cognition, 8*, 484–94.

Schon, D. A. (1963). *Displacement of concepts*. London: Tavistock.

Slaboda, J. (1976). Visual perception of musical notation: Registering pitch symbols in memory. *Quarterly Journal of Experimental Psychology, 28*, 1–16.

Soloway, E., & Ehrlich, K. (1984). Empirical studies of programming knowledge. *IEEE Transactions on Software Engineering, SE-10*(5), 595–609.

Sternberg, R. J. (1985). *Beyond I.Q.: A triarchic theory of human intelligence*. Cambridge University Press.

Thayer, A. W. (1921). *The life of Ludwig van Beethoven*. New York: The Beethoven Society.

Torrance, E. P. (1966). *The Torrance Tests of Creative Thinking: Norms-technical manual*. Princeton, NJ: Personnel Press.

(1972a). Career patterns and peak creative achievements of creative high school students twelve years later. *Gifted Child Quarterly, 16*, 75–88.

(1972b). Predictive validity of the Torrance Tests of Creative Thinking. *Journal of Creative Behavior, 6*, 236–52.

(1974). *The Torrance Tests of Creative Thinking: Norms-technical manual*. Bensenville, IL: Scholastic Testing Service.

(1980). Growing up creatively gifted: A 22-year longitudinal study. *Creative Child and Adult Quarterly, 5*, 148–59.

(1981). Predicting the creativity of elementary school children (1958–80) – and the teacher who "made a difference." *Gifted Child Quarterly, 25*, 55–62.

Torrance, E. P., & Wu, T. (1981). A comparative longitudinal study of the adult creative achievements of elementary school children identified as highly intelligent and as highly creative. *Creative Child and Adult Quarterly, 6*, 71–6.

Wallach, M. A. (1970). Creativity. In P. H. Mussen (Ed.), *Carmichael's manual of child psychology* (Vol. 1, pp. 1211–66). New York: Wiley.

(1976a). Psychology of talent and graduate education. In S. Messick & Associates (Eds.), *Individuality in learning*. San Francisco: Jossey-Bass.

(1976b). Tests tell us little about talent. *American Scientist, 64*, 57–63.

Wallach, M. A., & Kogan, N. (1965). *Modes of thinking in young children*. New York: Holt, Rinehart & Winston.

Wickelgren, W. A. (1974). *How to solve problems: Elements of a theory of problems and problem solving*. New York: Freeman.

Yamamoto, K. (1965). Effects of restriction of range and test unreliability on correlation between measures of intelligence and creative thinking. *British Journal of Educational Psychology, 35*, 300–5.

12 Teaching thinking and problem solving: illustrations and issues

Nancy J. Vye, Victor R. Delclos,
M. Susan Burns, and John D. Bransford

The contributors to this book provide a wealth of information about processes that underlie effective thinking, learning, and problem solving. It is possible, of course, that these processes are fixed at birth and that there is nothing one can do to change them. An alternative possibility is that people can be helped to improve their abilities to think, solve problems, and learn on their own. A number of theorists accept the latter hypothesis and have devised programs to facilitate thinking. As Mann (1979) notes, attempts to teach thinking and problem solving have been prevalent since the time of Aristotle. Furthermore, thinking programs have been devised for people ranging from preschool children to adults (see the Appendix for references to a variety of thinking skills programs).

In this chapter we focus on three innovative programs for teaching thinking:

1. Feuerstein and colleagues' Instrumental Enrichment
2. Lipman and colleagues' Philosophy for Children
3. Sternberg's Intelligence Applied

We have selected these programs because they are representative of some of the best among the many available thinking skills curricula. Each is grounded in theory, and each provides extensive training materials and teacher guides. At the same time, these programs exemplify the diversity of approaches that have been developed to teach thinking. They are designed to meet the needs of different age and ability levels, and they approach the fundamental issues in different ways.

We begin by describing each of the programs. We then discuss their similarities and differences, and we consider important issues that underlie any attempt to help people increase their abilities to think and learn.

Feuerstein's Instrumental Enrichment Program

Feuerstein's approach grew out of a real-world problem. After World War II, hundreds of displaced adolescents wanted to immigrate to Israel. Con-

Preparation of this chapter was supported by Contract MDA903-84-C-0218 from the Army Research Institute. We are indebted to Jackie Welch for her editorial help.

ventional test scores revealed that an unusually large number of these adolescents were functioning three to six years below their age norms, with IQ scores in the mentally retarded range. Feuerstein believed that these scores reflected the adolescents' deficiencies in problem-solving skills rather than their native ability. By means of his dynamic assessment technique (see Feuerstein, Rand, & Hoffman, 1979), he was able to demonstrate that many of these individuals had far greater potential to learn than their test scores predicted, and he identified a number of deficient "cognitive functions" that seemed to account for their poor cognitive performance. This led to the development of the Instrumental Enrichment Program, which is designed to provide students with critical cognitive functions and strategies and to help them realize their potential to learn on their own (see Feuerstein, Rand, Hoffman, & Miller, 1980).

Instrumental Enrichment is based on the concept of the mediated learning experience (MLE). This concept emphasizes the role of human agents (parents, teachers, peers) in the cognitive development of the child. Feuerstein's theory of MLE assumes that effective mediators are not simply sources of information, analogous to physical stimuli, that enrich the child's perceptual environment. Instead, effective mediators help the child focus on certain features, interpret various experiences, and so forth.

Why are some children deprived of sufficient MLE? Feuerstein emphasizes that a lack of MLE does not necessarily imply absent parents or significant others. He notes that the quality of MLE depends on characteristics of both the child and the mediating agent. A lack of MLE can occur when the agent fails to mediate to the child (e.g., in the case of an apathetic parent, a parent with diminished expectations, a parent who is too busy doing other things) or when the child poses barriers to mediation (e.g., emotional disturbance).

According to Feuerstein, the consequences for children who lack sufficient MLE can be severe. In general, they manifest 'a diminished level of cognitive functioning. In many cases their scores on conventional tests will fall within the mildly retarded or moderately retarded range. It is commonplace to refer to these individuals as retarded; the invited inference is that they are retarded *individuals*. Feuerstein rejects that inference and uses the term retarded *performers*; to Feuerstein poor performance does not necessarily mean a lack of capacity to think and learn.

Feuerstein notes that retarded performers generally exhibit a phenomenon that he refers to as an *episodic grasp of reality*:

In essence, grasping the world episodically means that each object or event is experienced in isolation without any attempt to relate or link it to previous or anticipated experiences in space and time. An episodic grasp of reality reflects a passive attitude toward one's experiences because no attempt is made by the individual to actively contribute to his experience by organizing, ordering, summating, or comparing events and thereby placing them within a broader and more meaningful context.

. . . An episodic grasp of reality is also responsible for the limited readiness of the individual to respond to incompatibilities in the field that provide the basis for the recognition of the existence of a problem. (Feuerstein, et al., 1980, p. 102–3)

Feuerstein warns that people commonly react to children with low test scores by creating simplified learning environments that do not require sophisticated thinking. He argues that this approach is self-defeating. It creates a self-fulfilling prophesy by depriving the children of the challenging learning experiences they need. He devised his Instrumental Enrichment Program in order to provide children with the tools, confidence, and motivation necessary to learn and solve problems independently. Feuerstein notes that his program is one of many possible ways to provide the kinds of mediation he envisions.

An overview of the instruction

Instrumental Enrichment (IE) was designed primarily for adolescents. Instruction in IE centers around a series of exercises divided into units, or *instruments*, that provide a context for mediating learning. Beginning students usually use the Organization of Dots I (ODI) instrument and the Orientation in Space I (OSI) instrument. Students work on one or the other on alternate days. Figure 12.1 illustrates problems from two different pages of the ODI instrument. (There are a total of 20 pages in this instrument.) The problems within each instrument are ordered by increasing difficulty. For example, the problems in Figure 12.1b are more difficult than those in Figure 12.1a.

Other illustrations of tasks from IE are provided in Figure 12.2. Like the Organization of Dots, many of these tasks are quite different from ones usually found in academic environments. Feuerstein wanted to create learning environments in which students would not have negative attitudes because of previous failures. In addition, he tried to devise environments that did not presuppose a great deal of domain-specific knowledge; otherwise, the students who did not have this knowledge would have a very difficult time.

A discussion of the ODI instrument will illustrate the type of mediation that occurs in IE. The basic task of ODI is to connect dots so that they form figures that match a model. The task has two basic rules: (a) Each dot must be used once and only once, and (b) the figures drawn by connecting the dots (e.g., square, triangle) must be identical to those in the model in size and shape but may differ from the model in orientation. Students usually find the task interesting and are highly motivated to complete the problems. However, the IE teacher does not simply hand out a page from the instruments and collect students' work when they are finished. The teacher's task is to provide MLE by encouraging cognitive activities relevant to the materia.

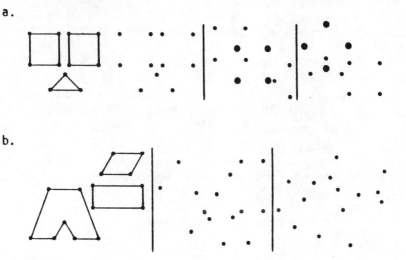

b.

Figure 12.1. Sample exercises from the Organization of Dots. From Feuerstein, Rand, Hoffman, and Miller (1980).

als. Four important elements of this mediation are (a) problem definition and use of strategies, (b) informed practice, (c) introduction of basic concepts, and (d) teaching for transfer. We consider each of these elements in detail.

Problem definition and use of strategies. An important component of each IE lesson involves problem identification and definition. Imagine that students have received a page from ODI. They are asked to define what they think the task is and to explain what led them to their definition. The students are also prompted to consider in what ways the present dot problems are similar to and different from previous problems. For example, students are urged to notice changes in the models (new forms, more complex forms, etc.), in the number and type of cues provided, in the density of dots, and so forth.

An additional step involves the anticipation of difficulties that may arise from changes in the problem format. For example, students may be helped to notice that, for some problems, the answer is readily apparent. At other times one confronts difficulty and must resort to a more systematic, analytic approach. Students are therefore prompted to evaluate different strategies for solving problems. For example, in ODI, students are prompted to consider which figure should be searched for first.

Informed practice. Nearly every IE lesson devotes a considerable amount of time to practice. Students are prompted to evaluate strategies by actually using them and then considering their effectiveness.

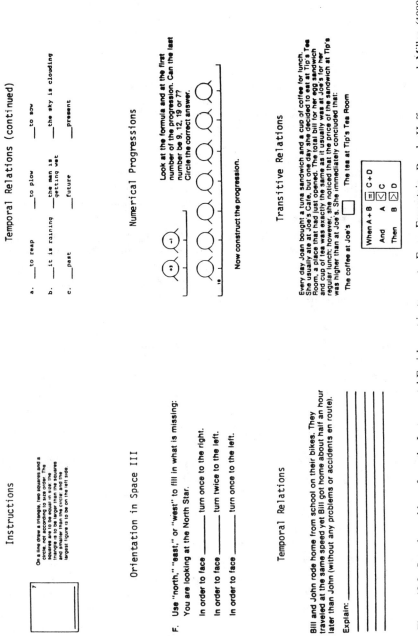

Figure 12.2. Sample problems from the Instrumental Enrichment instruments. From Feuerstein, Rand, Hoffman, and Miller (1980).

The instruments provide a great deal of practice, but each problem encountered is novel. An advantage here is the virtual impossibility of memorizing the answers to each problem. Even teachers who have taught for several years have to work most problems anew. In this way the teacher acts as
a problem-solving model for the students, not simply as someone who provides answers. Students who finish the problems quickly also act as
"teacher"; they are encouraged to help other students who are experiencing
difficulty. Once again, it is impossible simply to provide the correct answers.
The student–student dyads discuss strategies for solving the problem at
hand.

Introduction of basic concepts. A third component of most IE lessons involves the introduction of relevant basic concepts. Concepts such as *model*
and *rules* may be introduced in the context of defining the problem; concepts such as *planning, strategy,* and *checking* may be introduced in the context of attempts to work the problems. Students may also be helped to notice the importance of labeling various aspects of each page in order to
facilitate group discussion. At times, standard labels (e.g., *square, rectangle,
triangle*) are more appropriate; at other times students must confer about
the label ("Let's call this one a teepee").

Teaching for transfer. Two aspects of IE instruction are designed to help students understand how their experiences with the instruments are relevant to
other aspects of their lives.

First, each IE lesson focuses on one or two principles that have broad
generality. For example, the cover page of ODI does not include any dot
problems such as those in Figure 12.1; instead, it provides a view of stars
connected into familiar constellations such as the Big Dipper. Students are
encouraged to discuss whether these stars are actually connected or whether
we simply imagine them to be, and if the latter, why? Students can thereby
be introduced to a general principle such as "Organization is imposed on the
environment for certain purposes" before ever beginning to solve problems
involving dots.

Each of the subsequent lessons involving dots (and all the other instruments, for that matter) are organized around at least one major principle.
Sometimes one or two additional principles are introduced, although they
may not be developed to the same extent. The following are examples of
principles: "When cues diminish, we frequently have to change strategies";
"A good strategy for self-checking is to reverse an operation." A major
function of a principle is to organize the lesson so that it has a focal theme.

The second aspect of relating IE to other experiences involves the concept
of "bridging" to provide examples of situations in which a principle is applicable. Students are encouraged to generate their own examples and to eval-

uate the adequacy of examples suggested by others. Bridging is extremely important and serves four functions. First, it prompts the students to draw on their own experiences. Second, because there are an indefinite number of examples of the application of each principle, the teacher learns about the students' life experiences and knowledge and the students learn from one another. Third, the generation of examples shows whether a student has precisely understood a principle. Finally, instantiation in a variety of contexts encourages transfer to new domains.

The Instrumental Enrichment Program has been implemented extensively in Canada, Israel, the United States, and Venezuela, among other countries. Students classified as mentally retarded, learning disabled, emotionally disturbed, deaf, and gifted have participated in IE classes, as have educationally deprived adolescents and adults. The program has been evaluated extensively. Although it is beyond the scope of this chapter to discuss these evaluations, the interested reader will find many articles and chapters that report research with various populations (see Arbitman-Smith, Haywood, & Bransford, 1984; Bransford, Arbitman-Smith, Stein, & Vye, 1985; Savell, Twohig, & Rachford, 1986).

The Philosophy for Children Program

The Philosophy for Children Program (Lipman, 1985; Lipman, Sharp, & Oscanyan, 1980) is broad in scope. Lipman and colleagues envision a curriculum that will eventually extend from kindergarten through grade 12. In this chapter we focus on the part of the program designed for grades 5 through 8.

The program is not designed to each children *about* philosophy in the traditional sense; for example, children do not learn about famous philosophers and their particular theories or positions. Instead, Lipman and colleagues attempt to help children learn to think philosophically. They reject the assumption that "the learning process [consists] in nothing more than the transmission of the contents of human knowledge from the old to the young." They adopt an alternative position that emphasizes the importance of thinking. Lipman et al. argue that, just as there are differences between learning historical facts and learning to think historically, or between learning scientific facts and learning to think scientifically, there are important differences between learning philosophical facts and learning to think philosophically.

Lipman et al. (1980) emphasize that philosophical thinking does not simply involve thinking and reasoning; it involves thinking about thinking. In their words:

It is well to remember that when philosophy emerged in Greece in the sixth century, B.C., it did not burst suddenly out of the Mediterranean blue. The development of societies of reasoning creatures − what we call civilization − had been a process to be measured not in thousands but in millions of years. Human beings became civilized as they became reasonable, and for an animal to begin to reason and to learn how to improve its reasoning is a long, slow process. So thinking had been going on for ages before Greece – slowly improving itself, uncovering the pitfalls to be avoided by forethought, endeavoring to weigh alternative sets of consequences intellectually. What happened in the sixth century, B.C., is that thinking turned round on itself; people began to think about thinking, and the momentous event, the culmination of the long process to that point, was in fact the birth of philosophy. (p. xi)

When the early philosophers began to think about thinking, they emphasized criteria for evaluating the quality of thinking. For example, Socrates stated that each belief must be subjected to the tests of logic and experience. According to Lipman et al. (1980):

It does not matter whose opinions they are, or whose ideas they are – they must submit to the requirement that they be internally consistent, and their proponents must divulge the evidence that supports them. . . . Socrates does not deceive himself into thinking that, because he converses with a general, he is discussing strategy, or that, because he converses with a statesman, he is discussing statecraft. He knows he is dealing with the *assumption* of these disciplines, and these assumptions must be treated philosophically. (p. xiv)

Note that Socrates emphasized the existence of criteria for the evaluation of thinking. It is not *who* says something that makes arguments true or valid or reasonable; instead, these properties depend on people's initial assumptions and on the internal consistency of their arguments. Philosophical thinking therefore involves a concern for *coherence* (internal consistency), for the *correspondence* between ideas and available data, and for the *assumptions* that underlie one's arguments. Philosophical thinking is also *imaginative*; for example, one must often redefine problems and search for alternative sets of assumptions. Socrates encouraged people to imagine possibilities and to separate what is possible from what is momentarily true. He also emphasized the *relevance* of philosophical inquiry to the management of everyday activities; he argued that people can improve their lives by thinking things through.

Lipman and colleagues do not subscribe to the view that philosophical thinking is beneficial only for adults. They maintain that it is beneficial for children as well. For example, children are interested in concepts such as friendship and fairness; these ideas are relevant to their everyday lives. Lipman et al. also argue that children are interested in understanding reasons and in exploring alternatives. It is natural for children to ask about purposes and causes, and children are eager to examine assumptions and to explore alternative points of view.

An overview of the instruction

In Philosophy for Children, students read about groups of children and adults who discuss issues that arise in the course of everyday activities.

These models of dialogue and reflection are presented in novels. As explained by Lipman et al. (1980):

The books are works of fiction in which the characters eke out for themselves the laws of reasoning and the discovery of alternative philosophical views that have been presented through the centuries. The method of discovery for each of the children in the novels is dialogue coupled with reflection. This dialogue with peers, with teachers, with parents, grandparents, and relatives, alternating with reflections upon what has been said, is the basic vehicle by which the characters in the stories learn − by talking and thinking things out. (p. 82)

As an illustration of the novels, consider some excerpts from *Harry Stottlemeier's Discovery* (hereafter *Harry*). The major purpose of this 96-page novel is to help fifth and sixth graders discover information about the structure and function of formal and informal logic.

The excerpts that follow occur in the context of a science class. Harry has been daydreaming during a lecture on the solar system. Suddenly he realizes that the teacher, Mr. Bradley, is calling on him: "'What is it that has a long tail, and revolves around the sun every 77 years?'" (p. 1). Harry does not know the answer because he has not been listening; however, he does remember that earlier Mr. Bradley had said that all planets revolve around the sun. Because planets revolve around the sun and the thing with the long tail revolves around the sun, Harry decides that the answer to the teacher's question is "a planet."

He wasn't prepared for the laughter from the class. If he'd been paying attention, he would have heard Mr. Bradley say that the object he was referring to was Halley's comet, and that comets go around the sun just as planets do, but they are definitely not planets.

Fortunately the bell rang just then, signaling the end of school for the day. But as Harry walked home, he still felt badly about not having been able to answer when Mr. Bradley called on him.

Also, he was puzzled. How had he gone wrong? He went back over the way he had tried to figure out the answer. "All planets revolve about the sun," Mr. Bradley had said, very distinctly. And this thing with the tail also revolved about the sun, only it wasn't a planet.

"So there are things that revolve about the sun that aren't planets," Harry said to himself. "All planets revolve about the sun, but not everything that revolves about the sun is a planet."

And then Harry had an idea. "A sentence can't be reversed. It you put the last part of a sentence first, it'll no longer be true. For example, take the sentence "All oaks are trees." If you turn it around, it becomes "All trees are oaks." But that's false. Now, it's true that "All planets revolve around the sun." But if you turn the sentence around and say that "All things that revolve around the sun are planets," then it's no longer true − it's false!"

The story continues by describing Harry's fascination with his discovery. He tries it out on a few more examples (e.g., "All cucumbers are vegetables") and decides that it works.

Later in the first chapter we find Harry returning home and finding his mother talking with a neighbor, Mrs. Olson:

Mrs. Olson was saying, "Let me tell you something, Mrs. Stottlemeier. That Mrs. Bates who just joined the PTA, all she ever talks about is helping the poor. Well, I believe in that too, of course, but then I keep thinking how all those radicals keep saying that we ought to help the poor, and that makes me wonder whether Mrs. Bates is well, you know . . . "

"Whether Mrs. Bates is a radical?" Harry's mother asked politely.

Mrs. Olson nodded.

Suddenly something in Harry's mind went "CLICK!" "Mrs. Olson," he said, "just because, according to you, all radicals are people who say they want to help the poor, that doesn't mean that all people who say they want to help the poor are radicals."

"Harry," said his mother, "this is none of your business, and besides, you're interrupting."

But Harry could tell by the expression on his mother's face that she was pleased with what he'd said. So he quietly got his glass of milk and sat down to drink it, feeling happier than he had felt in days.

Note that this episode provides a model of inappropriate reasoning that is eventually corrected (and corrected by a child).

Harry Stottlemeier's Discovery covers much more than the rules of basic logic. Even the brief excerpts presented here provide a rich source of additional information; they mention daydreaming and attention, and they highlight some connections between reasoning processes, school performance, and everyday life. Personal reactions to being laughed at by the class are also emphasized; so is the excitement of discovery, the urge for experimentation, and the confrontation with counterexamples.

An important component of the Philosophy for Children Program involves philosophical discussion among students in the classroom. The idea of holding class discussion is hardly new, of course, but Lipman and colleagues emphasize the importance of *philosophical* discussions and attempt to differentiate these from other types of dialogue. Students are encouraged to reflect on their own contributions to the discussion. Have they barged in and hence violated rules of social etiquette? Are they contributing ideas that are relevant and not merely repetitions of what others have said? (Students therefore have to learn to listen.) Teachers in the Philosophy for Children Program provide mediation in an attempt to increase awareness of the importance of these endeavors and to improve use of each one. They also attempt to help children appreciate the cooperative nature of the enterprise and to realize the value of hearing other opinions and views.

The teacher's manual suggests various leading ideas that teachers can select for the purposes of discussion. (Ideally, these are congruent with the direction of the class discussion.) The episode about Harry's attempts to reverse the "planet" sentence, for example, can lead to a discussion of the general issue of "the process of inquiry." Are there general stages through which all kinds of inquiry proceed? A second leading idea is "discovery and invention." What are the differences between these? Why are they exciting? A third is "the structure of logical statements." What do we mean by rules of logic? When do they apply and when do they not apply?

Other leading ideas are more appropriate for other aspects of the first chapter of *Harry*. For example, at one point in the chapter Harry feels resentment toward Lisa because she shows him that his rule concerning the reversal of sentences does not always work. The teacher's manual includes a leading idea on "resentment": How does it differ from anger? Are there times when such feelings are justified? One could imagine another leading idea on "consistency," relating to the episode in which Harry's mother tells him he is interrupting the conversation yet seems pleased at his contribution. The important point is that the introduction of leading ideas is designed to help students view particular episodes as instances of more general issues. Lipman and colleagues make use of the philosophical literature in order to formulate general issues to be explored.

Philosophy for Children has been implemented in a variety of countries and has produced some promising outcomes at those sites where formal evaluations have been conducted. As we pointed out earlier, it is beyond the scope of this chapter to discuss evaluation results in great detail, and instead we refer the reader to papers by Lipman (1985), Lipman et al. (1980), and Bransford et al. (1985) for in-depth discussion. However, we should say that improvements following the introduction of the program have been documented in the areas of reading, reasoning, and mathematics, and hence optimism about the effectiveness of the program is warranted.

Intelligence Applied

Sternberg's approach to teaching thinking is based on his "triarchic" theory of intelligence (Sternberg, 1985, 1986). The program is designed to help people improve their abilities to perform the processes assumed to underly intelligent behavior. It is appropriate for students in secondary school and college and can be used as either a semester or a year-long course.

The triarchic theory, as its name implies, consists of three parts (see Table 12.1 for a sketch of the components of the theory). The first part specifies internal or mental processes that underlie intelligent behavior. According to Sternberg, three types of mental processes or components comprise intelligent behavior: metacomponents, performance components, and knowledge acquisition components. Metacomponents are used to plan, monitor, and evaluate problem-solving strategies. In other words, they are the executive processes that coordinate procedures used to solve problems. Some examples of metacomponents discussed in the program are defining the problem, selecting a mental representation, and allocating mental resources.

Performance components implement the plans that the metacomponents formulate. Although the number of performance components is assumed to be very large, Sternberg emphasizes a small subset thought to be relevant to many intellectual tasks. Processes such as inferring relations between stimuli, applying previously inferred relations to new stimuli, and mapping

Table 12.1. *Sketch of the components of the triarchic theory*

I. Information-processing components of intelligence	A. Metacomponents
	For example, defining problems, selecting strategy, solution monitoring
	B. Performance components
	For example, inferring relations between stimuli, applying previously inferred relations to new stimuli, mapping higher-order relations between stimuli, comparing attributes to stimuli
	C. Knowledge acquisition components
	  1. Processes used to determine meaning
	    a. Selective encoding
	    b. Selective combination
	    c. Selective comparison
	  2. Contextual cues that signal meeting
	  3. Textual cues that influence apprehension of contextual cues

II. Experience and intelligence	A. Processes for coping with novelty
	  1. Selective encoding
	  2. Selective comparison
	  3. Selective combination
	B. Automatization of information processing

III. Context of intelligence or practical intelligence	For example, skills for adapting to, shaping, and selecting environments

higher-order relations between stimuli are some examples of important performance components.

The instruction provided on the performance components places the greatest emphasis on the process of drawing inferences. Students in the program receive instruction on making various kinds of inferences (e.g., similarity, contrast, prediction, and subordination), as well as on identifying common inferential fallacies (e.g., irrelevant conclusion, representativeness, and labeling). For the most part, the practice items are typical of inductive-reasoning items that might be found on traditional intelligence tests such as verbal and figural analogies, series completion, and classification items.

Finally, knowledge acquisition components are the processes that enable people to learn new information. They are the processes that the learner uses to identify important information and to combine and compare new information with existing knowledge so as to make it more meaningful. Instruction on the knowledge acquisition component is conducted in the context of deriving the meanings of new words from text. Students are given short paragraphs containing unknown words whose meaning they must try to decipher. Three processes of knowledge acquisition are stressed: (a) *selective encoding*, or locating relevant information in the text; (b) *selective combination*, or combining this information into a meaningful whole; and (c) *selective comparison*, or interrelating information with what is already known. In addition, students are informed about cues in the text – setting cues, class membership cues, affect cues, to name a few – that can used to derive helpful information.

The second major part of the triarchic theory is concerned with the real-world contexts in which intellectual processes operate. This is the part of the program in which Sternberg trains students in "practical" intellectual skills. He describes important ways in which the individual can manipulate the environment to achieve certain ends. Essentially, this involves adapting to existing environments, shaping existing environments, or selecting new environments. This part of the theory is relatively unique among theories of intelligence. By attempting to understand how individuals manipulate their environment to meet their needs, one can gain important insights as to what contributes to individual difference in life success among people matched on other processing characteristics.

The topics included for instruction on practical intelligence are diverse. Sternberg suggests that there are many forms of practical intelligence, and the types of skills assessed and discussed in this section are testimony to this. Students practice decoding nonverbal cues from photographs, and they are presented with scenarios of real-world problems for which they must generate conflict resolutions. Finally, there is discussion of common reasons why intelligent people sometimes fail in career and interpersonal situations (e.g., lack of motivation, lack of product orientation, use of wrong abilities).

The third part of Sternberg's theory of intelligence deals with the role of novelty and automaticity in intelligent performance. Sternberg suggests that it is necessary to consider not only the processes of thinking, but the kinds of problems to which they are applied. Assessment of thinking is assumed to be most useful when the problems to which the processes are applied are relatively, not wholly, novel. Other things being equal, individuals who are able to use and acquire insights from new information, and who are able to perform operations smoothly and without much conscious effort, are likely to be more successful on tasks than individuals who do not have these skills. The training on coping with novelty is conducted with various forms of insight problems because Sternberg assumes that one of the most important mental skills for dealing with novelty is insight. The processes assumed to contribute to insight are the three knowledge acquisition processes discussed earlier, that is, selective encoding, selective combination, and selective comparison. Students practice each of these processes in solving insight problems.

An overview of the instruction

As already mentioned, Intelligence Applied is structured around the triarchic theory. Students are taught the component processes in the theory and practice these processes in solving an extensive set of relevant problems. The program consists of two elements: a student's text, which contains narrative material and exercises for students to complete, and a teacher's guide, which contains material teachers can use to maximize the effectiveness of the program.

The first several units of instruction review some theories of intelligence – including the triarchic theory – and other programs for training intelligence. This information is provided because Sternberg suggests that the success of a program depends at least as much on the *student's* understanding of what the program does, how it does it, and why, as it does on the teacher's understanding of this information. This suggestion is consistent with recommendations by Brown and others whose research on learning strategies points to the importance of "informed" practice during training for facilitating transfer (e.g., Brown, Campione, & Day, 1981).

Subsequent units of the program are devoted to components of the theory. The format of the instruction is similar in each unit. The unit begins with a description of a problem that is relevant to the component under discussion. For example, to introduce metacomponents, Sternberg begins with a description of the problems encountered by a friend who had to get from Connecticut to New York City to catch a plane. The friend was delayed by traffic en route to the terminal from which the airport limousines departed. The friend missed his designated limo, waited for a subsequent one, and hence missed his plane.

The anecdote provides an excellent example of poor planning, thereby setting the stage for a discussion of the nature and importance of metacomponents in problem solving. In other words, having created the need, Sternberg next provides a heuristic for solving the problem. He uses the airport example to discuss the importance of defining problems in ways that facilitate solution. From beginning to end, Sternberg's colleague had defined his problem as one of reaching the limo terminal in time to take a limousine to the airport. Sternberg points out that his friend might not have missed his plane had he redefined the problem as one of obtaining suitable transportation to reach the airport on time. If his friend had done this he might have considered alternative means of getting to the airport terminal (e.g., driving his own vehicle, driving to the next limo stop).

The sequence of presenting a problem in need of solution followed by a more formal discussion of the component process that facilitates solution is repeated throughout the program. Indeed, the program is rich in example problems. They are included not only to introduce parts of the theory, but also to illustrate various concepts and, of course, for practice purposes.

Following a discussion of each process, Sternberg provides examples of strategies that learners can adopt to improve their abilities to use the process. For example, to facilitate problem definition, he recommends rereading or reconsidering the question and/or simplifying goals. The practice of systematically providing explicit suggestions for improvement seems important.

Each unit concludes with a series of practice problems relevant to the topic of the unit. A variety of problem types are included, ranging from some of the classical problems in the psychological literature to relatively ill defined problems from everyday contexts. The variety and number of problem types are one of the strengths of the program, because they may facilitate transfer to contexts outside of the program. Examples of problems are presented in Figure 12.3.

Intelligence Applied is the most recently developed of the three programs we have described and hence has yet to be implemented and evaluated in as many sites. Nevertheless, the program, in large part developed in Venezuela, has been tested at two universities there. Sternberg (1986) notes that, although the statistical outcome data are not yet available, the clinical data are highly favorable.

Similarities among the programs

Our goal in this section is to discuss similarities and differences among the three programs by focusing on four issues that seem especially relevant to any attempt to teach thinking (see Sternberg, 1983, for discussion of additional issues). These issues involve the degree to which each program emphasizes

  1. "metacognitive" aspects of thinking and problem solving,
  2. the role of specific knowledge in thinking and problem solving,
  3. the importance of "knowledge by acquaintance" rather than merely "knowledge by description,"
  4. the need for special training to facilitate transfer.

Each of these issues is discussed below.

Metacomponents of thinking

A number of theorists argue that there are a variety of components of the problem-solving process that should be emphasized during training (e.g., Anderson, 1980; deBono, 1985; Hayes, 1981; Maier, 1930, 1931; Mayer, 1977; Newell & Simon, 1972; Sternberg, 1977, 1981; Whimbey & Lochhead, 1982; Wickelgren, 1974). For present purposes we emphasize five components: *i*dentify, *d*efine, *e*xplore, *a*ct, and *l*ook and *l*earn. These form what Bransfrod and Stein (1984) call the IDEAL approach to problem solving. We apply this framework to each of the three programs that we have discussed.

Metacomponents

Solution Monitoring

You are in a job interview and concerned that you make the best impression possible. During the course of the interview, you find yourself monitoring both your own behavior and that of the interviewer in order to determine how well the interview is going. What kinds of signs might you look for in the interviewer's behavior to get some indication of the interviewer's opinion of you?

Performance Components

Detecting Fallacies

Josh and Sandy were discussing the Reds and the Blues, two baseball teams. Sandy asked Josh why he thought the Reds had a better chance of winning the pennant this year than the Blues. Josh replied, "Every man on the Reds is better than every man on the Blues, so the Reds must be the better team." Determine whether the reasoning is valid or fallacious, and if it's fallacious, characterize the nature of the fallacy.

Verbal Analogies

Sonata : Composer :: Lithograph : (a) physicist, (b) artist, (c) sculptor, (d) author.

Misdemeanor : Crime :: Peccadillo : (a) stutter, (b) pretense, (c) amnesia, (d) sin.

Practical Reasoning Problems

Problem:
Mr. Peters owned an apartment building near the county airport. Some airplanes flew over the building at low altitudes, while others flew over at higher altitudes. One day Mr. Peters erected a tall television antenna on top of his building. A low-flying plane owned by Air Mideast hit the antenna with its wingtip, causing some damage to both the plane and the antenna.

Mr. Peters brought suit against Air Mideast for the damage to his property. Will Mr. Peters win?

Principles:
1. A landowner who in no way contributes to the injury of an uninvited trespasser is not liable to that trespasser.

2. The owner of land has the exclusive right to as much of the space above it as may be actually occupied and used by him and necessarily incident to such occupation and use, and anyone passing through such space without the owner's consent is a trespasser. The owner may recover damages for such trespass.

Facts:
1. Mr. Peters erected a television antenna on top of the apartment building that he owned, and a plane hit the antenna.

2. Airplanes had previously flown in the area occupied by the antenna.

3. The antenna was very tall.

4. The plane was damaged when it hit the antenna.

Outcomes:
1. Mr. Peters will win.

2. Mr. Peters will lose.

Knowledge Acquisition Components

Determining Word Meaning with Value/Affect Cues

In our mobile society, where families are often spread across the states and neighbors are strangers, eremophobia is a constant complaint. Mental-health professionals treat the condition primarily through extended counseling sessions, but when anxiety and nervousness are pronounced, tranquilizers may be necessary. Often, not only the immediate sufferers but also those close to them may require counseling. Sufferers of eremophobia may exhibit intense dependency behavior, adversely affecting those close to them. For instance, an older couple, who lost all their children but one in a car accident, placed unreasonable demands for emotional support on the remaining child. He complained that his parents overfocused on him to the point where the quality of his life had declined drastically. Can you find any affect/value cues and can you define the word?

Coping with Novelty

Selecting Encoding

A taxi driver picked up a fare at the Hyatt Regency Hotel who wanted to go to the airport. The traffic was heavy, and the taxicab's average speed for the entire trip was just 40 miles per hour. The total time of the trip was 80 minutes, and the customer was charged accordingly. At the airport, the taxi driver picked up another customer who wanted to be taken to the same Hyatt Regency Hotel. The taxi driver returned to the hotel along the same route that he had used just before, and traveled with the same average speed. But this time the trip took and hour and 20 minutes. Can you explain why?

Practical Intelligence

Real World Problems

Your 1969 Plymouth station wagon is about to give up the ghost. To avoid the inevitable breakdown, you decide to purchase a new car, a Ford Thunderbird, no less. The dealership in your town is well stocked with the new model, and it has a good reputation. After describing to the salesman just what you have in mind, you find out that the price is much higher than you expected. Do you:
   a) decide to haggle and bargain for the absolute lowest price possible?
   b) resign yourself to the purchase of a different type of auto?
   c) buy the car of your dreams, knowing that you will have to acquire a second job to supplement your income?

Figure 12.3. Sample problems from Intelligence Applied. From Sternberg (1986).

Instrument Enrichment. The Instrumental Enrichment Program places a strong emphasis on developing metacomponents of thinking and problem solving. Feuerstein et al. (1985) describe one of the goals of the program as the production of insight as to the importance of various metacognitive processes. This constitutes an effort to improve individuals' understanding of the relationships between particular strategic actions and problem-solving outcomes. This emphasis can be seen most clearly in the format of a typical IE lesson.

The first three phases of each daily lesson comprise an IDEAL problem-solving cycle. During the introduction (Phase 1), the teacher and students study the page(s) for the day. They compare the exercise with previously completed work and *identify* differences that may present problems. For example, on one page in ODI students encounter an exercise in which the model consists of two identical squares and an isosceles triangle whose sides are the same length as those of the squares. During the introductory discussion, this situation is noted and discussed as a potential source of errors. Once the problem is identified, the discussion moves on to *defining* the nature of the difficulty. In our example, the class would most likely define the problem as one of distinguishing between the dots that will form the triangle and the dots that will form the square, since each of the squares contains two isosceles triangles.

The final phase of the discussion is devoted to *exploring* strategies for dealing with the problem as it has been defined. In the example of two squares and a triangle, one strategy might be to search for and draw the squares first so that the dots needed to make up those squares are not mistaken for the dots to be used for the triangle.

During the independent work phase (Phase 2) of the IE lesson, students *act* on the strategies they developed during the exploration phase of the introduction. Individual items increase in complexity and difficulty on the page(s), and students must apply the strategies with increasing care. As they solve problems on their own, they are encouraged by the teacher to continually *look* at the results of their work to gauge whether they have been successful.

The group discussion (Phase 3) is the formal conclusion to the IDEAL cycle. The teacher invites the students to share their experiences in applying the strategies and the class evaluates the entire problem-solving process they have just experienced.

Philosophy for Children. Lipman and colleagues also focus on important metacomponents of problem solving. For example, in *Harry Stottlemeier's Discovery*, Harry *identifies* the existence of a number of problems. Some involve student's reactions to his behavior (in the excerpt provided earlier the students laugh at an answer he gives to a teacher's question, which indicates to him that he has somehow made an error). Other illustrations of problem identification involve Harry's abilities to detect flaws in arguments (e.g., Mrs. Olson's; see the illustration from *Harry* provided earlier). One of the major strengths of the program is that examples of problem identification are present throughout the novels that the students read.

Philosophy for Children also sensitizes children to the importance of different *definitions* of problems and the effects of problem definitions on potential solutions. For example, in the early part of *Harry* (see the illustration provided earlier), Harry spends a considerable amount of time trying to define the nature of his error with respect to the teacher's question. Similarly, in another part of *Harry* a boy decides not to salute the American flag and give the pledge of allegiance. Classmates wonder why. In this situation there are a number of ways to define the issue to be explored. One is to ask, "Why is this boy so stupid (or unpatriotic) to refuse to salute the American flag?" A very different way is to ask, "What kind of courage does it take to stand by one's convictions even though they may be unpopular?"

The Philosophy for Children Program also helps students *explore* a variety of strategies. In *Harry*, for example, children frequently construct examples or simple cases that exemplify a principle they are trying to test.

Finally, the Philosophy for Children Program provides a great deal of emphasis on *acting* on the basis of ideas or hypotheses and looking at the effects. Thus, in *Harry* we see many instances in which students formulate a test case and ask friends, parents, and teachers for counterexamples. The latter are readily found. Rather than giving up, however, the students in *Harry* continually revise their ideas and test them again.

Intelligence Applied. Of our three programs, Sternberg's Intelligence Applied places the strongest emphasis on the issue of metacognition or metacomponents. Metacomponents form a crucial part of Sternberg's theory of intelligence, and much of his training is aimed at increasing students' abilities to identify potential problems during the planning stages of problem solving, to understand how different definitions of problems lead to different strategies, to select appropriate strategies, and to monitor the effects. As part of the training, Sternberg explicitly describes each metacomponent. He also provides example problems that have been carefully selected in such a way that application of the metacomponent under discussion facilitates problem solution.

The relationship between the IDEAL model and Sternberg's approach to problem solving can be seen in his example of the colleague who missed his plane. The following is an analysis consistent with that presented by Sternberg: First, the colleague failed to *identify* potential problems that might arise during his trip to the airport. More specifically, he did not plan for the extra time that might be spent in traffic. Furthermore, once the problem arose − once he missed the first airport limousine − he *defined* the problem in a way that led him to *explore* an ineffective solution strategy. As discussed earlier, he defined his problem as one of too little time rather than one of needing an alternative mode of transportation. Hence, he *acted* on the strategy of waiting for the next limousine, instead of the strategy of taking a taxi, using his own car, and so forth. One would hope that the friend *looked* at the effects of his strategy and *learned* something that would help him next time.

Concerns with the role of knowledge in problem solving

The discussion of the previous section emphasized the importance of helping students develop general skills such as the ability to identify problems, to define them from various perspectives, and to select and evaluate potential strategies. Activities such as these seem to be important components of thinking and problem solving irrespective of the domain in which the thinking occurs. However, it also seems clear that the ability to think about issues and solve problems is highly dependent on the availability of specific knowledge. A large body of research provides strong support for the notion that effective problem solvers rely heavily on domain-specific knowledge (e.g., see Bransford, Sherwood, Vye, & Rieser, 1986; Glaser, 1984; Newell, 1980). An important issue involves the extent to which our three programs − and any program for that matter − deal with the issue of domain-specific knowledge and skills.

Instrumental Enrichment. Among the goals of Feuerstein's Instrumental Enrichment Program is the acquisition of (a) concepts, labels, and operations and (b) an understanding of relationships, strategies, and skills required to work with those concepts, labels, and operations. Indeed, Feuerstein argues that one of the "deficient cognitive functions" that commonly hamper performance is the lack of conceptual and verbal tools necessary to think effectively about particular domains of inquiry. He also emphasizes the importance of "efficiency" in being able to access and use these tools.

Feuerstein's method of dealing with the importance of domain-specific knowledge is unique among the three programs being discussed. One way in which the Instrumental Enrichment Program manages the knowledge problem is to try to eliminate it as a bottleneck in problem solving. Many of the instruments in IE are designed to involve knowledge that most children already have. When task-specific knowledge is required, there is an attempt to keep it to a minimum, and there are specific procedures for teaching it. In Organization of Dots, for example, the problems are quite challenging, yet the prerequisite knowledge is easy to teach. An advantage of this approach to teaching is that students have the opportunity to engage in significant problem-solving activities even though they may lack a number of verbal and conceptual tools necessary to do well in more traditional academic areas. The sense of pride and achievement that students can gain from such opportunities is extremely important for future learning experiences (e.g., see Dweck & Elliott, 1983, for excellent work on the importance of self-concept and learning).

One potential disadvantage of a format that reduces the demands of domain-specific knowledge rather than attempts to teach it is that many tests of achievement require such knowledge. The effects of IE may therefore seem to be less than optimal when one uses such tests to evaluate the program (see Arbitman-Smith et al., 1984). Another potential disadvantage of using "content-free" or nonspecific materials is that applications of strategies and skills learned in these environments may not be transferred to specific academic areas. Feuerstein and his colleagues are well aware of this problem and attempt to deal with it by encouraging students to discuss the ways in which strategies and concepts used in the IE exercises would apply to content areas such as reading, mathematics, and organization of their time. These "bridging" exercises, as they are called, seem to be especially important if one wants to facilitate achievement in specific academic areas. It seems likely that the effects of IE will become stronger to the extent that bridges to the students' other classes are explicitly developed and emphasized (see Bransford, et al., 1985).

Philosophy for Children. Lipman and colleagues' program also emphasizes the role of specific knowledge in problem solving. Indeed, a major part of this program involves the teaching of core concepts that must be clarified in order for students to think more effectively about important issues in their lives. A number of concepts are explored throughout the program. For example, children are helped to clarify concepts such as *fairness, friendship*, and *patriotism*. Concepts such as these can create confusion in thinking if they are not adequately understood. Thus, a child may state, "John would do what I ask if he were my friend, but he didn't do it so I guess he isn't my friend." The child's fuzzy understanding of the concept of friendship must be clarified in order for the child to think more effectively about this issue.

The Philosophy for Children Program also emphasizes the importance of values and ethics. An important goal of the program is to help students analyze and evaluate their own values rather than to teach them values they ought to hold. This is an especially valuable part of the program, and it illustrates another way in which Philosophy for Children deals with the issue of knowledge. By helping students develop procedures for analyzing the assumptions inherent in their own concepts, ideas, and values, the program attempts to provide tools for clarifying information in any knowledge domain.

Intelligence Applied. Sternberg's program also acknowledges the important role of specific knowledge in problem solving. When discussing the solution to formal analogy problems, for example, he helps students understand that many tests of analogy are really tests of vocabulary rather than of general reasoning processes. He also helps students analyze the semantic relationships among items in analogy problems, and he emphasizes that a number of possible relationships exist. In addition, when discussing components such as inferencing, Sternberg notes that the degree of difficulty of these activities depends on the problem to which they are applied (e.g., see Baron & Sternberg, 1987).

An important part of Sternberg's program — and one that is unique in comparison with IE and Philosophy for Children — is the emphasis on the acquisition of new knowledge. Sternberg argues that, because knowledge is so important in problem solving, it is imperative that students learn how to acquire new knowledge on their own. Sternberg discusses the acquisition of new knowledge in the context of learning new vocabulary, although the strategies and processes he teaches are assumed to be generalizable to other situations.

He emphasizes three processes that are important for acquiring new information: locating the important information to be learned, and combining and comparing it with existing knowledge in order to make it more meaningful. By engaging in these activities, the learner will be better able to learn new concepts and procedures. Sternberg also teaches students the types of textual cues (e.g., setting cues, affect cues) that contain information that will enable them to locate, combine, and compare. A final part of the instruction on knowledge acquisition concerns the use of effective memory techniques such as interactive imagery and categorical clustering. Although there are other aspects of learning that one might emphasize (e.g., see Bransford & Stein, 1984; Hayes, 1981), Sternberg has chosen to emphasize knowledge acquisition strategies that are valuable in a wide variety of domains.

Emphasis on knowledge by experience versus description

A third feature of the three programs discussed in this chapter involves the degree to which they help students *experience* important aspects of thinking and problem solving rather than simply tell students *about* thinking.

The opportunity to experience something versus simply being told about it has been described as the difference between knowledge by acquaintance and knowledge by description. Any set of events probably contains aspects of each of these, so the distinction is fuzzy. Nevertheless, it can be useful, even if oversimplified. For example, it is one thing to let people experience their inability to comprehend Bransford and Johnson's (1972) washing-clothes passage and then experience the difference when given the title – this is knowledge by acquaintance. It is another matter simply to present people with the washing-clothes passage, as well as its title, and *tell* them that it would be difficult to comprehend the passage without the title – this is knowledge by description. Similarly, it is one thing to try to tell people what it would be like to live for a year in another culture and quite a different thing for them to experience the difference for themselves.

As another illustration, consider the difference between letting people experience a momentary block in their ability to solve a problem and simply telling them about the notion of blocks to problem solving. Many authors of problem-solving books attempt to create situations in which such experiences can occur (e.g., see Bransford & Stein's, 1984, treatment of the cannonball problem, p. 21).

All three of the programs that we have discussed provide students with information *about* effective thinking and problem solving – hence, they involve knowledge by description. Nevertheless, they do much more than this. For example, in the Instrumental Enrichment Program, students do not simply learn about problems and strategies; they practice problem solving. In Philosophy for Children, the emphasis is on thinking philosophically rather than on descriptions of what philosophers have said. In Intelligence Applied, students are introduced to theories of intelligence and hence learn about the area; nevertheless, they have the opportunity to experience the processes of problem solving as well.

The kinds of experiences provided for students are heavily influenced by the exercises in each program, of which there are many. One advantage of these carefully constructed exercises is that they allow students to experience a momentary sense of difficulty, the degree to which appropriate strategies can help them solve problems, and so forth. They therefore experience problem solving for themselves.

It is important to note that students in the three programs are not simply provided with sets of problems and eventually given feedback about the correct answers. Instead, they are helped to *notice* and analyze important aspects of their experiences – aspects they might otherwise miss. For example, students who are attempting to solve a series of problems may be encouraged to reflect on their initial feelings of difficulty and frustration, the effects of various strategies on these feelings, and the sense of satisfaction that comes from having performed a task well.

Students's opportunities to experience problems and resolutions for themselves probably play an important role in enabling them to learn from others' descriptions. For example, in all three programs students are often encouraged to discuss the strategies they used to solve a problem. When a student has attempted to solve the same problem that others are discussing, the significance of the other students' descriptions is magnified. The student is much more capable of appreciating the advantages and disadvantages of another approach.

Emphasis on transfer

A fourth criterion for evaluating programs involves the degree to which they facilitate transfer. A number of researchers report that, even when a new situation is analogous to one encountered earlier, individuals often fail to notice the analogies and hence fail to utilize previously acquired knowledge that is relevant (e.g., Bransford, Vye, Adams, & Perfetto, in press; Gick & Holyoak, 1980). Similarly, many experimenters report that concepts learned in one context may have to be "decontextualized" in order for transfer to be achieved (Nitsch, 1977) and that strategies learned in one context often are not used in new situations even though they would improve performance to a considerable degree (e.g., Brown, Bransford, Ferrara, & Campione, 1983).

Researchers have also found that the way in which information is presented can affect the degree to which it will be thought about outside the classroom. For example, Vye and Bransford (see Bransford, in press) presented information about human attention to different groups of college students. Those in one group learned about experimental techniques for studying attention (e.g., the use of dichotic listening tasks); those in the second group were encouraged to think about lapses of attention and the need to control attention (e.g., when studying for a test, listening to a lecture, talking on the phone while conversing with someone in the room).

After having received this information, all students were asked to recall what they had learned about attention, and all did quite well. However, more interesting data were collected two days after the initial experiment. Students were asked to estimate how often they had thought about the concept of attention once they had completed the initial experiment and to state the conditions under which these thoughts had occurred. Few of the students in the group who had explored the problem of designing and interpreting experiments for studying attention reported thinking about the concept once they had completed the experiment. In contrast, those who had been prompted to think about lapses of attention reported that they had thought about the concept of attention quite frequently – usually in the context of studying or listening to lectures. These data suggest that it may be possible to keep ideas alive by paying more attention to the types of social situations that students naturally encounter once they leave the classroom. For example, because the college students who participated in the Vye and Bransford study frequently encountered problems involving studying and listening to lectures, it was possible to increase the probability of their thinking about the concept of attention.

Instrumental Enrichment. We noted earlier that in the Instrumental Enrichment Program there is an emphasis on the importance of "bridging." For example, a particular strategy that was used to solve problems in the instruments might be analyzed and described; students might then be asked to explain how a similar strategy would be valuable in other areas, such as mathematics, reading, or their everyday lives. This emphasis on bridging reflects Feuerstein and colleagues' concern for transfer. It also represents an excellent way to assess the quality of individual children's learning. The examples children generate during bridging can tell one a great deal about the degree to which they have understood something (see Bransford et al., 1985).

Philosophy for Children. The philosophy for Children Program includes several ways to facilitate transfer. The program revolves around novels that describe the experiences of students as they interact in school and at home. The students in the program think about thinking in these contexts, and the issues considered (e.g., the nature of friendship) are ones that are important to them. The novels should have effects similar to those demonstrated in the Vye and Bransford experiment described earlier. Once students leave the classroom, ideas from Philosophy for Children should come to mind because they were presented in a context that is similar to the world in which the children live.

Philosophy for Children also emphasizes the importance of discussions among students and teachers. These discussions provide a natural opportunity to consider the relevance of various issues and principles to a variety of contexts. This type of experience is similar to the bridging exercises provided by Feuerstein et al.

Intelligence Applied. Intelligence Applied is also concerned with transfer. The program helps students learn something about different concepts of intelligence so that they can clarify and refine their own ideas about it. Changes in the way that people think about their own intelligence may have a pervasive influence on their lives.

Sternberg also increases the probability of transfer by emphasizing skills and procedures that should have a great deal of generality. Two excellent examples occur in his section on knowledge acquisition. One involves teaching mnemonic techniques − techniques that are useful in a wide variety of settings. An example that is more unique to his program involves teaching students to infer the meanings of new words from context. This is a situation that most people encounter throughout their lives.

Finally, Sternberg places a strong emphasis on the need to understand relationships between internal mental processes and people's everyday environment, and a great deal of effort is directed toward helping students learn about practical intelligence. This part of the program, especially, seems to have great potential for helping students transfer from the course to their everyday lives.

Speculations about the future

We noted earlier that the three programs discussed in this chapter seem especially promising. There are a number of other programs as well (see the Appendix). What can we expect from such programs? Will they have a significant impact on people's abilities to think and learn?

We suspect that any of the three programs we have discussed could be very beneficial, and there are at least some data to back this claim (e.g., Arbitman-Smith et al., 1985; Savell et al., 1986; Bransford et al., 1985). Nevertheless, it also seems clear that thinking and problem solving are evolving processes that can be improved and refined throughout one's lifetime – they are not simply skills that, once mastered, never have to be refined. Furthermore, it seems certain that problem solving is heavily knowledge dependent and that the ability to think effectively about various issues involves a lifelong ability to learn (e.g., Bransford, Sherwood, Vye, & Rieser, 1986).

Because the need for thinking and problem solving is both ubiquitous and knowledge dependent, many authors argue that thinking should be infused throughout the curriculum and taught in all subject areas. Furthermore, these authors argue that thinking should be taught at all grade levels, not just during a single course. (Note that Philosophy for Children includes programs from kindergarten to grade 12 and IE is frequently taught over a period of two to three years.) In an excellent article entitled "How to keep thinking skills from going the way of all the frills," Carl Bereiter (1984) makes a cogent argument for the need to permeate the entire curriculum with an emphasis on thinking. We agree with his argument and suspect that Feuerstein and colleagues, Lipman and colleagues, and Sternberg do too. Nevertheless, there is a need to begin somewhere. The programs discussed in this chapter provide excellent illustrations of principles that might eventually be extended to a variety of content domains.

We also agree with another arguement advanced by Bereiter (1984), namely, that many curriculum developers and textbook publishers claim that their materials teach thinking and problem solving when, in fact, they mainly teach aspects of thinking but do not really help students improve their own abilities to think and learn. Bereiter ends his article by describing two ways of exploring the effectiveness of a program's capacity to teach thinking. One is to ask a curriculum or textbook supplier, "Where do you teach such-and-such cognitive skill?" This is not the question that Bereiter recommends. Instead, he suggests the following strategy: Open the program text to any page and ask, "How is your approach to teaching thinking represented on this page?"

Appendix: Selected thinking and learning skills programs and books

Thinking and learning skills programs

Blank, M. (1973). *Teaching learning in the preschool: A dialogue approach.* Columbus, OH: Merrill.

Burns, M. S., Haywood, H. C., Brooks, P., Cox, J., & Willis, E. (1983). *Cognitive curriculum for young children: Experimental version.* Unpublished manuscript, Vanderbilt University, George Peabody College, John F. Kennedy Center, Nashville, TN.

Copple, C., Sigel, I., & Saunders, R. (1984). *Educating the young thinker: Classroom strategies for cognitive growth.* Hillsdale, NJ: Erlbaum.

Covington, M., Crutchfield, R. S., Davies, L. B., & Olton, R. M. (1974). *The Productive Thinking Program: A course in learning to think.* Columbus, OH: Merrill.

Dansereau, D. (1985). Learning strategy research. In J. W. Segal, S. F. Chipman, & R. Glaser (Eds.). *Thinking and learning skills: Relating instruction to research* (Vol. 1, pp. 209-39). Hillsdale, NJ: Erlbaum.

deBono, E. (1973). *CoRT thinking materials.* London: Direct Education Services.

Feuerstein, R., Rand, Y., Hoffman, M., & Miller, R. (1980). *Instrumental Enrichment.* Baltimore: University Park Press.

Gagne, R. M. (1967). *Science − A process approach: Purposes, accomplishments, expectations.* Commission on Science Education, Association for the Advancement of Science.

Herber, H. L. (1985). Developing reading and thinking skills in content areas. In J. W. Segal, S. F. Chipman, & R. Glaser (Eds.), *Thinking and learning skills: Relating instruction to research* (Vol. 1, pp. 297−316). Hillsdale, NJ: Erlbaum.

Jones, B. F., Amiran, M., & Katims, M. (1985). Teaching cognitive strategies and text structures within language arts programs. In J. W. Segal, S. F. Chipman, & R. Glaser (Eds.), *Thinking and learning skills: Relating instruction to research* (Vol. 1, pp. 259−95). Hillsdale, NJ: Erlbaum. (Chicago Mastery Learning Reading Program with Learning Strategies.)

Kopp, K. (1985). *Cognitive enrichment workbook.* Unpublished manuscript, University of Tennessee, Knoxville.

Lipman, M., Sharp, A. M., & Oscanyan, F. S. (1980). *Philosophy in the Classroom.* Philadelphia: Temple University Press. (Philosophy for Children Program.)

Meeker, M. N. (1969). *The structure of intellect: Its interpretation and uses.* Columbus, OH: Merrill.

Nickerson, R. S., Perkins, D. N., & Smith, E. E. (1985). *The teaching of thinking.* Hillsdale, NJ: Erlbaum. (Project Intelligence.)

Olson, C. B. (1984). Fostering critical writing skills through writing. *Eductional Leadership, 11,* 28−39.

Regan, E. M., & Harris, M. (1980). *To learn/to think: Curriculum materials for the kindergarten.* Toronto: OISE Press.

Rubinstein, M. (1975). *Patterns of problem solving.* Englewood Cliffs, NJ: Prentice-Hall.

Shure, M. B., & Spivak, G. (1979). Interpersonal cognitive problem solving and primary prevention: Programming for preschool and kindergarten children. *Journal of Clinical Child Psychology, 2,* 89−94.

Sternberg, R. (1986). *Intelligence applied.* Hillsdale, NJ: Erlbaum.

Walberg, F. (1981). *Puzzle thinking.* Hillsdale, NJ: Erlbaum.

Wales, C. E., & Stager, R. A. (1977). *Psychology of reasoning: Structure and content.* Cambridge, MA: Harvard University Press. (Guided design.)

Weinstein, C., & Underwood, V. L. (1985). Learning strategies: The how of learning. In J. W. Segal, S. F. Chipman, & R. Glaser (Eds.), *Thinking and learning skills: Relating instruction to research* (Vol. 1, pp. 241−58). Hillsdale, NJ: Erlbaum. (Cognitive Learning Strategies Project.)

Whimbey, A., & Lochhead, J. (1982). *Problem solving and comprehension.* Philadelphia: Franklin Institute Press.

Whimbey, A., & Lochhead, J. (1984). *Beyond problem solving and comprehension: An exploration of quantitative reasoning*. Hillsdale, NJ: Erlbaum.

Books on thinking and learning skills

Anderson, B. F. (1980). *The complete thinker*. Englewood Cliffs, NJ: Prentice-Hall.
Bransford, J. D., & Stein, B. S. (1984). *The IDEAL problem solver*. New York: Freeman.
Brown, S. I., & Walter, M. I. (1985). *The art of problem posing*. Hillsdale, NJ: Erlbaum.
Halpern, D. F. (1984). *Thought and knowledge: An introduction to critical thinking*. Hillsdale, NJ: Erlbaum.
Hayes, J. R. (1981). *The complete problem solver*. Philadelphia: Franklin Institute Press.
Nickerson, R. S. (1986). *Reflections on reasoning*. Hillsdale, NJ: Erlbaum.
Nickerson, R. S., Perkins, D. N., & Smith, E. E. (1985). *The teaching of thinking*. Hillsdale, NJ: Erlbaum.
Perkins, D. N. (1986). *Knowledge as design*. Hillsdale, NJ: Erlbaum.
Polya, G. (1957). *How to solve it*. New York: Doubleday.
Wickelgren, W. A. (1973). *How to solve problems: Elements of a theory of problems and problem solving*. New York: Freeman.

References

Anderson, B. F. (1980). *The complete thinker*. Englewood Cliffs, NJ: Prentice-Hall.
Arbitman-Smith, R., Haywood, H.C., & Bransford, J. D. (1984). Assessing cognitive change. In C. McCauley, R. Sperber, & P. Brooks (Eds.), *Learning and cognition in the mentally retarded*. Baltimore, MD: University Park Press.
Baron, J., & Sternberg, R. (Eds.) (1987). *Teaching thinking skills: Theory and practice*. New York: Freeman.
Bereiter, C. (1984). How to keep thinking skills from going the way of all frills. *Educational Leadership, 42*, 75–7.
Bransford, J. D. (in press). *Enhancing thinking and learning*. New York: Freeman.
Bransford, J. D., Arbitman-Smith, R., Stein, B. S., & Vye, N. J. (1985). Improving thinking and learning skills: An analysis of three approaches. In J. W. Segal, S. F. Chipman, & R. Glaser (Eds.), *Thinking and learning skills: Relating instruction to research* (Vol. 1, pp. 133–206). Hillsdale, NJ: Erlbaum.
Bransford, J. D., & Johnson, M. K. (1972). Contextual prerequisites for understanding: Some investigations of comprehension and recall. *Journal of Verbal Learning and Verbal Behavior, 11*, 717–26.
Bransford, J. D., Sherwood, R., Vye, N., & Rieser, J. (1986). Teaching thinking and problem solving: Suggestions from research. *American Psychologist, 41*, 1078–89.
Bransford, J. D., & Stein, B. S. (1984). *The IDEAL problem solver*. New York: Freeman.
Bransford, J. D., Vye, N. J., Adams, L. T., & Perfetto G. A. (in press). Learning skills and the acquisition of knowledge. In R. Glaser & A. Lesgold (Eds.), *Handbook of Psychology and Education*. Hillsdale, NJ: Erlbaum.
Brown, A. L., Bransford, J. D., Ferrara, R. A., & Campione, J. D. (1983). Learning, remembering and understanding. In J. H. Flavell & E. M. Markman (Eds.), *Carmichael's manual of child psychology* (Vol. 1, pp. 77–166). New York: Wiley.
Brown, A. L., Campione, J. C., & Day, J. D. (1981). Learning to learn: On training students to learn from text. *Educational Researcher, 10*, 14–21.
deBono, E. (1985). The CoRT Thinking Program. In J. W. Segal, S. F. Chipman, & R. Glaser (Eds.), *Thinking and learning skills: Relating instruction to research* (Vol. 1, pp. 363–88). Hillsdale, NJ: Erlbaum.

Dweck, C. S., & Elliott, E. S. (1983). Achievement motivation. In P. H. Mussen (Ed.), *Handbook of child psychology* (Vol. 4, pp. 643–91). New York: Wiley.

Feuerstein, R., Jensen, M., Hoffman, M. B., & Rand, Y. (1985). Instrumental Enrichment, an intervention program for structural cognitive modifiability: Theory and practice. In J. W. Segal, S. F. Chipman, & R. Glaser (Eds.), *Thinking and learning skills: Relating instruction to research* (Vol. 1, pp. 43–82). Hillsdale, NJ: Erlbaum.

Feuerstein, R., Rand, Y., & Hoffman, M. (1979). *The dynamic assessment of retarded performers: The learning potential assessment device, theory, instruments, and techniques.* Baltimore, MD: University Park Press.

Feuerstein, R., Rand, Y., Hoffman, M. B., & Miller, R. (1980). *Instrumental Enrichment.* Baltimore, MD: University Park Press.

Gick, M. L., & Holyoak, K. J. (1980). Analogical problem solving. *Cognitive Psychology, 12,* 306–65.

Glaser, R. (1984). Education and thinking. The role of knowledge. *American Psychologist, 39,* 93–104.

Hayes, J. R. (1981). *The complete problem solver.* Philadelphia: Franklin Institute Press.

Lipman, M. (1985). Thinking skills fostered by Philosophy for Children. In J. W. Segal, S. F. Chipman, & R. Glaser (Eds.), *Thinking and learning skills: Relating instruction to research* (Vol. 1, pp. 83–108). Hillsdale, NJ: Erlbaum.

Lipman, M., Sharp, A. M., & Oscanyan, F. S. (1980). *Philosophy in the classroom.* Philadelphia: Temple University Press.

Maier, N. R. F. (1930). Reasoning in humans: 1. On direction. *Journal of Comparative Psychology, 10,* 115–43.

(1931). Reasoning in humans: 2. The solution of a problem and its appearance in consciousness. *Journal of Comparative Psychology, 12,* 181–94.

Mann, L. (1979). *On the trail of process: A historical perspective on cognitive processes and their training.* New York: Grune & Stratton.

Mayer, R. E. (1977). *Thinking and problem solving: An introduction to human cognition and learning.* Glenview, IL: Scott, Foresman.

Newell, A. (1980). One final word. In D. T. Tuma & F. Reif (Eds.), *Problem solving and education: Issues in teaching and research.* Hillsdale, NJ: Erlbaum.

Newell, A., & Simon, H. A. (1972). *Human problem solving.* Englewood Cliffs, NJ: Prentice-Hall.

Nitsch, K. E. (1977). *Structuring decontextualized forms of knowledge.* Unpublished doctoral dissertation, Vanderbilt University, Nashville, TN.

Savell, J. M., Twohig, P. T., & Rachford, D. L. (1986). Empirical status of Feuerstein's "Instrumental Enrichment" (FIE) technique as a method of teaching thinking skills. *Review of Educational Research, 56,* 381–409.

Sternberg, R. J. (1977). *Intelligence, information processing, and analogical reasoning: The componential analysis of human abilities.* Hillsdale, NJ: Erlbaum.

(1981). Intelligence as thinking and learning skills. *Educational Leadership, 39,* 18–20.

(1983). Criteria for intellectual skills training. *Educational Researcher, 12,* 6–12.

(1985). *Beyond I.Q.: Toward a triarchic theory of intelligence.* Cambridge University Press.

(1986). *Intelligence applied.* Orlando, FL: Harcourt Brace Jovanovich.

Whimbey, A., & Lochhead, J. (1982). *Problem solving and comprehension.* Philadelphia: Franklin Institute Press.

Wickelgren, W. A. (1974). *How to solve problems: Elements of a theory of problems and problem solving.* New York: Freeman.

13   The development of thinking

Linda B. Smith, Maria Sera, and Bea Gattuso

"Mother, who was born first, you or I?"
"Daddy, when you were little, were you a boy or a girl?"
"The sun sets in the sea. Why is there no vapor?"
    (Chukovsky, 1971)

There are obvious differences in the ways that children and adults think. Adults know that mothers must have been born before their children, that fathers must have been boys when they were little, and that when the sun sets, it does not plunge into the earth. Although children make many such mistakes in thinking about the world, they are not completely ignorant; very young children do know some things. Three-year-olds, for example, know that Daddy is alive but dreams are not (Keil, 1979), and even younger children, 20-month-olds, appear to know, for example, that one dries oneself with a towel *after* a bath and not before (O'Connell & Gerard, 1985). The goal of developmental cognitive psychology is to document the nature of emerging thought and knowledge, to explain why children seem to know some things and to think like adults in some ways but not in others, and finally to explain how immature thought becomes transformed into mature thought. We begin our consideration of these issues with an examination of the data: What is the developmental trend in thinking?

The phenomena: early partial competence

Jean Piaget, perhaps the most influential developmental theorist, emphasized major qualitative shifts in thought. In his view, children are not miniature adults, but rather think according to rules that are different from adults.[1] For the past 15 years, researchers have investigated many of Piaget's claims. His account appears to have exaggerated the differences between "immature" and mature thought. We now know that there are many commonalities between the thinking of young children and that of adults. In general,

This chapter was supported by grants from the National Institute of Child Health and Development, KO4 HD 00589 and RO1 HD 19499. Comments by Susan Scanlon Jones on an earlier draft are greatly appreciated.

the evidence suggests considerable but partial competence in the young child's thinking that becomes elaborated into mature form with development.

Infancy

Early theorists, including Piaget, characterized the infant's experience of the world as one of unconnected and constantly changing information. Infant thought was said to be limited to the here and now – to current perceptions and actions. Consider Piaget's (1954) description of his seven-month-old daughter and her apparent forgetting of an object once it was out of sight:

> Jacqueline tries to grasp a celluloid duck on top of her quilt. She almost catches it, shakes herself, and the duck slides down beside her. It falls very close to her hand but behind a fold in the sheet. Jacqueline's eyes have followed the movement, she has even followed it with her outstretched hand. But as soon as the duck has disappeared – nothing more! It does not occur to her to search behind the fold of the sheet, which would be very easy to do (she twists it mechanically without searching at all). . . . I then take the duck from its hiding-place and place it near her hand three times. All three times she tries to grasp it, but when she is about to touch it I replace it very obviously under the sheet. Jacqueline immediately withdraws her hand and gives up. The second and third times I make her grasp the duck through the sheet and she shakes it for a brief moment but it does not occur to her to raise the cloth. (pp. 36–7)

To Piaget, infant experience consisted of a succession of unconnected, fleeting percepts and actions, and because of this the infant was said not to possess the object concept – not to understand that objects have a permanent, stable existence in time and space. "Everything occurs as though the child believed that the object is alternately made and unmade" (Piaget, 1954, p. 31).

We now know that infants' experiences are not so disconnected and not populated by magical objects that come and go. Baillageron, Spelke, and Wasserman (1985) reported evidence showing that young infants, five-month-olds, conceive of their world as populated by stable objects. Their experiment was ingenious. In the first phase, all of the infants watched a rectangular figure rotate 180 degrees toward and then away from them, as shown at the top of Figure 13.1. After watching this event for some time, the infants watched either the possible or impossible sequence shown in the figure. In the possible sequence, infants saw the rectangular figure lying on the table with a block behind it. The figure was then rotated (obscuring the block when it was rotated) until it was stopped by the block. This possible sequence was repeated several times. The remaining infants saw a sequence that was identical to the possible one except that the figure was rotated 180 degrees and (apparently) *through* the position held by the block. This is an *impossible* event given the persistence of objects in time and space. These five-month-old infants apparently found it odd because they watched this sequence much more frequently and for a much longer time than their coun-

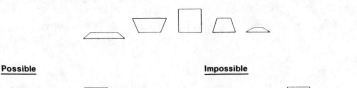

Figure 13.1. The three sequences of *continuous* object motion in the experiment by Baillageron, Spelke, and Wasserman.

terparts watched the possible sequence. That these infants found the impossible event "unusual" suggests that infants know that objects (e.g., blocks) persist in space and time and are not just "alternately made and unmade."

Infants also appear to possess other abstract concepts, such as concepts of number. Starkey, Spelke, and Gelman (1982), for example, showed that six- to eight-month-olds are able to detect intermodal correspondences in numerosity between sounds and sights. The infants were presented with two pictures to look at (one on the right and the other on the left). One picture contained two objects, the other three. At the same time, infants heard either two or three drumbeats. The babies looked at the picture that matched the sounds in number! Apparently, infants can *think* about the abstract commonality that exists between two objects and two sounds.

These two examples of early knowledge of the persistence of objects and of number are tantalizing. Clearly infants can think and indeed do think about some rather complex things. Unfortunately, we do not yet know all that infants are capable of thinking about. The problem is that it is difficult to determine precisely what infants do think and know, given their limited response systems. However, as experimenters develop new techniques, such as the preferential looking used in the present two examples, we will continue to refine what we know about thought in infancy. On the basis of what is currently being discovered, it appears that infants can represent ideas and clearly do think in ways that are beyond those Piaget proposed. Thus, thought in the child seems to begin with a base of considerable competence in infancy.

Thought in the child

The suggestion of the competent infant contrasts with the seeming incompetencies of preschool children. It is remarkably easy to find evidence of inabilities, confusions, and "errorful" thought in preschoolers. From these inabilities, Piaget developed his theory of qualitative shifts in the structure of thought. However, despite the frequency with which preschoolers fail seemingly simple cognitive tasks, it is also possible — by structuring the measuring task — to show considerable latent abilities in young children. The current evidence suggests that young children possess many adult-like competencies that are somehow severely limited in their use. There are many examples of early partial competence. We sample a few.

Transitive inferences and seriation. One domain in which we see provocative early competence is transitive inference making. In a transitive inference task, we might be told, for example, "Sam is taller than Henry" and "Henry is taller than Fred." From these premises, adults easily infer that "Sam is taller than Fred"; young children do not. According to Piaget, the young child's difficulty stems from a lack of the critical operations or "rules for thought" that are necessary for thinking about quantitative relations. In support of this claim, Piaget pointed to other difficulties that the young child has with quantitative dimensions — for example, difficulties in seriation tasks that require objects to be ordered along some dimension (e.g., from tallest to shortest).

Research indicates that preschool children can think about quantitative relations and can make transitive inferences, at least in certain situations. Specifically, Bryant and Trabasso (1971) showed that preschool children make transitive inferences *if* they correctly remember the premises. If children for some reason do not remember the premises or remember only parts of them (e.g., "Sam is tall"), they have no basis on which to make an inference. To ensure that the children in their experiment remembered the premises, Bryant and Trabasso trained the children on the premise information until they could answer all the premise questions correctly; only then were they asked to make an inference. Figure 13.2 provides an example of Bryant and Trabasso's tasks, including the sets of premise statements the children learned and the inference questions they were asked. In this context, Bryant and Trabasso found that four- to seven-year-olds were well able to correctly answer the inference questions. Young children possess the abilities necessary for making transitive inferences but may not show this ability because their recall of premises is poor.

Trabasso and Riley (1975; see also Trabasso, 1977) subsequently found a "distance" effect in inference making. Using a task like that of Bryant and Trabasso, they found that both children and adults take more time to judge which of two items is longer (or shorter) if the items are close to each other in the series. Relative to Figure 13.2, they found that both children and adults took less time to judge the blue segment to be longer than the yellow than to judge the blue segment to be longer than the green. This distance effect makes sense if one is answering the inference question from an *imagined* series. Preschool children, then, may not successfully seriate real objects, but they apparently can seriate objects mentally given practice at

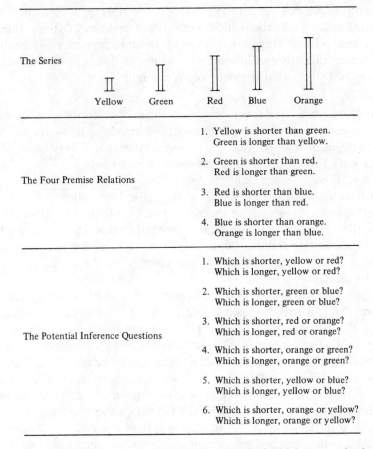

Figure 13.2. Illustration of the kind of stimulus series (which is not seen by the child), premise relations, and inference questions used in studies of the transitive inference making of children.

remembering verbal descriptions of the relations between pairs of objects. Moreover, given that both children and adults show a distance effect, both seem to be making inferences in much the same way.

What are we to make of these results? Should we conclude that the child's thinking in this area is just like the adult's? The data do not allow us to draw such a simple conclusion. In subsequent research, Trabasso and Riley (1975) showed that for young children to make transitive inferences they must learn the premises in both directions during the training phase of the experiment. One cannot simply teach a child that red is shorter than blue and blue is shorter than orange; rather, one must explicitly teach the child that red is shorter than blue, blue is longer than red, blue is shorter than orange, and orange is longer than blue. The premises must be learned in both directions because of the young child's strong tendency to interpret and remember comparative adjectives categorically. Without explicit training of the premise information in both directions, the child encodes and remembers that red is short instead of encoding and remembering that red is shorter than blue and therefore has no basis on which to make transitive inferences.

This fact is important. It is not that young children have difficulty remembering the premises as we might have difficulty remembering a list of facts. Rather, young children systematically misremember the information (see Halford, 1984, for further limitations on children's success in transitive inference making). Because of this systematic misremembering and the need for very special input, preschool children probably rarely make transitive inferences in their daily lives. Children's transitive inference making is thus a case of "can but do not." Under only very special circumstances do children make transitive inferences. There is competence but the use of that competence is severely limited.

Number. Reasoning about number provides another case of children having a competency but being generally unable to exercise it. Preschool children typically fail Piaget's number conservation task. In the standard version of this task, two rows of objects are placed in front of the child. Each row contains, for example, 10 objects and the child agrees that the rows have the same number of objects. The experimenter then makes one row longer than the other by increasing the distance between the objects. When the child is asked which row has more objects, or if both rows still have the same number of objects, preschool children answer that the longer row has more objects. Older children, in contrast, assert that the rows have the same number of objects, as long as nothing has been added or taken away. According to Piaget, younger children fail because they do not yet possess the knowledge that spatial arrangement is irrelevant to numerosity.

However, Gelman (see Gelman & Gallistel, 1978) has shown that children as young as two and three years old do know that spatial arrangement is irrelevant to numerosity. They show this knowledge when the numerosities involved are small (i.e., 1, 2 or 3). Furthermore, three- to five-year-old children possess the principle that addition and subtraction (as opposed to spatial arrangement) are the relevant transformations when the numerosities involved are small; they know, for example, how to turn "two" into "three" and "three" into "two." Again, we see an early understanding that is severely limited. Children who conserve "threeness," who know that $3 = 3$ regardless of spatial arrangement and who know that $2 + 1 = 3$ and $3 - 1 = 2$, nonetheless perform in the precise manner described by Piaget when confronted with sets of 10 objects. In reasoning about number as in transitive inference making, we see early competence that does not extend very far.

Categories and classes. Categorization provides another example of early partial competence. According to the traditional view, the preschooler cannot classify (Inhelder & Piaget, 1964; Werner, 1948; Vygotsky, 1962). In a wide variety of tasks, regardless of procedure, preschoolers seem consistently unable to sort objects by a criterion − to put red objects in one pile, blue in another, or animals in one pile and vehicles in another. Despite these well-documented and easily replicated failures to classify, we now know that there are contexts in which the preschooler is well able to classify. Although the preschool child will not readily put a car and boat in one pile and a cat and horse in another, that same child will consistently group a sedan and stationwagon together and apart from a sailboat and a rowboat (Rosch, Mervis, Gray, Boyes-Braem, 1976).

The categories by which preschool children easily classify are predicted by a theoretical view of the structure of natural categories put forth by Rosch (1973). Rosch suggested that there is a certain level of categorization that is more basic or simpler than other levels. The basic level is that at which consistent motor routines are applied to objects and at which objects are easily segregated by *overall* perceptual similarity. For example, the category *car* is said to be a basic-level category − cars are said to be similar to one another in many ways, no one similarity being critical. In classification tasks, preschool children easily classify objects into *basic* categories (e.g., cars, boats, cats, horses) − categories highly determined by overall similarity. The same children, however, fail to classify objects into *superordinate* categories (animals, vehicles) that are not as well structured by overall similarity. These superordinate categories, however, are the ones that were typically examined in the traditional studies of early classification skill.

One should not conclude from these results that young children possess basic categories but not superordinate ones. Young children may not easily classify by superordinate categories (e.g., animals), but they do know something about them. Keil (1979), for example, has shown that young children systematically know which predicates apply to animate entities (walks, sleeps) and which apply to inanimate objects (broken). More recently, S. Gelman (1985) and Carey (1978) have shown that very young children have "theories" about superordinate classes; they expect, for example, that all animals have the same insides and that these differ from the insides of machines. Regardless of their difficulties in performing classification tasks, young children possess some superordinate categories.

The classification and categorization results thus present another picture of partial competence. Young children can classify, but not at all levels within the hierarchy of categories. And young children have knowledge of some levels of categories that they do not show in categorization tasks. Again, then, we have a case of partial limited competence − clear evidence for some knowledge that shows itself only in certain situations.

Remembering. Earlier, we saw that memory of premises was critical for children's success in making transitive inferences. In general, children do not remember as well as adults (Flavell, 1977). However, memory is not a simple or single ability. Rather, it involves all one's knowledge as well as the processes by which one interprets, stores, and remembers, that knowledge. Memory, in other words, is a series of processes. How, then, do children's memories differ from adults'? Studies in which *no* developmental differences are found help to answer this question.

In one landmark study, Ann Brown (1973) showed that young children remembered as well as adults in a task requiring that they recognize complex visual scenes as either "old" (seen before) or "new" (not seen before). The lack of developmental differences in Brown's task contrasts sharply with the usual result of young children remembering much less than older children and adults. What is special about Brown's study is that it involved memory of visual scenes, and memory of complex scenes is not benefited by the use of strategies. We now know that strategies for remembering are a critical source of developmental differences. If older (e.g., 10-year-old) and younger (e.g., 6-year-old) children are asked to remember a list of items, the older children do a number of things, such as rehearse, to ensure that they will; the younger children do not. Furthermore, if older children are prevented from rehearsing, they remember about as much as younger children. However, we *cannot* easily teach younger children to remember as much as older children by teaching them to rehearse. Attempts to teach strategies such as rehearsal to preschool children have not been very successful (see, e.g., Flavell, 1977).

Memory development, then, is like the development of inference making, number reasoning, and categorization. Aspects of the immature memory system are much like the mature one; if the strategies pay no role in performance, young children's memories seem much like those of older children. However, strategy differences are often involved, and there are usually very large performance differences between younger and older children in remembering. Thus, younger children have memory competence, but it is not well used.

Summary

In this section we presented the principal phenomenon to be explained in cognitive development: the phenomenon of "can but don't" − that is, early, but highly limited competence in a variety of domains. What should we make of these early competencies? On one hand, young children show many mature-like abilities. On the other hand, they do not perform as well as adults on *most* tasks.

What limits children's thinking?

If children are partially competent, what are they lacking such that they are not fully competent? Three general notions about developmental change have been offered to account for the "can but usually don't" nature of early thought: (a) changes in processing capacity, (b) changes in accessibility of knowledge, and (c) changes in the knowledge base itself.

Processing capacity

Several developmental theorists have proposed limits on children's information-processing systems (e.g., Case, Kurland, & Goldberg, 1982; Pascual-Leone, 1970). The notion is that developmental growth reflects changes in "capacity" or processing space. Capacity (also called resources or attention) is a pervasive construct in theories about adult cognition; the assumption is that mental operations draw on some finite amount of processing capacity and that the level of performance and the number of mental tasks that can be jointly conducted are limited by available capacity. The developmental hypothesis is that there is an age-related increase in functional capacity and that young children often fail when older children succeed because younger children lack the necessary amount of capacity (rather than the necessary abilities) to do the task.

According to one account (Case, 1972), functional capacity does not increase with maturation per se but rather increases with specific experience at various mental tasks. It has been well demonstrated in adults that the amount of processing capacity required to perform some mental task declines dramatically with practice in performing the task (Schneider & Shiffrin, 1977; Shiffrin & Schneider, 1977). A common-experience example of a task that demands less capacity with practice is learning to drive. At first, learning to drive takes a great deal of mental effort. We cannot remember to shift, brake, turn on signals, and at the same time carry on a conversation or listen to the radio. With practice, however, the components of driving demand less mental capacity and we are able to drive and do other mental tasks (e.g., talk) as well. The developmental hypothesis, then, is that many mental tasks require more capacity for children than for adults. Adults may be more facile and better able to accomplish more when reasoning, for example, because many of the components of the task are well practiced and not highly demanding. Young children, in contrast, may often fail because many tasks require more capacity than is available. According to this view, however, young children may possess the necessary abilities and be able to succeed if the processing demands (i.e., the capacity demands) of a task have been sufficiently reduced.

How might children's partial competencies be described by this capacity-limitation view? Consider, for example, young children's difficulties in making transitive inferences. Young children may often fail standard transitive inference tasks because they require more capacity to encode comparatives correctly than do adults. Given their relative inexperience with comparatives, encoding the premises correctly could exceed available capacity such that children would often misremember the information and encode the adjectives categorically (e.g., *tall* instead of *taller*). Adults who are more practiced at encoding relational adjectives would require less capacity to do so correctly and therefore would have more capacity available for remembering the premises and/or for reasoning from them (i.e., by mentally seriating). This proposal about developmental changes in the amount of capacity needed to perform tasks captures the general flavor of preschool thought: It is better than one might expect, in some ways adult-like, but it is fragile and collapses under seemingly small increases in task difficulty. The proposal also suggests a clear source and mechanism of changes in thinking. As the child comes to know more and becomes more practiced at various subtasks (e.g., word knowledge, remembering), more mental resources become available such that more complex tasks can be performed.

Some evidence suggests that there may be maturational growth in capacity as well as increased efficiency in the performance of specific mental tasks. Roth (1983) examined the processing speed of child and adult chess experts and novices in a task requiring the comparison of chessboards. Amount of knowledge about chess was a critical determinant of speed of comparison but, nonetheless, child experts were slower than adult experts and child novices were slower than adult novices. Thus, age differences in processing time were *not* eliminated when task-relevant knowledge was comparable at the two age levels. Further support for the possibility of maturational increases in capacity have been reported by Kail (1986). He reasoned that, if performance on *any* speeded task is limited by capacity and that if capacity increases with development, the same pattern of growth should be observed across tasks irrespective of degrees of practice in the tasks. Kail obtained supporting evidence. Thus, capacity itself may increase.

Regardless of whether capacity increases owing to general developmental growth or to practice in specific cognitive tasks or both, limits on capacity seem a likely source of the child's partial, limited competence. The young child may in some ways think very much as adults do, but the young child's performance may not reflect the underlying competence because of capacity limits. A specific ability may be seen only in very special task contexts that require minimal mental effort. With development, increases in capacity may allow that same ability to come into play in an ever wider array of tasks of increasing complexity and difficulty.

Accessibility

A second proposal about the development of children's thinking concerns the accessibility of knowledge (e.g., Brown, Bransford, Ferrara, Campione, 1983; Rozin, 1976). Again, the focus is on the fragility of children's thinking as compared with the cross-situational strength of older children's and adults' thinking. The young child possesses the critical knowledge but is not in full control of it and has only limited access to it. An everyday example of limited access is the case of tying one's shoe. Adults' knowledge of how to tie a shoe appears inaccessible in the sense that adults have little conscious awareness of the procedure. What, for example, is the *third* step in tying one's shoe? To answer this question, most people have to go through the entire process of tying their laces. Tying one's laces is a whole unit, not easily divisible into components. One's access to the third step in lace tying is thus limited in two ways: in the manner of retrieving the information (one has only one route – start at the beginning) and in one's awareness of the steps (one knows how to go through the steps of lace tying but does not consciously know the steps).

Much of the young child's knowledge may be difficult to access just as shoe-tying knowledge is difficult to access for adults, and much of the developmental growth in thinking may be growth of access to knowledge (Pylyshyn, 1978; Rozin, 1976). Children might possess the ability to solve a particular problem, but that knowledge may be tied to a particular situation or routine and thus children may show their knowledge in only some situations. *Welded knowledge* is the term used to refer to knowledge limited to a specific situation. Children's access may be limited in another sense as well. They may know how to do things but not know what they know; they may have little awareness of, and therefore little conscious control over, their knowledge.

Findings by Bullock and Gelman (1977) concerning children's reasoning about numerosities provide an example of tacit knowledge – knowledge without conscious awareness. Their experiment consisted of a game in which children picked winning plates of mice. The children were shown two plates of mice – one plate might contain one mouse and the other two mice – and were told that either the one-mouse or the two-mouse plate was the winner. There was no mention of number of mice. In a second phase of the experiment, the children were shown plates with, for example, three mice and four mice and asked which was the winner. Consider the case in which in Phase 1 (with two objects vs. one) the children were told that the two-mouse plate was the winner. If in Phase 2, the children chose the four-mouse plate in the context of four mice versus three, they would be showing knowledge of the abstract relation of *more than* – an understanding that the relation between 1 and 2 was the same as that between 3 and 4. Bullock and Gelman reported that 4- and 5-year-olds applied such an abstract ordering rule, choosing the plate with more mice (or fewer, depending on the direction of the winner in Phase 1). However, despite their clear use of an abstract ordering relation of *more than*, the children could not correctly explain their choices and did not describe the winner in terms of *more* or *less*. Indeed, most of the children justified their answers by making reference only to the number in the set they chose, giving such reasons as "because there are four" but not explaining how 4 in the case of three mice versus four was similar to 2 in the case of one mouse versus two mice. This experiment indicates that children have knowledge of ordinal relations and at some level "know" that the relation between 4 and 3 is the same as between 2 and 1, but they apparently have little awareness of that knowledge.

Additional findings by Bullock and Gelman provide an example of situational limits on access to knowledge. In their original task, the 2-year-olds, in contrast to the older children, did not choose relationally in Phase 2. Bullock and Gelman suggest that the 2-year-olds' failures were due to the children's not accessing knowledge they did have. Specifically, they suggest that the 2-year-olds' Phase 1 knowledge was not accessed by the Phase 2 task. It is as if the 2-year-olds thought they were playing two separate, unrelated games. Bullock and Gelman conducted a second study and found support for this notion. They were able to make the 2-year-olds choose relationally simply by leaving the original Phase 1 plates in view (but covered so that the children could not see the actual number of mice). It seemed as though the youngest children had to be reminded that they were involved in the same task and that the original rule (*more* or *less*) was relevant. Clearly, these very young children possessed the critical knowledge; however, they did not spontaneously access it and needed a specific prompt to do so.

Developmental changes in the use of strategies for remembering also point to the possible importance of the accessibility of knowledge. The consistent use of strategies for rote memorization of verbal material (e.g., rehearsal) may depend on the child's being aware of the workings of his or her own memory. Metamemory, or knowledge about memory, does change with development. Young children, unlike older children, are often unable to predict how well they will remember (Markman, 1973). For example, when given a set of 10 items versus a set of 3 items to remember, preschool children cannot predict which set will be more difficult to remember. Furthermore, older but not younger children know what they can do to increase the likelihood of recall (e.g., rehearse). Increased awareness of how one's own memory works, then, might be a major factor in children's development of specific strategies for remembering.

Overall, the suggestion of increased accessibility of knowledge captures one aspect of the developmental trend in thinking: from passive context-specific to increasingly strategic, active, and consciously directed thought. Notice that the capacity and accessibility accounts are not mutually exclusive. Both accessibility and available capacity may depend on practice at performing component processes (Mandler, 1983). Furthermore, accessing knowledge may require capacity, and functional capacity might well increase with the increased accessibility of knowledge structures. Both notions also capture well the partial competence that appears to be the hallmark of developmentally immature thought.

The role of the knowledge base

Children and adults differ greatly in what they know. Adults have at their disposal years of experience and knowledge, which includes factual information (e.g., Paris is the capital of France), relational information (e.g., the ways in which fathers and boys are alike), and procedural information (e.g., how to add). Increases in knowledge may be a major source of many changes in cognitive development. Although, as we have seen, equating older and younger subjects' expertise in chess, for example, does not eliminate all developmental differences, some performance differences between children and adults do decrease or even reverse when children's knowledge is not, as it usually is, impoverished relative to that of adults. Another study of experts and novices in chess emphasizes this point. Chi (1978) compared the performance of 10-year-olds and adults. One task was a digit span task. Both 10-year-olds and adults listened to a series of numbers and were asked to recall them immediately. It is not surprising that the adults outperformed the 10-year-olds. The second task involved memory of legal arrangements of chess pieces on a chessboard. In this case, the 10-year-olds outperformed the adults. This result is not surprising when one knows that the 10-year-olds were chess experts and the adults were novices. Level of expertise – that is, one's knowledge in a content area – greatly determines the efficiency of one's processing in that area. One reason that adults' and older children's processing is more efficient than that of younger children's may be the fact that older subjects know more than younger subjects.

Greater processing ability may result not just from more knowledge, but from more *organized* knowledge. Chi and Koeske (1983) tested a single child on knowledge and subsequent memory performance of better known and lesser known groups of dinosaurs. They contrasted two types of "more knowledge." In one case, "more knowledge" referred to knowledge of more properties about a concept, for example, knowing that a particular dinosaur was a plant eater, lived in water, and was horned versus knowing only that that dinosaur was a plant eater. In another case, "more knowledge" referred to the pattern and number of links between concepts, for example, knowing that two dinosaurs were alike in being both horned and plant eaters. Chi and Koeske concluded that differences in the patterns of the links and not the property knowledge per se were the source of the differences in memory performance. The better known (and remembered) dinosaurs shared more links with each other than did the lesser-known dinosaurs, even though the child's knowledge of properties in the two cases was equal. This demonstration suggests that it is not simply what is known but how knowledge is organized that determines the ease with which it is accessed and actually used.

Summary: what develops?

Thinking appears to develop from partial competence that is situationally specific and fragile into more complete, flexible, and robust abilities that are applied across situations. Developmental increases in processing capacity, in the accessibility of knowledge, and in the knowledge base are all likely aspects of growth. In the next section we consider developmental changes in the knowledge base in more detail, since growth of knowledge may be a major source of growth of capacity and the accessibility of knowledge.

Developmental changes in organization of knowledge

The development of the knowledge base involves both the accumulation of facts and the organization and reorganization of those facts. Changes in the organization of knowledge in particular provide a potential explanation of partial competence. Much may be known by the young child, but the various pieces may not be organized into a coherent system. Studies of child language provide several examples of reorganization of what is in some sense already known (see Bowerman, 1982). One example concerns knowledge of plural forms. Very young children appear to distinguish between many singular and plural forms of nouns. That is, they apply *cat* to a single cat, and *cats* to more than one cat (similarly, *dog−dogs, child−children,* etc.). Their performance with these words is thus like adult performance; they have knowledge of singular forms and plural forms. When children first use the plural, however, they do not seem to realize that a systematic relationship exists between many singular and plural forms of nouns, that there is a general rule (as well as exceptions). Instead, early organization seems to consist of a set of unanalyzed item-by-item correspondences. It is as if the child has a set of separate facts: *dog−dogs, child−children, cat−cats, foot−feet.* The correspondence between *cat* and *cats* has no more special status than the one between *foot* and *feet.* That children have abstracted the plural rule (*-s*), and thus have reorganized the information in this domain, is evident when they overregularize and say such things as *foots.* Only after children have abstracted that rule do they attach the *s* to forms that do not take them (e.g., *childs*) − forms that they had used correctly during a previous, rule-free period. Evidence in other areas also suggests developmental changes of just this sort, early piecemeal knowledge that is subsequently organized into a *system.*

Relational knowledge

One domain in which developmental changes in the organization of a knowledge system can be seen is the development of relational knowledge – the
knowledge that underlies transitive inference making and seriation. When
we discussed preschool children's transitive inference making, we noted that
young children sometimes interpret relative adjectives in their comparative
form (e.g., *taller*) categorically (e.g., as *tall*). These errors appear to stem
from the incomplete nature of what is ultimately a very complex knowledge
system. In particular, the development of relational knowledge in early childhood appears to consist in children's integrating various bits and pieces of
knowledge they already possess about relations and relational language into
a coherent system.

One demonstration of growth in children's organization of relational
knowledge concerns their use of the adjectives *high* and *low*. Smith,
Cooney, and McCord (1986) reported that younger children (three-year-
olds) interpret *high* and *low* as referring to the extremes of height values.
Thus, for these children there were many intermediate heights that were
neither *high* nor *low*. More specifically, given variation from zero to six feet,
objects were *high* only between five and six feet and *low* only between zero
and one foot. In contrast, older children and adults interpreted *high* and *low*
as referring to two mutually exclusive categories such that all heights were
either *high* or *low*. Thus, the two categories were negations of each other; if
a height was not high, it was low. These results suggest a change in the
organization of *high* and *low*. For younger children, the terms refer in a
fixed way to distinct, unconnected categories; for the older subjects *high* and
low are defined in terms of each other; the meanings are unified into one
system.

The separateness of *high* and *low* for young children is also seen in their
interpretations of *higher* and *lower* (Ratterman & Smith, 1985). Children
who have disjointed categories for *high* and *low* do not correctly interpret
higher and *lower* across the entire range of comparisons. Rather, they correctly judge which of two objects is higher if they are both high (e.g., at five
and six feet), but they refuse to judge which of these two categorically high
objects is lower. When asked which of two high objects (e.g., objects at five
and six feet) is lower, they answer, "They are both high." Analogously,
children can judge which of two low objects (one and two feet) is lower but
they refuse to judge which is higher – as if this question were nonsensical
since both objects are low. Older children, of course, accurately judge which
of two objects is higher or lower regardless of the actual height of the objects. Older children know that, if six feet is higher than five feet, then five
is lower than six feet, and their judgments of higher and lower do not depend on the heights involved. Older children clearly have *higher* and *lower*

organized as opposing directions of difference that apply across the continuum; younger children, in contrast, restrict *higher* and *lower* to their respective separate categories.

The young child's restricted use of *higher* and *lower* is particularly interesting because it seems analogous to the correct use of comparatives referring to disconnected nominal categories, such as color. We can judge, for example, which of two red objects is redder but we cannot judge which of two red objects is greener. Early in development, then, *high* and *low* appear to be organized as separate categories like *red* and *green* but become reorganized as negations of each other with development.

In summary, young children may have many bits and pieces of relational knowledge. They have polar adjectives linked to the proper ends of their continua. They can even correctly interpret comparatives. What they do not have, however, is a system that integrates all this knowledge. Children then may be partially competent in dealing with relations because they are working from an incomplete knowledge system. The situations in which young children show their knowledge may depend on the specific structure of their partial competence. For example, in the transitive-inference-making task, the reason that premises may have to be stated in both directions (e.g., "A is taller than B" *and* "B is shorter than A") may be precisely because young children do not integrate the meanings of the opposing terms. An explanation of specific findings of "can but don't," then, may require very detailed accounts of knowledge growth in specific domains.

Number knowledge

R. Gelman's (1977) investigations of children's understanding of number provide another example of growth in a knowledge system. According to Gelman's view, very young children possess some universal principles about number. These principles include (a) one-to-one correspondence (counting by putting one number name to one object), (b) stable ordering of number names, (c) cardinality (the last number named is the number in the set), and (d) order irrelevancy (the order in which objects are counted does not matter). The evidence for this knowledge is found in children's early counting behavior. Children show evidence of one-to-one correspondence by showing that they know that one number name goes with one object. Young children show evidence of the stable ordering principle by developing stable, if erroneous, lists (e.g., 1, 2, 3, 4, 7, 11, bipple). Very young children show evidence for a cardinality principle by giving as the number in a set the last number named when in the count of a set. They show evidence of an order irrelevancy principle by counting a set in more than one order (object 1 in 1−2−3 can be object 2 in a second count). Even two-and-a-half-year-olds show evidence of these principles – at least in counting to 2. Given this early competence, this beginning of a knowledge system, what develops? The stable list of number names develops, and error-free counting develops with practice. Early on, children may know not to double count or miss an item but they have trouble not doing so. What is most interesting, however, is that from these early principles and practice at error-free counting, new knowledge may emerge and be organized into a complex system.

One example of knowledge emerging from these early counting principles concerns the abstract knowledge that the spatial arrangement of items is irrelevant to its numerosity, that is, number conservation. Gelman and Gallistel (1978) have shown that preschool children "conserve" (show evidence that spatial arrangement is irrelevant) up to the numerosity that they can count. A child who can count to 5 knows that $4 = 4$ even if one row is longer than another. However, if presented with 10 items in the standard conservation task, the same child will maintain that one row now has more objects if it is lengthened. If young children truly understand that only addition and subtraction are relevant to numerosity, they should conserve regardless of whether or not they can count the set; two sets that are equal remain equal, if nothing has been added or subtracted. Children demonstrate this abstract knowledge and conservation with sets too large to count once they are able consistently to count to 10. This fact suggests an interesting hypothesis. Perhaps, children have to prove to themselves that spatial arrangement is irrelevant and do so by counting. By counting, children may discover that as long as nothing is added or subtracted $1 = 1, 2 = 2, 3 = 3, \ldots$ Once they have demonstrated, by counting, the irrelevance of spatial arrangements across a wide enough variety of numerosities (i.e., up to 10), they make the induction that spatial arrangement is irrelevant for all n.

Counting also appears to play a critical role in children's understanding of infinity – in their knowledge that there is no largest number. Evans (1982; see also Gelman & Gallistel, 1978) asked young school-age children to name the largest number. Many named a large number (e.g., 1,000), but upon questioning, many discovered that there was no largest number. The key to the children's *discovery* of infinity was the question Evans asked them: "What if I added one?" From knowledge of the way in which the numbers in the number sequence are generated, many children were able to prove to themselves that there is no largest number. Which children were able to discover infinity in this way was predictable from their ability to count to 100 and their concomitant knowledge of the manner in which the number sequence is generated. They took what knowledge they had and upon questioning reanalyzed it and moved to a new level of competence.

These examples of the development of number knowledge may be particularly informative of the way in which thinking develops. The child may begin with a few principles that enable and constrain the discovery of new knowledge. From early partial competence, a complex knowledge system may emerge.

Concepts and categories

Children's acquisition of object categories provides a final example of developmental changes in the knowledge system. How natural categories such as *dog, chair,* or *animal* are organized has long been a perplexing problem to philosophers and psychologists. Two general classes of proposals about the structure of concepts have been offered (see Smith & Medin, 1981). According to one, the traditional or classical account, concepts are structured logically by defining properties, that is, by necessary and sufficient features. "A closed figure is a triangle if and only if it has three sides" is an example of a category organized by a defining property. Rosch's (1973) overall similarity account of the structure of basic categories is an example of the second kind of proposal. According to this view, no one property or set of properties is necessary and sufficient for an object to be a member of a category; chairs, for example, are not all alike in any one way (or several ways). Rather, there is a set of noncriterial but characteristic features of chairs such that most chairs are alike in terms of a large number of features, none of which is criterial or possessed by all chairs. As we noted earlier many basic categories, the first categories named by children (e.g. *dog, chair*), appear to be organized by overall similarities or characteristic properties. In general, there appears to be a developmental trend from categories organized by characteristic to defining features, the former (e.g., *dog*) being acquired earlier than the latter (e.g., superordinate categories such as *animal*).

There also appears to be a *reorganization* of individual concepts with development. Keil and Batterman (1984) showed that younger and older children differed in their understanding of various words, the younger children defining the words in terms of characteristic properties and the older in terms of necessary and sufficient properties. For example, to children under seven, an island was land near water with palm trees and sand – properties characteristic of a prototypical island. For older children, however, an island was a body of land surrounded by water; one criterial property determined membership in the category. This shift from characteristic to defining properties does not occur at a particular age. Keil and Batterman showed that the shift occurs at different times for different concepts, depending on the structure of the concepts and the individual's experience with them. In other words, when we learn concepts, either as an adult or as a child, we may first organize them in terms of characteristic properties and then later *reorganize* them as we determine the defining features. This point raises the important possibility that many changes in thought are not, as is often assumed, age-related but rather knowledge-related.

Summary: Changes in the knowledge base

Growth of knowledge is not simply the accumulation of facts. Rather, a critical aspect of development appears to be the organization and integration of pieces of knowledge into highly structured systems. Within such systems, organization of knowledge may give rise to new knowledge. For example, children may figure out infinity simply by applying what they know. Indeed, children (as well as perhaps adults) may be internally motivated to acquire, organize, and master domains. As an example, De Loache, Sugarman, and Brown (1985) have studied 18- to 24-month-olds' ordering of nesting cups in free play. With no encouragement, external pressure, or motivation other than the task itself, the children worked long and hard at ordering cups, stopping and starting and trying again. There appears to be an inner drive to master and to understand.

Other issues in the study of the development of thought

The evidence and ideas we have considered in this chapter suggest that the acquisition and organization of knowledge play the major role in the development of thinking. Our emphasis on this topic leaves some important issues about development unresolved. We shall briefly consider some of them.

The child as novice

An essential difference between older and younger children is that, by virtue of having lived longer, older children have probably learned more about the world; they have had more time and experience with which to organize that knowledge and to become practiced at using it. So in a sense, the young child is a novice in the world. But how far should we push this analogy? Are there age-related differences in thinking independent of knowledge?

These questions are not easily answered. It is difficult to equate all relevant knowledge in a child and an adult. Attempts to do so in the examples of knowledge of chess discussed earlier suggest that domain-specific knowledge is a critical determinant of performance (Chi, 1978) but that there may be age-related differences even when the knowledge of children and adults is comparable (Kail, 1986; Roth, 1983). Another weakness of the analogy between the child in general and the novice in some specific domain is that the knowledge systems at issue are not truly comparable. Knowledge systems like relational knowledge, number knowledge, and knowledge of categories differ from knowledge of chess or dinosaurs in a very important way. Knowledge about relations, number, and natural categories are instances of knowledge that *all* human beings acquire from their daily interactions with the world and require to understand their world in the most basic ways. Knowledge of chess or dinosaurs does not have such universality or biological importance. One unresolved issue, then, is whether universally acquired knowledge systems differ from more culturally specific knowledge systems, and if so, how do they differ?

Readiness

Readiness is a traditional notion in developmental psychology. The idea is that training in some domain will not result in mature performance unless the child is sufficiently developed to benefit from the training. In other words, there may be conditions within the child that allow experiences to have their effect.

Readiness has often been considered a critical factor in learning to read. Reading skill in children learning an alphabetic system such as that of written English is clearly related to the ability to segment spoken speech into phonemes – to judge, for example, that *bat* and *beak* begin with the same sound or that *cute* and *salt* end in the same sound. Although the relation between reading skill and phoneme-segmentation skill is clear, the causal direction has been debated. Must one be able to segment speech into phonemes to learn to read, or does learning to read teach phoneme segmentation? The latter seems to be the case, at least for adults. Adult illiterates (even when similar to literates in other cognitive skills) are poor at segmenting speech into phonemes (Morais, Cary, Alegria & Bertelson, 1979; Read, Zhang, Nie, & Ding, 1986) but may acquire this skill if taught to read (Read et al., 1986). Thus, age alone seems not to be the sole determinant of phoneme-segmentation skills. However, these results do not show that some age-related ability is not critical. Adult illiterates of normal intelligence can be taught to segment speech into phonemes; four-year-old children are not so easily taught. Young children may have to wait to learn to read until they are perceptually "ready" to learn to segment spoken speech into its constituents, and that perceptual readiness may be independent of training in this domain. There may be a developmental boundary on learning to read and to segment spoken speech, a lower limit that cannot be passed and is, perhaps, determined by the development of some general (possibly biological) ability.

However, it can also be argued that there are virtually no developmental boundaries that one has to pass in order to acquire some knowledge. All apparent readiness boundaries may simply be insufficient prior acquisition and organization of knowledge. A compelling example of this possibility derives from the history of arithmetic (Evans, 1982). During the Middle Ages, Arabic numerals were not used in Europe; Roman numerals were. As a result, multiplication and division were extremely difficult operations to perform. The techniques were cumbersome, roundabout, and known only by very few specialists with much training. With the advent of the Arabic numeral system and its decimal organization and place holders (i.e., zero), multiplication and division became much easier to perform. The point is that during the Middle Ages multiplication and division could not be readily learned by many. There was a lack of readiness for learning these operations, but the lack of readiness stemmed from the existing knowledge system. Now, with another, learnable knowledge system, multiplication and division are easily learned. Perhaps with more knowledge of the psychological nature of reading and learning, we would also find that there are no age limits on learning to read.

Changes in what is learned

Related to the issue of readiness are *general* developmental changes in the kind of knowledge acquired from experience. Consider the balance-scale problem. In this task, the child has to figure out which side of the scale goes down as differing weights are placed at differing distances from the fulcrum. Siegler (1978) found that 5-year-olds tend to induce one-factor rules (e.g., only weight matters). Somewhat older children induce a *simple* two-factor rule (weight matters unless the weights on each side are equal; then distance from fulcrum matters). Finally, 17-year-olds induce rules about the interaction of the two relevant factors. In brief, from the same experiences, older subjects develop more systematic and more complex knowledge structures. These developmental changes in rule formation appear to be *general*; they are not specific to specific problems. The source of these developmental changes is unclear; they could reflect an accumulation and organization of general knowledge, or they could be due to age-related processing limits.

Domain specificity

The emphasis placed on the growth of knowledge in particular content areas in order to account for developmental changes in cognition raises another issue — whether "thought" is a unitary aspect of mind or whether the mind is composed of separate, independent domains. According to one current view the mind is composed of separate modules, each developing according to a different set of principles. First and most explicitly put forth by Fodor (1975, 1983), this view of thinking was intended to account for the *diversity* in development. The basic notion is that since different knowledge domains have different and unique properties, general abilities cannot be expected to explain the progression within each of these domains. For example, number reasoning depends on specific knowledge about numbers; an understanding of infinity reflects the growth of domain-specific knowledge.

Although growth of thinking depends to some degree on growth of domain-specific knowledge bases, the separation of these domains is debatable. Too strong an emphasis on domain specificity is problematic in that it lends itself to the possibility of a separate module being proposed for every cognitive task. What is needed is a theory of domains, a principled means of segregating cognition into domains. Such a theory will presumably grow out of more complete descriptions of various knowledge systems. However, even if separate domains do exist and are identifiable, developments in one domain might influence developments in another, and single concepts may be involved in more than one domain.

Some cognitive psychologists have argued for separate knowledge-specific domains on biological grounds. The notion is that, in order for cognitive development to be as rapid and as universal as it is, there must be strong constraints on the outcome of development. These constraints would be built in and would determine the course of development. Gelman's number principles are a good example of specific constraints that might both enable and constrain the acquisition of a specific knowledge system.

Although cognitive psychologists with a nativist bent argue for separate domains in development, psychobiologists studying biological growth and the growth of species-typical behavior emphasize cross-domain dependencies and interactions (Fentriss, 1984). This approach has been called systems theory. Thelen and Fogel (in press) have applied these notions to the development of human walking. The idea is that walking depends on a number of abilities, each with its own developmental growth rate and each serving a variety of systems. Some of these abilities seem central or specific to the domain of "walking skill." For example, the pattern generation system that controls organized stepping would seem to be the central skill in walking. Other relevant factors are not as central to the ability to walk and include such things as the strength of various muscle groups and body shape and mass. Thelen has shown that pattern generation is intact at birth and remains so. In a sense, then, the infant has the ability to walk but will not walk until the less central factors of body shape and mass vis-á-vis muscle strength develop sufficiently.

The point is that the emergence of an ability, even a biologically preprogrammed one like walking, may well depend on developments in other domains or the emergence of enabling conditions. An interactional systems approach to cognitive development might provide a way of integrating domain-specific and general developments in cognition. Growth of capacity per se, for example, could be critical for the appearance of various domain-specific abilities that are to some degree "in place" before they are exhibited.

Stages of development

Piaget's theory posited successive, qualitatively distinct stages that were invariantly ordered, each successive stage being built from the prior stage.

The notion was of an all-pervasive manner of thought and successive, massive reorganizations of thought that affected performance across domains. The findings of very early partial competencies and the importance of learning and domain-specific knowledge would seem to counter Piaget's grand theory of stages.

However, we may not want to abandon the notion of stages, only to redefine them (see Brainerd, 1978). If one looks at children of different ages and their approach to a variety of tasks, ignoring all the details of the tasks and the subtleties of performance, what does one see? One sees children who are qualitatively different from what they were at an earlier age. In his or her interactions with the world a 1-year-old is not at all like a 3-year-old, who is not at all like the individual he or she will be at age 8 or 18. And on a global level, the intellectual differences between children at each of these ages seem to match Piaget's descriptions. Recall that, if we present children with the same tasks that Piaget did, we get the same results. Children have not changed since Piaget studied them, nor has their level of performance. What has changed is our understanding. Underneath the large global changes are many specific, stepwise, perhaps domain-specific areas of growth and reorganization.

Systems theory as it has been used to explain the development of walking provides a potential way of integrating findings of continuous growth patterns in specific abilities and global qualitative shifts in behavior. An infant who does not yet walk is different in his or her manner of getting about from one who does; and the shift in means of getting about from, say, crawling to walking takes place rapidly within several weeks, sometimes within days. But the specific developing abilities that underlie this shift do not change qualitatively. Rather, some (e.g., the stepping pattern) may be fully developed from the beginning. Others (e.g., motivation, body constraints, postural control) may mature slowly and continuously; they may be fully developed months before walking but are not used until one final component, such as extensor strength, reaches a certain level of development. At that juncture, there is a qualitative shift in motor behavior, and walking becomes the central means of getting about. The point is that stages and qualitative changes probably ought to be retained as useful theoretical constructs at one level of analysis. The more we know about underlying abilities, about growth in specific domains, the less "stagelike" development will probably seem in detail. However, at another level of analysis, that of the whole child, stages still seem to be useful concepts.

Summary

What develops in the development of thinking? In this chapter, we considered evidence principally concerning children's thinking about relations, number, and classes. In each domain, we saw the beginnings of mature-like thought in very young children. These early aspects of thought appear to enable the acquisition of new knowledge. The acquisition and organization of knowledge have a major impact on the speed and efficiency of basic processes and may in this way enable more sophisticated and more context-independent uses of knowledge. Unresolved issues in the development of thinking center on the way in which knowledge is organized in different domains, on the interaction between domains, and whether areas or aspects of growth independent of knowledge acquisition constrain knowledge acquisition and utilization across domains.

References

Baillargeron, R., Spelke, E., & Wasserman (1985). Object permanence in the 5-month-old infant. *Cognition, 20,* 191–208.

Bowerman, M. (1982). Reorganizational processes in lexical and syntactic development. In E. Wanner & L. R. Gleitman (Eds.), *Language acquisition: The state of the art* (pp. 319–425). Cambridge University Press.

Brainerd, C. J. (1978). The stage question in cognitive-developmental theory. *Behavioral and Brain Sciences, 2,* 173–213.

Brown, A. L. (1973). Judgments of recency for long sequences of pictures: The absence of a developmental trend. *Journal of Experimental Child Psychology, 15,* 473–80.

Brown, A. L., Bransford, J. D., Ferrara, R. A., & Campione, J. C. (1983). Learning, remembering, and understanding. In P. H. Mussen (Ed.), *Handbook of child psychology: Vol. 3. Cognitive development* (pp. 77–166). New York: Wiley.

Bryant, P. E., & Trabasso, T. R. (1971). Transitive inferences and memory in young children. *Nature, 232,* 456–8.

Bullock, M., & Gelman, R. (1977). Numerical reasoning in young children: The ordering principle. *Child Development, 48,* 427–34.

Carey, S. (1978, November). *The child's concept of* animal. Paper presented to the Psychonomics Society, San Antonio, TX.

Case, R. (1972). Validation of a neo-Piagetian mental capacity construct. *Journal of Experimental Child Psychology, 14,* 287–302.

Case, R., Kurland, D. M., & Goldberg, J. (1982). Operational efficiency and the growth of short-term memory span. *Journal of Experimental Child Psychology, 33*(3), 386–404.

Chi, M. T. H. (1978). Knowledge structures and memory development. In R. S. Siegler (Ed.), *Children's thinking: What develops?* (pp. 73–95). Hillsdale, NJ: Erlbaum.

Chi, M. T. H., & Koeske, R. D. (1983). Network representations of knowledge base: Exploring a child's knowledge and memory performance of dinosaurs. *Developmental Psychology, 19*(1), 29–39.

Chukovsky, K. (1971). *From two to five.* Berkeley & Los Angeles: University of California Press.

De Loache, J., Sugarman, S., & Brown, A. (1985). The development of error-correction strategies in young children's manipulative play. *Child Development, 56,* 928–39.

Evans, D. (1982). *Understanding infinity and zero in the early school years.* Unpublished doctoral dissertation, University of Pennsylvania, Philadelphia.

Fentriss, J. C. (1984). The development of coordination. *Journal of Motor Behavior, 16,* 99–134.

Flavell, J. H. (1977). *Cognitive development.* Englewood Cliffs, NJ: Prentice-Hall.

Fodor, J. A. (1975). *The language of thought.* New York: Crowell.

(1983). *Modularity of mind: An essay on faculty psychology.* Cambridge, MA: MIT Press.

Gelman, R. (1977). How young children reason about small numbers. In N. J. Castellan, D. B. Pisoni, & G. R. Potts (Eds.), *Cognitive theory* (Vol. 2, pp. 219–38). Hillsdale, NJ: Erlbaum.

Gelman, R., & Gallistel, C. R. (1978). *The child's understanding of number.* Cambridge, MA: Harvard University Press.

Gelman, S. (1985). *Reasoning about categories: The development of induction within categories named by language.* Unpublished doctoral dissertation, Stanford University, Stanford, CA.

Halford, G. S. (1984). Can young children integrate premises in transitivity and serial order tasks? *Cognitive Psychology, 17,* 65–93.

Inhelder, B., & Piaget, J. (1964). *The early growth of logic in the child.* New York: Norton.

Kail, R. (1986). Sources of age differences in speed of processing. *Child Development, 57,* 969–87.

Keil, F. C. (1979). *Semantic and conceptual development: An ontological perspective.* Cambridge, MA: Harvard University Press.

Keil, F. C., & Batterman, N. (1984). A characteristic-to-defining shift in the development of word meaning. *Journal of Verbal Learning and Verbal Behavior, 23,* 221–36.

Mandler, J. M. (1983). Representation. In John H. Flavell & Ellen M. Markman (Eds.), *Cognitive development,* Vol. 3 of *Handbook of psychology* (Paul Mussen, Series Ed., pp. 420–94). New York: Wiley.

Markman, E. M. (1973). Factors affecting the young child's ability to monitor his memory. Unpublished doctoral dissertation, University of Pennsylvania.

Morais, J., Cary, L., Alegria, J., & Bertelson, P. (1979). Does awareness of speech as a sequence of phones arise spontaneously? *Cognition, 7,* 323–31.

O'Connell, B. G., & Gerard, A. B. (1985). Scripts and scraps: The development of sequential understanding. *Child Development, 56,* 301–45.

Pascual-Leone, J. (1970). A mathematical model for the transition rule in Piaget's development stages. *Acta Psychologica, 63,* 301–45.

Piaget, J. (1954). *The construction of reality in the child.* New York: Basic.

Pylyshyn, Z. W. (1978). When is attribution of beliefs justified? *Behavioral and Brain Sciences, 1,* 592–3.

Ratterman, M. J., & Smith, L. B. (1985, April). *Children's categorical use of "high" and "low."* Paper presented at the biennial meeting of the Society for Research in Child Development, Toronto.

Read, C., Zhang, Y., Nie, H., & Ding, B. (1986). The ability to manipulate speech sounds depends on knowing alphabetic writing. *Cognition, 24,* 31–44.

Rosch, E. (1973). On the internal structure of perceptual and semantic categories. In T. E. Moore (Ed.), *Cognitive development and the acquisition of language* (pp. 112–44). New York: Academic Press.

Rosch, E., Mervis, C. B., Gray, D., & Boyes-Braem, P. (1976). Basic objects in natural categories. *Cognitive Psychology, 3,* 382–439.

Roth, C. (1983). Factors affecting developmental change in the speed of processing. *Journal of Experimental Child Psychology, 35,* 509–28.

Rozin, P. (1976). The evolution of intelligence and access to the cognitive unconscious. *Progress in Psychobiology and Physiological Psychology, 6,* 245–80.

Schneider, W., & Shiffrin, R. M. (1977). Controlled and automatic human information processing: Detection, search and attention. *Psychological Review, 84,* 1–66.

Shiffrin, R. M., & Schneider, W. (1977). Controlled and automatic human information processing: Perceptual learning, automatic attending, and a general theory. *Psychological Review, 84,* 127–90.

Siegler, R. S. (1978). The origins of scientific reasoning. In R. S. Siegler (Ed.), *Children's thinking: What develops?* (pp. 109–47). Hillsdale, NJ: Erlbaum.

Smith, E. E., & Medin, D. L. (1981). *Categories and concepts.* Cambridge, MA: Harvard University Press.

Smith, L. B., Cooney, N., & McCord, C. (1986). What is "high"? Development of implicit reference points for "high" and "low." *Child Development, 57,* 583–602.

Starkey, P., Spelke, E., & Gelman, R. (1982, April). *Detection of intermodal numerical correspondence by human infants.* Paper presented at the International Conference on Infant Studies meetings, Austin, TX.

Thelen, E., & Fogel, A. (in press). Toward an action-based theory of infant development. In J. Lockman & N. Hazen (Eds.), *Action in social context.* New York: Plenum.

Trabasso, T. (1977). The role of memory as a system of making transitive inferences. In R. V. Kail & J. W. Hagen (Eds.), *Perspectives on the development of memory and cognition.* (pp. 333–65). Hillsdale, NJ: Erlbaum.

Trabasso, T., & Riley, C. A. (1975). The construction and use of representations involving linear order. In R. L. Solso (Ed.), *Information processing and cognition: the Loyola Symposium* (pp. 381–409). Hillsdale, NJ: Erlbaum.

Vygotsky, L. S. (1962). *Thought and language.* Cambridge, MA: MIT Press.

Werner, H. (1948). *Comparative psychology of mental development.* New York: International University Press.

14 Methodology for laboratory research on thinking: task selection, collection of observations, and data analysis

K. Anders Ericsson and William L. Oliver

Most people have little understanding of their own thought processes even though they are constantly thinking. One might suppose that, simply by drawing on our vast personal experience as thinkers, we would come to know everything about thinking that is worth knowing. However, the mere practice of thinking apparently does not make us experts on the subject, just as daily exercise does not make us experts on the physics of motion and the eating of food does not make us experts on the biochemistry of digestion. In fact, it is difficult to identify general principles for all the different types of thought we engage in. After all, the term *thinking* encompasses a huge variety of mental activities. We are thinking when we solve problems, daydream, remember facts, and so on. Is it reasonable that there is a *single* method or even several methods for understanding these different types of thinking?

This chapter reviews many of the methods for studying thinking that modern researchers believe to be of general use. These methods provide knowledge that is thought to be suitable for scientific analysis. Since some of the brightest people have for centuries been struggling with the way the mind should be studied, we begin with a description of their earlier attempts along with an account of the problems and criticisms they encountered.

Introspection and early theorizing about the mind

The earliest speculations about the human mind were closely related to religious and philosophical questions about the nature of human beings. The human mind was often viewed as divine and therefore inherently incomprehensible. However, some philosophers began to ask how the mind acquired new knowledge and how faithfully this knowledge represented the true state of the world. Their basic source of information was the observation of their own thought processes by means of introspection. These analyses were directed toward very general issues and were speculative, there being little

We are very grateful for the thoughtful comments and suggestions on earlier drafts of this chapter by Peter Foltz, Alice Healy, Peter Polson, Kurt Reusser, Robert Sternberg, and Michael Wertheimer.

concern to support them with firm empirical data. Although many of the ideas about thinking that emerged from early theorizing became influential, this type of introspective inquiry gradually became suspect because the methods employed were not considered scientific. Before we discuss the first scientific psychological studies, let us examine the methods used in intro-spective studies of thought and a few of the findings that emerged.

One of these findings was that thought seems to proceed sequentially, as illustrated by an introspective report of James Mill (1829/1878):

> I see a horse: that is a sensation. Immediately I think of his master: that is an idea. The idea of his master makes me think of his office; he is minister of state: that is another idea. The idea of a minister of state makes me think of public affairs; and I am led into a train of political ideas; when I am summoned to dinner. This is a new sensation, followed by the idea of dinner, and of the company with whom I am to partake it. The sight of the company and of the food are other sensations; these suggest ideas without end; other sensations perpetually intervene, suggesting other ideas: and so the process goes on. (pp. 70−1)

In this report Mill describes a sequence of connected thoughts. One can elicit similar experiences, or reports, by asking students to introspect while they answer the following question: How many windows does your parents' house have? All students report counting the windows sequentially and nearly all of them report visualizing the rooms in the house in an orderly fashion. Demonstrations that all observers agree on the way they think argue forcefully for general processes involving sequences of images and thoughts. Demonstrations such as this convinced early philosophers that thought is always sequential.

Another question philosophers asked was; How many things can be thought of or attended to at a given instant? Aristotle argued that only one thing at a time could be attended to, and many subsequent philosophers agreed. Yet the intriguing possibility remained that one could hold more than one thing in one's attention at a time. Hamilton (1870) suggested that the issue could be resolved by an experiment:

> You can easily make the experiment for yourselves, but you must be aware of group-ing the objects into classes. If you throw a handful of marbles on the floor, you will find it difficult to view at once more than six, or seven at most, without confusion; but if you group them into twos, or threes, or fives, you can comprehend as many groups as you can units; because the mind considers these groups only as units − it views them as wholes, and throws their parts out of consideration. (p. 254)

Hamilton's experiment suggests that people can attend to only a few units at once − an important finding. Note that Hamilton simply assumes that this experiment on himself provides a measure of the attentional capacity of all humans. In fact, the assumption that basic characteristics of the mind are shared by all humans was taken for granted by many philosophers.

Although modern scientific psychology relies very little on self-observa-tions as evidence, the practice of using introspection to generate hypotheses and ideas for experiments continues. The origin of many, if not most, psychological concepts in current research is self-observation. Even during the height of behaviorism the importance of introspection was acknowledged, as evidenced by Lashley's (1923) famous remark that "introspection may make the preliminary survey, but it must be followed by the chain and transit of objective measurement" (p. 352).

Toward a scientific analysis of thinking

Although introspection may convince individuals of the validity of general principles of thought, it is still necessary to evaluate these principles in an objective and unbiased way. At least such is the dictum of the modern scientific method, which was originally developed to counter naïve but highly plausible notions about the world. A combination of skepticism and careful observation enabled early scientists to dispel beliefs that people had held for centuries. Scientists are well aware that initially plausible theories may turn out to be completely wrong in the light of new evidence. Thus, when scientists try to understand natural phenomena they maintain a certain skepticism about current ideas and look for evidence that either refutes or supports these ideas. Methodology, as we define it here, is this process of obtaining observations or facts that can critically influence what we are willing to believe.

In order to develop a deep understanding of the mind, we must find general laws of thinking that hold for all humans. A general characteristic of thought should be observable whether we study farm workers in China or American college students. Hence, the laws of thought that we seek should not vary with culture or individual experience. It is important to keep this challenging goal in mind when we consider how we are to go about the study of thinking.

There are many ways to perform psychological research on thinking. In all cases one has to choose a task or a collection of tasks and select a group of subjects to study. One also has to choose an experimental procedure and to decide what observations will be collected for each subject. Finally, one has to analyze one's data in a manner that allows one to draw general conclusions. In subsequent sections we will discuss some issues involved in making these decisions and describe some alternatives. We will argue that these decisions are made on implicitly or explicitly theoretical grounds. Influential theories of thinking are not developed in isolation, but are constrained by broad theoretical frameworks that are generally agreed on by groups of researchers. In order to understand these broad constraints on theorizing, let us turn to a brief description of the major theoretical frameworks used to study thinking.

Theoretical approaches to thinking

The first approach to the study of thinking, structuralism, concentrated on describing the structure and content of thoughts. When people observe themselves as they think and daydream they usually experience visual and auditory images that lack any correspondence to the external situation. It was assumed that these images are similar to perceptions of external objects, but are not as strong and vivid. Observers were trained to describe their thoughts in detail by referring to the sensory elements of each image. Considerable controversy arose between different groups of psychologists over the nature of these sensory elements and over whether all thoughts can be adequately described as sensory images. Disagreements among trained observers made theorizing particularly difficult because there was no means to confirm the correctness of any one subject's descriptions (Humphrey, 1951; Woodworth, 1938). With the emergence of behaviorism, the detailed analysis of thinking was deemed unscientific.

The second major theoretical framework we will consider, behaviorism, was developed largely as a negative response to introspective approaches to thought. According to behaviorism the only valid evidence about thinking is observable behavior. Because thinking is not often associated with any observable behavior, investigators were diverted from the study of thinking and focused instead on other psychological phenomena, such as learning. By defining clear criteria for deciding whether or not people (or rats) learned, the behaviorists were able to amass an immense amount of data about variables that influence the learning process. The theories accounting for these data, however, were simplistic and had essentially nothing to say about the mental processes involved in learning. The impoverishment of these theories was a consequence of a very deliberate emphasis on finding direct relationships between observable events and behaviors and on avoiding the introduction of any theoretical (nonobservable) entities. Nevertheless, some research was directed toward finding observable behavior that accompanied thinking and could thus be studied objectively. Watson (1920) suggested that thinking could best be described as subvocal speech and that this speech could be observed as small movements of the tongue and larynx. A method introduced by Watson (1920) was to instruct subjects to think aloud, that is, simply vocalize their subvocal speech. Since then, other behavior (e.g., eye movements) and many physiological measures (e.g., the electroencephalogram) have been related to thought activity.

A third theoretical framework was provided by the Gestalt psychologists, who criticized both the behaviorists and the structuralists for describing behavior and mental processes as combinations of very simple elements and processes. They argued that complex objects are not simply a sum of their parts. In the domain of perception they showed that recognition of a complex familiar object is not attained by identification of its features and then its parts. Instead, the complex object is immediately identified and then decomposed into its parts. For example, we usually recognize a caricature of a famous politician before we are aware of such features as the eyebrows or the nose. Similarly, in the domain of thinking Duncker (1945) and Wertheimer (1945) demonstrated that insight and understanding depend on the recognition of complex patterns. Their method of argument was to show that simple processes could not account for individuals' responses to particular visual stimuli or for their means of solving particular problems. They chose their examples (e.g., Wertheimer's parallelogram problem) carefully so that the reader was sure to notice the role of the complex processes they proposed. It was not until computers were developed that these complex processes could be explicitly characterized and modeled.

The dominant contemporary theoretical framework, information processing (Anderson & Bower, 1973; Atkinson & Shiffrin, 1968; Newell & Simon, 1972), attempts to explain human thought with simulation models that can be implemented on computers. For a given task, one must have a description of the thinking process that is so complete it can be handed to a skilled computer programmer, who then can write a computer program. Ideally, this program should be able to generate the correct answers when it is given the same description of the task as is given to human subjects. These simulation models usually perform only certain types of tasks, such as those used in the psychology laboratory. The relevant facts and methods that the subjects know before the experiment must be represented in computer models. This requirement makes these models quite complex. Furthermore, a model implemented as a computer simulation is not necessarily an accurate model of human behavior simply because it can mimic certain aspects of human behavior, such as providing the correct answer to a problem. Instead, the model must be *psychologically plausible* by being consistent with known constraints on thinking and mental capacities. The model also has to be consistent with empirical findings gathered from subjects who perform the task that is being modeled. We will first discuss the criteria for psychological plausibility.

In accepting that human cognition is information processing, one assumes that cognitive processes are a sequence of internal states or mental representations successively transformed by a series of information processes. An important and more specific assumption is that information is stored in several memories having different capacities and accessing characteristics: several sensory stores of short duration, a short-term memory with limited capacity and/or intermediate duration, and a long-term memory with large capacity and relatively permanent storage, but with slow storage and access times compared with the other memories.

An information-processing model for a specific task domain (a collection of related tasks) consists of a sequence of processes that generates the same responses as people generate. Any reasonable model must be constrained by several additional considerations that exclude outlandish explanations. For instance, the model can draw only on knowledge that human subjects would also have and must have available to it the same information that is presented to the subjects. For example, a reasonable model of the way people understand stories written in English would require, at the very least, a vocabulary of English words. Models satisfying these criteria will generate explicit sequences of processing steps that differ for different tasks in the task domain. It is possible for investigators of thinking to examine these sequences of steps and judge on introspective grounds whether a model is consistent with their intuitions. Although these judgments are of value, they are not a valid substitute for empirical studies of subjects' actual thought processes. In this chapter we will show how one can obtain a wide range of observations on thought processes.

Methodology of thinking research: an overview

There is no agreed-upon general methodology for the study of thinking. In fact, the use of specific experimental procedures is often confined to a particular subarea of research on thinking. It is fortunate that these specialized procedures are usually well documented (e.g., Puff, 1982). In this chapter we will attempt to identify the general methods that are widely used for the study of thinking.

We have already described the relatively uncontroversial core assumptions of information-processing theory. From these we will derive implications for three methodological questions that must be asked when one designs studies of thinking:

1. What makes the task under study particularly suitable for the study of thinking? (task selection)
2. What types of observations on thinking do we have at our disposal, and how can the experimental situation be adapted to provide clean data on thinking processes? (collection of observations)
3. How can one aggregate and pool observations from different individuals and tasks and still obtain interpretable measurements on cognitive processes and their components? (data analysis)

Laboratory study of thinking: selection of tasks

The first step in an experimental study is to elicit interesting phenomena under controlled circumstances in the laboratory. The primary method for getting subjects to think on demand is to instruct them to perform a task, such as solving a problem. As in any type of laboratory study, it is essential that the instructions to subjects and other aspects of the procedure be determined in advance so that all subjects are given the same task. Let us now consider which tasks are suitable for studies of thinking.

The earliest studies of thinking were primarily descriptive and relied on a wide range of tasks. Considerable research was done on the free-association task, in which subjects are instructed to say the first word that comes to mind after hearing or seeing a word like *needle* or *father* (Jung, 1910). This task was thought to involve a single associative step (from the stimulus word to the response word) and hence to correspond to the simplest from of thinking that could be studied by means of introspective reports. In comprehension tasks designed by Karl Buehler (see Humphrey, 1951) subjects were asked to indicate as quickly as possible whether they did or did not understand sentences such as "We depreciate everything that can be explained." Other types of questions testing general knowledge were also used, for example, "Do you know where our other stopwatch is now?" After responding to these sentences, the subjects told the experimenter what they remembered thinking about.

At first sight these tasks seem useful for the study of basic thought processes. But this research was, perhaps legitimately, criticized for placing too much trust in the subject. Imagine a devious subject who decides what response to give in the free-association task or the comprehension task before the stimulus word or the sentence is presented. There is no way for experimenters to identify these subjects with any certainty, because any response given by a subject is acceptable – some associations may be unusual for legitimate reasons.

More modern methodology eliminates these problems of interpretation by determining the correct answer a priori. For example, the question "Is Stockholm the capital of Sweden?" has only one correct answer – yes. However subjects can guess the correct answers when tasks require choosing among a few alternatives. If there are only two possible responses – "yes" and "no" – correct answers will be obtained about half of the time purely by chance. In many studies of thinking, only correct responses are analyzed and the data from subjects with high error rates (more than 10 to 20%) are discarded. An alternative approach requires that subjects give more informative answers or responses; the correct response to the task "Name the capital of Sweden" – "Stockholm" – is not easily guessed.

Recent studies of thinking have primarily used tasks in logic (Guyotte & Sternberg, 1981; Johnson-Laird & Steedman, 1978) mathematics (Ginsberg, 1983), probability (Estes, 1976), and other domains in which a given task has a single correct answer. Using tasks in formalized domains has many advantages. It is especially easy in these domains to generate problems that differ from one another only in their surface elements. By drawing on a a pool of similar problems, the investigator can observe individual subjects performing the same task, or very nearly the same task, trial after trial. In addition, formal domains permit investigators to carry out careful analyses of tasks. Task analyses are invaluable because they may suggest the kinds of theories to be considered before observations of people performing the tasks are gathered.

Task analysis

When we know the correct answers to a task, we are also likely to know a fair amount about the knowledge and procedures that the subjects must use to answer correctly. A systematic analysis of this information for a task or a domain of tasks is called a *task analysis*. A task analysis should always be made before the collection and analysis of observations.

Although the term *task analysis* is relatively new, experimental psychologists have always been concerned with the way subjects generate responses. They have attempted to eliminate the possibility of a subject performing a task in a way that is unanticipated by the investigator. For example, nonsense syllables, such as *qub* or *teg*, were used to prevent subjects from relying on previous knowledge when committing syllables to memory (Ebbinghaus, 1885/1964). It was later learned that subjects actually draw on their knowledge of words and common spelling patterns when they memorize nonsense syllables (Montague, 1972). Thus, empirical evidence showed that the initial task analysis was inadequate, since subjects used information not considered by the investigators to be important. This example shows that task analyses are always provisional and should be modified in the light of new findings.

It is particularly important to explicate the knowledge necessary to generate successful solutions when we study tasks that cannot be easily performed with simple strategies. In such task domains as mathematics and logic, clearly defined procedures exist for generating correct solutions. These procedures can be described as a sequence of steps, which in turn can be described with flow charts or even computer programs. Let us consider the simple example of mental multiplication of three digits $- n_1 \times n_2 \times n_3$. The subjects are asked to give the product of three digits as quickly as possible. This task has not been used, to our knowledge, in any previous studies, so our task analysis represents our best efforts to understand the task before using it in an actual study.

A reasonable procedure for solving this problem would be to multiply the first two numbers $n_1 \times n_2$ and then multiply this intermediate result by the last number n_3. Implicit in this procedure is the knowledge that the multiplication of three numbers can be broken down into these two steps. Drawing on our knowledge of multiplication (laws of associativity and commutativity) we find that the three-digit multiplication task can be solved in several equivalent ways: $(n_1 \times n_2) \times n_3 = (n_1 \times n_3) \times n_2 = (n_2 \times n_3) \times n_1$, and so on. In this way we can enumerate possible sequences of behavior for solving this task, but for all sequences the multiplication of two numbers serves as a basic process. Any task analysis of a complex task must make similar assumptions about basic processes that can occur in a number of possible sequences.

Because this task is to be performed mentally by a human subject, the possible solution sequences may be constrained in important ways. Drawing on the theory of human information processing that we presented earlier, we know that subjects must solve problems like this one sequentially and, in addition, that the information about intermediate values must be stored in an available memory store. Before the subjects can start to solve the task they have to look at, recognize, and encode at least two digits. Next they must generate the product of these two numbers, store this product, look at and encode the final digit, and, finally, multiply the intermediate value with this last digit. The exact sequencing of these events ought to be reflected in the way the subjects look at the three digits. In a later section we will describe in more detail how observations of eye movements can be used to study the cognitive processes involved in task performance.

What other knowledge might be used by subjects in performing this task? Beyond the knowledge necessary for breaking the problem into subparts, there appears to be little more that subjects need to know. Most adults know the multiplication table for numbers less than 10. Answers to multiplications such as 2×28 are usually not retrieved from memory and must be calculated by a series of steps, such as $2 \times 8 = 16$; carry 1; $2 \times 2 = 4$; $4 + 1 = 5$; 56. Because in some cases subjects will directly retrieve intermediate answers from memory and in other cases have to compute answers, the multiplication of different triplets of numbers may require different numbers of steps.

The difficulty of certain problems may depend on the way they are broken down into sequences of steps. For example, $4 \times 7 \times 2$ can be solved by $4 \times 7 = 28$ and 28×2, where the last multiplication must be separately computed. But this problem could also be solved by $4 \times 2 = 8$ and $8 \times 7 = 56$; here the sequence of operations is altered so that answers to all of the multiplications can be retrieved from memory. Hence, a good strategy would be to find two digits that yield a single digit when multiplied and proceed from there. For the example $7 \times 4 \times 5$, it is easier to solve $4 \times 5 = 20$ and $7 \times 20 = 140$ than to solve $7 \times 4 = 28$ and $5 \times 28 = 140$. As people gain experience in the task, they may adopt this strategy, so that types of problems that were once difficult for them are now easy.

A search for other strategies, such as a strategy that would be required if one of the digits were zero, can extend the task analysis, and we see from our simple example how we can anticipate a subject's behavior. Although the example we have used is a simple one, it illustrates how we might out-line reasonable sequences of cognitive processes in advance. It is important to note that a task analysis is useful only if we restrict ourselves to plausible scenarios that are constrained by what we know about human information processing and by the knowledge the subjects are likely to use.

There are many ways to use a task analysis in research. It can be used, for example, to identify a subset of tasks for which no shortcuts are available. The subjects' performance on these tasks should be very similar since they would all use the same, or at least very similar, strategies. Task analysis has also been used to identify a single plausible solution method or a small num-ber of such methods that can be focused on in empirical studies. Finally, task analysis can be used to provide a description of intermediate steps, which serves as a kind of first-order theory to be tested and later refined (Resnick, 1976).

By necessity our description of task analysis is limited and our goal has been merely to convey a sense of its aims and methods. In the following sections we will give many examples of research that demonstrate the use of task analysis. The interested reader should consult the classic work on this topic of Newell and Simon (1972).

Discussion

We recommend that tasks be selected that have predetermined correct re-sponses and that are also amenable to extensive a priori task analysis. How-ever, many important research efforts on thinking use tasks without these characteristics, such as studies of daydreaming (Pope, 1978) of creativity (for a review see Gilhooly, 1982), of judgment involving personal preference (Svenson, 1979), of written composition (Hayes & Flower, 1980), and of expertise in many domains, such as chess (de Groot, 1978). All of these studies represent major contributions to our understanding of thinking. Our point, nevertheless, is that investigators face far fewer methodological prob-lems when they select tasks with characteristics that make them easier to study than other tasks that are not as well specified. For any task selected, many different types of observations can be recorded.

Selecting types of observations to be recorded

Once a task is selected for study, the investigator must decide what kind of observations will provide information on the cognitive processes used in that task. The central issue concerns the way in which these observations reflect underlying cognitive processes. Within the framework of information-process-ing theory, a wide range of observations provide information about the order and duration of processing steps. Figure 14.1 schematically illustrates the temporal sequence of thought processes in generating an answer to a task.

We assume for our discussion that the cognitive processes used to perform tasks can be described by a sequence of processing steps or thoughts (see Figure 14.1). The reaction time, which is measured from the beginning of the task to the end, will then consist of the sum of the times required to complete individual processing steps. If the generated response or answer is correct, we can safely assume that one of the sequences of processes specified by a task analysis was used. If the generated answer is incorrect, the subject either lacked some crucial knowledge or made an error in executing one or more of the processing steps. We call observations that bear on the total performance of a task (i.e., reaction time and accuracy of the response) *performance observations*.

Some observations reveal information about individual processing steps, such as spontaneous verbalizations and eye-movement sequences that occur when a task is performed. As subjects think aloud during the solution of the task, one records the sequence of verbalizations corresponding to the sequence of generated thoughts. We call observations of this type *process observations*. Many investigators are reluctant to collect process observations because they are concerned that the collection procedures might alter the subjects' normal thought processes.

We can also collect observations after a task is completed by asking subjects to remember the thought processes they used during the task or to remember information that was presented to them. We can even interview the subjects about the strategies they remember using. We call observations such as these *postprocess observations*.

We have indicated above how different types of observations reflect the underlying cognitive processes or processing steps used in a task. In the following sections we will discuss methods for collecting observations that accurately reflect the important properties of cognitive processes.

Performance observations

Investigators typically record the speed and accuracy of a response by having subjects respond verbally or press a button the instant they have completed a task. Depending on the task, reaction times range from 150 milliseconds to hundreds of seconds. Reaction time has been a particularly important measure in studies of performance on tasks that are completed in about one second. We will describe how reaction times have been analyzed for specific studies of thinking in later sections of this chapter. Provided that the investigator takes several precautions, reaction times give relatively pure estimates of the time necessary to perform a task correctly.

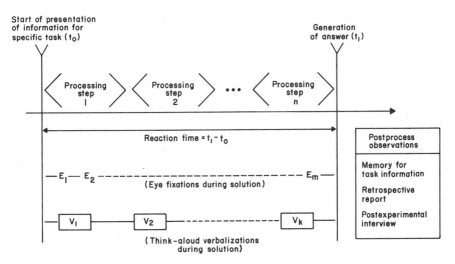

Figure 14.1. Different types of observations on a thinking process for a given task.

Reaction times are unreliable if subjects take longer than necessary to respond because they suffer lapses of attention or hesitate when checking the accuracy of an answer. In these cases the observed reaction times are not pure estimates of the durations of the processing steps the investigator wishes to measure, but reflect the durations of extraneous cognitive activities as well. Problems in interpreting the speed and accuracy of responses also arise if the subjects are so intent on reponding rapidly that they guess or respond prematurely. Therefore, in studies measuring reaction time, subjects are usually instructed to respond as rapidly as possible without making errors. The investigator should then obtain reasonably accurate reaction times for correct responses that are uncontaminated by extraneous processing.

The investigator must also note whether subjects drastically change the way they perform a task as they become more proficient. Clearly, the correct answers to some tasks can be generated by a wide variety of methods and strategies, and subjects may use different methods and strategies at different times. To reduce this source of variability, subjects are usually given some initial practice (warm-up) on the types of tasks used in the experiment. It is often assumed that the subjects use this warm-up period to adopt a strategy that is most efficient for them. Practice also gives them a chance to determine how careful they must be in order to be both accurate and fast. It is assumed that reaction times at the end of the warm-up phase reflect the time necessary to perform *stable* sequences of cognitive processes.

The responses given by subjects can also be viewed as summary observations for sequences of cognitive processes. From a correct answer we can infer correct processing of all the individual steps, and from an error we can infer incorrect processing of at least one of those steps. These inferences apply only to an entire sequence of steps.

Process observations

Certain additional precautions should be taken when process observations are collected. Subjects are almost always aware that process observations are made and as a consequence may alter their behavior. For some types of process observations the instructions given to subjects are changed, and for other types of observations the physical situation or the task must be changed. For example, when eye-movement recordings are made, subjects must deal with an unfamiliar device. As long as we are convinced that we are not disrupting normal reading processes by introducing this equipment, the interpretation of eye-movements is straightforward.

Concurrent verbal reports. In many cognitive tasks subjects have been found to speak to themselves softly or silently with lip and tongue movements. By instructing subjects to vocalize their silent speech (talk aloud), we can transcribe their speech for further analysis. An example of the kinds observations these talk-aloud instructions yield is illustrated in Table 14.1. These observations consist of a sequence of verbalizations in which each verbalization can be segmented on the basis of brief pauses and intonation patterns. The verbalizations are relevant to a previous task analysis, which would predict different intermediate steps depending on the solution process. By matching these logically possible intermediate states with the verbalizations we can discover how the subject performs this task.

A different verbalizing instruction requires subjects to think aloud. They are asked to say out loud everything that passes through their mind as they perform a task. This instruction differs from the previous instruction in that subjects are asked to articulate thoughts they otherwise would not say silently to themselves. Relying on similar methods, we can identify a sequence of thoughts from these observations that provide insight into the solution process.

Concurrent verbal reports have been used extensively for many types of thinking. A criticism leveled at verbal report instructions used in many of these studies is that they probably alter the cognitive processes of subjects. Ericsson and Simon (1984) reviewed a large number of studies comparing the performance data of subjects who gave concurrent reports with the performance data of control subjects who gave no reports. They found that performance is changed only by some kinds of verbal report instructions. The first type of instruction (talk-aloud) does not appear to influence either reaction time or the accuracy of responses. The second type of instruction (think-aloud) does not influence accuracy, but it does systematically increase

Table 14.1. *Thinking-aloud protocol for a subject mentally multiplying 36 times 24*

Thinking-aloud protocol	Traditional method
OK	
36 times 24	36
um	24
4 times 6 is 24	144
4	720
carry the 2	864
4 times 3 is 12	
14	
144	
—	
2 times 6 is 12	
2	
carry the 1	
2 times 3 is 6	
7	
720	
720	
144 plus 72	
so it would be 4	
6	
864	

the time required to generate an answer or solution. This increase is to be expected because additional time will be required to verbalize each thought. In both of these verbalization procedures it is assumed that subjects go through the same sequence of thoughts as in the silent procedure but that the thoughts are verbalized as they arise. Ericsson and Simon (1984) found that the verbal report instructions that change performance do not merely require that subjects verbalize their thoughts, but also require that subjects give reasons or motives for their thoughts and actions. It is not surprising that there are changes in thought processes as well as in performance when subjects must think of rationalizations, which they would not normally do when performing the task silently.

Eye-movement recordings. In many tasks subjects must extract information from pictures or a text by a process of visual scanning. Because of the optics of the eye, people must look directly at detailed objects (e.g., words, symbols) in order to perceive them. Simply by looking at someone's eyes we can determine the general direction of their gaze, and with eye-movement recorders the direction of the gaze can be determined quite accurately. We can infer what information subjects are processing at a given instant by examining where their gaze is is directed. In normal situations there are usu-

ally several objects in the general area being looked at, which makes it difficult to determine which of the objects a person is perceiving. Such ambiguity can be avoided if objects are separated spatially so that the subjects
can look at only one thing at a time. Shift of attention from one location to
another under these conditions is clear-cut, because eye movements are de-
marcated by quick jumps (or *saccades*). Research has shown that visual processing is confined to the periods between saccades when the eyes are fixated on a single spatial location.

Let us illustrate the eye-movement methodology with a simple example
provided by Rosen and Rosenkoetter's (1976) research on the way people
decide which of two gambles to take. The arrangement of information displayed for the subjects is shown in Table 14.2. By recording the order in
which the subjects looked at the displayed information, Rosen and Rosenkoetter (1976) identified two different strategies the subjects used. In the
first strategy, shifts in eye fixation were primarily horizontal or between
pieces of information in the same row. These eye movements suggested pair-
wise comparisons between Gamble A and Gamble B with respect to the
amount to be won, probability of winning, and so on. In the other strategy,
the shifts were vertical or between pieces of information in each column,
suggesting that all attributes of a gamble were integrated into a holistic judgment. Eye-movement recordings have been used in a great variety of studies
on thinking, such as studies of reading comprehension (Raynor, 1983),
memory for pictures (Loftus, 1982) and spatial ability (Just & Carpenter,
1985).

Externalized thinking. When subjects require more than a few seconds to
perform a task, their behavior may clearly reflect the steps their thought is
taking. For instance, we may observe a subject writing down intermediate
values when trying to solve a physics or word arithmetic problem. We can
safely infer that the subject was thinking about these intermediate values
and ask how this behavior corresponds to the processing stages we can expect on the basis of a task analysis. It is clear that for some tasks subjects
will show great variability in the way they externalize their thinking. For
example, when solving problems, not all subjects may write down intermediate values; some subjects may instead draw diagrams representing the
problems. With a task analysis it is possible to describe different types of
mental representations of task information that might account for the different ways subjects take notes and draw diagrams while solving problems
(Hayes & Simon, 1977).

The structure of some tasks can force subjects to perform externalized
thought sequences, which can then be recorded and analyzed. For instance,
tasks that require subjects to solve puzzles or play games often provide excellent data in the form of sequences of moves. It is assumed that move

Table 14.2. *Arrangement of displayed information for two gambles*

	Gamble	
	A	B
Amount to be won	+$4.29	+$2.85
Probability of winning	.44	.72
Amount to be lost	−$1.29	−$2.80

Source: Adapted from Rosen and Rosenkoetter (1976).

sequences reflect the subjects' understanding of the task and are a direct consequence of the stategies they use. For example, blocking moves in tic-tac-toe are easy to identify, and repeated use of these moves shows that a person knows how to defend against losing on the next move. Process models have been developed to account for move sequences in such tasks as cryptarithmetic (Newell & Simon, 1972) and water-jug problems (Atwood & Polson, 1976).

Post process observations

Once subjects have performed a task, it might seem that no further information about cognitive processes used in the task could be recorded. However, testing subjects' memory can provide three additional types of observations. In experiments on thinking, the same information may not be continuously available. For instance, instructions may be given only once to subjects, who must then rely on their memory of the instructions to perform the task. After an experiment, therefore, subjects' memory of the instructions or their memory of other types of task information (memory for task information) can be tested. Observations of another kind are obtained when subjects are instructed to remember the specific thoughts they had while generating the response (retrospective reports). A final category of observations is obtained when the subject is questioned after the experiment about the strategies and representations they remember using (postexperimental questioning).

Memory for task information. By testing subjects' memory for task information, it is sometimes possible to draw inferences about their thought processes during a task. According to our simple information-processing model, subjects should remember best those things they focused on during the solution process. What was never perceived should not be remembered at all, and what was treated as incidental to the task should be poorly remembered. Furthermore, information that is processed in an automatic way, that is, without much awareness, should also be poorly remembered. Finally, systematic errors in recall may indicate how solution attempts went awry. A number of studies have tested subjects' memory for task information. A study from the problem-solving literature will serve as an example.

Dellarosa, Weimer, and Kintsch (1985) asked why children consistently fail to solve certain types of word arithmetic problems. Following up work by Riley (1979), they asked children to solve a sequence of word arithmetic problems and later asked them to recall these problems. They found that the children could remember many of the problems. Furthermore, the children better recalled the problems they had solved correctly than they recalled the problems they had missed. The children's recall errors indicated that they very often missed problems not because of errors in arithmetic, but because they misunderstood the problems and set up the wrong initial equations. This example illustrates how memory for task information may help in identifying the mental representations subjects use to solve problems.

Retrospective reports. Instead of asking subjects to recall what was presented to them, we can ask subjects to recall what they were thinking as they performed the task. A typical procedure (Ericsson & Simon, 1984) is to ask subjects immediately after their response is given to recall everything they can remember thinking during the solution of the task. Since we want to recapture the subjects' exact thought sequences, the subjects should be instructed to report thoughts they can remember with confidence and not include thoughts they believe they must have thought or might have thought. This instruction often results in retrospective reports that contain only parts of a thought sequence, especially when tasks require a long time to solve. Retrospective reports, however are suitable for studying tasks with shorter reaction times. Retrospective reports should be preferred over concurrent reports for these tasks because concurrent verbalization of thoughts would be too slow to capture rapid thought processes.

Retrospective reports can be requested after some or all trials of an experiment. It is important to instruct subjects to respond accurately and as rapidly as possible and not to think about the retrospective report until they have finished the task. Subjects should be asked to recall as much as they can, but without being given any clues about the nature of the experiment. Questioning of subjects about selected aspects of their thoughts might bias them toward being attentive to particular features of the task and might change their thought processes on subsequent trials.

Postexperimental questioning. There is a long-standing tradition in psychological research of interviewing subjects at the end of an experiment. On occasion, investigators use the results of these informal interviews to support their theories. For instance, subjects sometimes deny being aware of rules they have clearly learned during the course of an experiment (for a review see Brewer, 1974). This denial is taken as evidence of learning without awareness. Unfortunately, subjects' responses in these interviews are easily biased by leading questions. Studies that use different procedures for questioning subjects, but are in other respects the same, sometimes yield different results (Brewer, 1974).

If we want to tap subjects' memories of their actual thought processes during individual episodes in an experiment, it is not a good idea to question them at the end of a long experimental session. By then they will have forgotten a great deal, and recalling information may require considerable effort. Ericsson and Simon (1984) noted that postexperimental reports of subjects are often inconsistent with the actual behavior recorded in the experiments. They argue that these reports are inconsistent because they are sometimes based on memory of only a few unrepresentative trials and sometimes based purely on speculation.

It has been traditional in many experiments to ask subjects to give reasons for their behavior. In a very important review, Nisbett and Wilson (1977) showed that subjects' reasons frequently do not account for the variables that actually influence their behavior. The article raised a number of methodological issues, which have been discussed in detail elsewhere (Ericsson & Simon, 1980; Nisbett & Ross, 1980; Smith & Miller, 1978; White, 1980). For our current purposes it is sufficient to note that giving a reason for one's thoughts (ideally a cause relating to external stimuli) is quite different from reporting the thoughts as actually remembered. Let us illustrate this point with an example.

When asked to generate a word starting with the letter *A* most undergraduates respond with *apple*. If asked for a retrospective report they say that *apple* simply "popped out" or "came," and they are unable to report any intermediate thoughts. When asked why they thought of *apple* rather than some other word beginning with *A* they are quite willing to speculate: "I had an apple for lunch," "In grade school I learned 'A as in apple,' " and so on. Similarly, in many tasks used in thinking research, subjects report thinking of ideas without any relation to previous thought. Subjects' reported sequence of thoughts in these instances are nevertheless valid observations of the task. Subjects' retrospective analysis of *why* certain thoughts were elicited is a different source of information that may or may not be useful. The cognitive processes used by subjects in these retrospective analyses or rationalizations are not well understood.

Discussion

We have described many kinds of observations that are useful in studies of thinking. We noted that performance observations provide information about the speed and accuracy of entire sequences of cognitive processes leading up to a response. These observations are reliable only if subjects respond as quickly as possible and do not make many errors. It is important that the subjects be given practice before the observations are recorded so that they learn to perform the task consistently.

It is a good policy to instruct subjects to respond as quickly as possible when process observations are being collected. The experimenter can then be fairly confident that the subject is trying to be efficient and task-directed, and it is less likely that the methods for collecting data will intrude on the normal thought processes used to perform the task. Studies have shown that several methods for collecting process data do not cause subjects to perform a task differently than control subjects. Nevertheless, researchers should examine their methods, or their variations of previously used methods, to make sure that they are not unwittingly perturbing the behavior under study. Despite these dangers, process data are particularly useful because they provide detailed information on the intermediate steps involved in thinking.

Postprocess observations are collected after a task has been performed. To collect these observations, the experimenter may ask subjects to remember task information or to report what they thought about when they performed a task. Subjects may also be asked to give reasons for their behavior. All of these observations rely on the subjects' memory of what they thought about during a task. These observations will be uninformative if subjects cannot remember these thoughts. Furthermore, a distinction should be made between verbal reports that are restricted to what subjects remember actually thinking and reports that include subjects' rationalizations for their behavior. Research has shown that these rationalizations may be unreliable.

Other types of observations could also be recorded and related to the sequences of cognitive processing steps. For example, we did not discuss physiological measures. We are aware of only a few attempts to use these measures to validate cognitive theories (Kahneman, 1973; McGuigan, 1978), but we are convinced that the intensive research efforts in neuroscience and neuropsychology will ultimately provide important physiological variables.

Of greater concern is our deliberate omission of studies of individual differences based on psychometric testing. We believe that pretesting for knowledge and abilities will be essential for understanding the strategies used by subjects in task domains. However, at the current time, little is known about the general aspects of cognitive processes that are actually measured by standard ability tests (Hunt, 1978; R. J. Sternberg, 1977). Without a better understanding of what these tests measure, it is difficult for us to recommend how they should be used in studies of thinking.

Analysis and description of observations

In the first part of our discussion of methodology we described how task analyses can provide a set of possible sequences of cognitive processes or processing steps. In the next part we discussed many types of observations that could be interpreted to reflect aspects of the underlying processes. In this part we discuss how one can summarize and analyze a large number of observations of different tasks and from different subjects.

An important question that concerns us here is the extent to which different tasks elicit the same cognitive processes for all subjects. This question is perhaps easiest to answer when subjects repeatedly perform the same task or very similar tasks. A good example of this approach is provided by Ebbinghaus's (1885/1964) classic research on list learning, which we will briefly describe. Then we will describe attempts to use analyses of reaction times to identify processing steps in tasks of thinking. Next we will describe in detail the well-known analysis of sentence−picture verification by Clark and Chase (1972). These investigators proposed an information-processing model for the exact sequence of processes used to generate answers under different conditions. They assumed that all subjects would go through exactly the same sequence of processing steps (i.e., use the same strategy). This assumption was later shown to be incorrect by Hunt and his colleagues, who demonstrated two distinct strategies for the sentence verification task. By reviewing subsequent research we will evaluate the original theoretical assumption. We will also discuss how other observations, like retrospective reports, reveal different strategies as well as indicate which subjects use these strategies. Finally, we will describe how process observations directly measure the durations of component processes or processing steps. We will start with Ebbinghaus's classic analyses.

Ebbinghaus's (1885/1964) pioneering work on memory is generally recognized as the first "application of precise scientific method to the study of the higher mental processes" (p. xi). Ebbinghaus generated a pool of nonsense syllables by randomly assorting letters into 2,300 different consonant−vowel−consonant combinations. In one experiment, he generated from this pool separate lists, each with the same number of nonsense syllables. He measured the time it took him to memorize perfectly eight series of 13 syllables each. During 1879−80 he memorized different lists of nonsense syllables a total of 92 times. During each session, the time required to memorize all the lists was different, but the similarity between study times was apparent. The average study time was 1,112 seconds, half of the recorded study times falling within the range of 1,036 to 1,188 seconds. In fact, Ebbinghaus found that the frequency distribution of study times was remarkably similar to the normal distributions shown in Figure 14.2.

Memorization times of similar nonsense-syllable lists on 84 different occa-

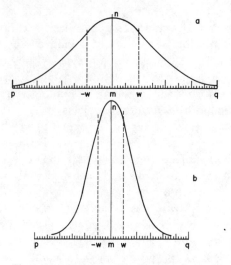

Figure 14.2. Frequency distributions of observations theoretically expected by Ebbing-haus, where m is the mean. For each of the distributions half of the observations fall between $-w$ and $+w$. Adapted from Ebbinghaus (1885/1913).

sions during 1883−4 showed the same close correspondence to the normal curve. Ebbinghaus (1885/1964) argued that the average study time was the best estimate of the true study time for a given amount of material and that deviations from the mean were due to random influences. By relying on statistics, Ebbinghaus derived an interval of study times that would with very high likelihood contain the true study time for memorizing a particular series of nonsense syllables. His times for the memorization of lists of different lengths showed that different numbers of nonsense syllables in a list led to distinctly different study times. He also showed that the relearning of a list memorized earlier was affected by the time that had elapsed since it had been previously memorized.

Ebbinghaus was explicitly concerned with maintaining the same cognitive processes or processing steps throughout the entire period of memorization. It seemed reasonable to assume that the fast presentation caused him to adopt a strategy of rapid rehearsal that did not differ from one list to another. By making this assumption he was able to use the number of repetitions instead of study time as the major variable.

Ebbinghaus's method of statistical analysis was adopted in later research. Most of these studies were conducted with several subjects whose average performance under various conditions was compared separately for each individual. From the fact that the pattern of results was the same for several different individuals, a general relation holding true for most or all adults was inferred.

These within-subject designs, in which the same subjects' performance under various conditions were directly compared, were found, however, to be inadequate. In 1904 Ebert and Meumann reported a study that measured subjects' memory ability both before and after they had been given training in the rote memorization of nonsense syllables. Ebert and Meumann (1904) concluded that memory training improved general memory performance. This conclusion was challenged by Dearborn (1909), who showed that similar general improvement could be obtained by retesting of subjects on memory tests *without* any intervening practice. Since then, experimental studies have used control groups and between-subjects designs, in which individual subjects participate in only one condition and performances under the different conditions are compared statistically. With a "between-groups" design it almost impossible to determine whether all subjects are influenced in the same manner by an experimental manipulation because we have no knowledge of the performance of the same subjects under all the conditions.

Analysis of reaction times

As we pointed out earlier, reaction times provide estimates of the overall amount of time necessary to perform a task. Ideally, we can draw inferences from these estimates about the specific mental processes used in the task. A method of collecting and analyzing reaction times was developed in the nineteenth century in an attempt to decompose reaction times into sequences of processing steps. We will briefly describe this early research before giving a detailed account of a more recent study involving similar methods.

By the middle of the nineteenth century a number of investigators had measured reaction times for what were considered to be the simplest possible tasks. For instance, it was known that subjects could respond to a bright flash of light by pressing a button or by giving a vocal response within 200 milliseconds (msec), whereas they could respond to an auditory stimulus within 150 msec. The time taken to respond to a simple stimulus came to be called *simple reaction time*. Although it is remarkable that people can respond so quickly, these results provide only an upper bound on the elementary mental processes that were presumed to take place before a response was made. Until F. C. Donders (1868/1969) published his "Speed of mental processes" in 1868 there was no method of estimating the times required to perform such elementary processes as perceiving the stimulus, deciding on a response, or actually carrying out the response. The *subtractive method* developed by Donders was extensively used to estimate the times required for these processing steps until the method fell into disfavor at the turn of the century (for reviews see Bartlett, 1958; Chase, 1978; Woodworth, 1938).

Donders measured reaction times for tasks that involved only one pro-

cessing step or two beyond the simple reaction-time task. He then subtracted the average reaction times for these tasks to derive an estimate of
the additional steps. In one experiment, subjects were to say out loud the
nonsense syllable, *ki* the instant they heard that syllable presented to them
(simple reaction-time task). In a second experiment, Donders presented five
nonsense syllables (*ki, ko, ke, ku, ka*) at random to the same subjects and
asked them to repeat the sounds the moment they heard them (choice reaction-time task). The second task took about 74 msec longer to perform than
the first one, and Donders reasoned that this time reflected additional processing steps. To perform the second task the subjects not only had to perceive the stimulus but had to *discriminate* one sound from another and then
decide which of two responses to make. A third task (c-reaction-time task)
was devised to omit the decision process so that the discrimination time
could be estimated. For this task, subjects had only to listen for the specific
sound *ki* and respond out loud by repeating that sound, though they did not
know ahead of time whether they would hear *ki, ko, ke, ku,* or *ka.* Note
that this task differs from the simple reaction-time task only in that the
subjects must discriminate the *ki* sound from the other sounds. The average
reaction time for this task was about 52 msec longer than that for the corresponding simple reaction-time task, giving what appears to be a reasonable
estimate of the discrimination time.

Unfortunately, Donders's subtractive method failed to provide consistent
results. Different results were obtained at different laboratories, and on occasion, tasks that were considered simple yielded longer reaction times than
tasks that were considered more complex. Verbal protocols indicated that
the method was flawed because it was not possible to add processes without
drastically changing the way subjects performed the entire task. For instance,
subjects reported being prepared to respond at the slightest sound for the
simple reaction-time task, but being far less prepared to respond during the
c-reaction-time task. This subjective state of preparedness could differ depending on the instructions or the inclinations of the subject and thus caused
large variability in the reaction times.

Modern variations of the subtractive technique require that subjects follow the same instructions throughout the experiment. The stimuli are then
varied over trials so that the subjects cannot predict what will be presented
to them on a given trial. For instance, in a memory scanning task, the subjects may be asked on different trials to remember lists of digits and then
indicate whether a digit presented to them is in those lists. On any given
trial, the subjects do not know, however, the length of the list they will have
to memorize or whether the letter subsequently presented will be among the
members of that list. Using this approach, Saul Sternberg (1966) showed
that average reaction time increases by a constant amount as the length of
the list to be remembered is increased one digit at a time. The time required

to scan items in short-term memory is extremely rapid, about 40 msec, and could not have been measured without Sternberg's careful application of the subtractive technique.

Other current methods for analyzing reaction time, such as the additive factor method (Posner, 1978; S. Sternberg, 1969), also rely on continuous variation of the stimulus properties of a task without the prior awareness of the subject. Inferences are drawn about the underlying mental processes if the reaction times vary with changes in the stimuli in a way that is consistent with theoretical expectations.

Let us now turn to research that illustrates how analyses of reaction times can provide evidence for process models of thinking. During our account of this research we will raise issues about the aggregation of data.

In a pioneering research effort, Clark and Chase (1972) studied the way subjects answer yes-or-no questions about very simple diagrams in an experimental procedure. Their experimental paradigm came to be known as the sentence–picture verification paradigm. Table 14.3 lists examples of the questions and the diagrams they used. In one variation of Clark and Chase's (1972) task, subjects first see a picture and then a sentence. Upon seeing the sentence, the subjects are to press one of two buttons indicating whether the sentence properly describes the picture. It is clear that the task is simple and that people should have no difficulty in responding without making errors.

The original research of Clark and Chase (1972) included sentences with negation (e.g., "Star is not above plus"), but we will consider only the four sentences in Table 14.3 without negation. Clark and Chase proposed that when the pictures are presented they are recoded into a relationship or proposition (e.g., "star above plus"). They assumed that the subjects prefer the "above" relation because previous work had shown that people prefer to describe the pictures as "star above plus" and "plus above star" rather than "plus below star" or "star below plus."

In order to judge whether a picture and a sentence match in meaning, their *encodings* have to be compared. In the first case of Table 14.3 the encodings are identical and the response is an immediate "yes." Clark and Chase (1972) assumed that this simplest case would require a reaction time of t_0 representing the base time required to do the task. In the second case in Table 14.3, the subjects encode the picture as "star above plus" and encounter the sentence "The plus is above the star." Clark and Chase assumed that the subjects recode the sentence into "star below plus" in order to see and act on the inconsistency. In this additional step, it is assumed that time a is taken to recode and time b to see and act on the mismatch. In the third case in Table 14.3, the subjects encode the picture as "plus above star" and then encounter the sentence "The plus is below the star." The subjects can see the inconsistency immediately after encoding the sentence. Clark and Chase (1972) assumed that encoding sentences with the "below" instead of

Table 14.3. *Sentences and pictures for four cases in the sentence–picture verification experiment*

	Case			
	1	2	3	4
Sentence presented	Star is above plus	Plus is above star	Plus is below star	Star is below plus
Picture presented	★ +	★ +	+ ★	+ ★
Correct response	Yes	No	No	Yes
Sentence encoding	(Star above plus)	(Plus above star)	(Plus below star)	(Star below plus)
Picture encoding	(Star above plus)	(Star above plus)	(Plus above star)	(Plus above star)
Predicted reaction time	t_0	$t_0 + a + b$	$t_0 + b + c$	$t_0 + a + c$

Source: Adapted from Clark and Chase (1972).

the "above" relation takes additional time, represented by the parameter c. Hence, the latency for the third case is time t_0 (base time) plus time c (extra time for "below") plus time b (for seeing and acting on the mismatch). The fourth and final case requires additional time to encode the "below" relation for the sentence "The star is below the plus" (time c) and to recode ("star below plus" becomes "plus above star") taking time a. These hypothesized processing steps were identified by means of multiple regression, a statistical technique, which gave reasonable results of 1,793 msec for the base time t_0, 2112 msec for the recoding time (a), 91 msec to note and act on the mismatch (b), and 128 msec to deal with the "below" relation as opposed to an "above" relation (c) (Experiment 2, Clark & Chase, 1972). The estimates were used in the model to account for the average reaction times observed for each case in Table 14.3. The model's predictions closely matched the average reaction times. It is important to realize that these estimates were identified for the "average" subject since the average reaction time was calculated across different trials and different subjects.

In tasks such as the sentence–picture verification task, the reaction times differ noticeably among subjects. Robert Sternberg (1977) suggested that these differences could be accounted for by assuming that different subjects require different amounts of time to carry out the processing steps. By analyzing the reaction time for each subject separately one can estimate the time corresponding to recoding and to falsification in the example discussed above. Analyses of individual subjects are particularly interesting because they show whether a given processing model is appropriate for all subjects.

Research by Hunt and his associates (MacLeod, Hunt, & Mathews, 1978;

Mathews, Hunt, & MacLeod, 1980) indicated that subjects in fact used very different strategies for the sentence−picture verification task. One group's data fit a "linguistic" model like the one proposed by Clark and Chase (1972), whereas the data of a second group fit a "pictorial" model. The pictorial model assumed that both the pictures and the sentences were transformed into mental images with picture-like properties. It was assumed that subjects whose strategy conformed to the pictorial model could easily compare the pictorial representation of the sentence with their representation of the picture subsequently presented. Note that this pictorial strategy would lead to few difficulties during the comparison stage but might require additional processes (and models). However, Hunt and his associates found evidence that corroborates their account. First, the average encoding and judgment times for the two groups showed the expected pattern. Subjects who fit the pictorial model spent more time reading sentences and made judgments much faster than subjects who fit the linguistic model. Second, performance on tests that measured the subjects' verbal and visual aptitude predicted in advance of the experiments which strategy the subjects would use! For instance, the experimental data for subjects whose test scores indicated aptitude for visual problem solving fit the pictorial model best. Third, Hunt and his associates found that training in one strategy or the other (verbal or pictorial) biased the subjects so that their subsequent performance was best explained by the model that conformed to the type of training they were given (Mathews et al., 1980). This finding suggests that subjects could change strategies fairly easily though they may have been predisposed toward a particular strategy.

We see from this example that we should not assume that all subjects will perform the same way on a task. If evidence is being sought for a particular model or explanation, the aggregation of data when different strategies are used might obscure the results or lead the investigator to make generalizations that are too broad. We also see the advantages of specifying explicit models of behavior that predict differences in performance data. A model can then be tested if experimental manipulations can be expected a priori to affect one or several of the model's components.

The identification of different strategies and the subjects who use them is quite difficult when one relies exclusively on performance data. In the next section we will demonstrate that other types of data are more informative and allow for a more direct assessment of the strategies used by subjects.

Assessing strategies with verbal reports

Retrospective reports may be particularly useful for identifying the strategies that subjects use. By the standard procedure, reaction time and correctness of solution, in addition to verbal reports, are recorded. Immediately after having given an answer, the subjects are asked to tell the experimenter what they can remember thinking during the task.

Retrospective reports typically contain a sequence of reported thoughts, often intermediate steps in the solution process. In Table 14.4 we have presented two verbal protocols from a study by Svenson and Hedenborg (1980) in which school children gave retrospective reports after adding two numbers. From these reports we can identify thoughts or intermediate sums, as illustrated in Table 14.4. Svenson and Hedenborg found that the process of direct memory retrieval was evidenced in protocols by remarks like "I know it by heart," "It just came to me" (Svenson & Sjoberg, 1983, p. 119) and "I knew it," "I knew it directly" (Svenson & Hedenborg, 1980, p. 97). They also observed a counting procedure, whereby the smaller number is counted up from the larger number. For example, to add 4 and 3, the children might count to themselves "four, five, six, seven," noting that they have counted three times after they have started with "four." In fact, these two processes accounted for more than half of the verbal reports. Protocols like those in Table 14.4 could not be accounted for by these processes since they imply a counting process with steps larger than 1 (normally steps of 2). About 20% of the retrospective reports contained evidence for counting with steps larger than 1 (Svenson & Hedenborg, 1980). Regression analyses that were designed to predict solution times resulted in a poor fit when it was assumed that subjects counted in steps of 1 (regardless of what they reported). However, when the number of steps reported in the protocols was entered as an additional variable, the fit was dramatically improved. This additional variable accounted for more variance than any other variable and was statistically significant for all subjects (Svenson & Hedenborg, 1980). This example illustrates how a model can be supported by convergent findings based on what have been traditionally viewed as very different types of data. Svenson and Hedenborg's (1980) research also shows that initially unknown processes can be uncovered to provide a more detailed account of the data.

In our next example, retrospective reports provided information about the intermediate processing steps in an alphabetic retrieval task that subjects could perform very rapidly. Two English investigators, Hamilton and Sanford (1978), studied subjects who made simple judgments of whether two letters, such as *RP* or *MO*, were in alphabetical order. In accord with previous investigators, they found that the reaction times were longer when the two letters occurred close together in the alphabet than when they were far apart. From the reaction-time data alone, one would infer a uniform retrieval process that varies as a simple function of the number of intervening letters. Retrospective verbal reports of subjects making individual decisions indicated, however, two types of cognitive processes. In some of the trials, subjects reported having had no intermediate thoughts before responding; they had direct access to their order judgments. In the other trials, subjects

Table 14.4. *Retrospective reports from grade school students solving mental addition problems*

Task	Retrospective report	Sequence of intermediate steps
6 + 4	Started with 6 and then 8, 10	6−8−10
8 + 3	First 8 and then 10 and 11	8−10−11

Source: The protocols are from Svenson & Hedenborg (1980).

reported that they ran through brief segments of the alphabet before making a decision about the order of the letters. For example, when the letter pair *MO* was presented, a subject reported retrieving *LMNO* before reaching the decision that the letters were in alphabetical order. In another case a subject reported retrieving *RSTUV* before deciding the letter pair *RP* was not in alphabetical order. In a subsequent analysis of the reaction times, Hamilton and Sanford (1978) found that the distance between letters in the alphabet had very different effects on reaction time depending on whether order judgments were directly accessed or preceded by retrieval of letter strings from the alphabet. During trials when segments were retrieved, the observed reaction time was a linear function of the number of retrieved letters. The estimated rate of retrieval per letter was about the same rate at which people are able to recite the alphabet out loud. During trials with reports of direct access, the number of intervening letters in the alphabet did not influence the reaction time. Hamilton and Sanford (1978) concluded that the original effect was due to a mixture of two quite different processes and that closeness of the letters influenced the probability that recall of intervening letters would be necessary before an order decision could be made.

The two preceding examples were selected to illustrate cases in which the thought processes are relatively easy to identify and generalize. For example, in the case of letter-order judgments, we can readily accept that mental scanning of consecutive letters is the same process regardless of what letters are scanned. We can in this instance give the process a name, such as *letter scanning*, and specify when it is applied. As long as the process is manifested by clear behavioral criteria (in this case a fixed amount of time per letter scanned) we can feel confident about its role in our model. Abstracting and identifying such underlying general processes, however, is difficult in many tasks, as illustrated by the following studies.

Three-term series problems are often used to study reasoning (R. Sternberg, 1980). In such studies, the subject sees two premises, such as "The square is lighter than the circle" and "The triangle is darker than the circle" and is asked a question, such as "Is the square lighter than the triangle?" The subject is then expected to respond with the correct answer − in this case "yes." Egan and Grimes-Farrow (1982) collected retrospective verbal reports to assess the cognitive processes used by subjects in this task. The retrospective reports suggested that the premises were mentally represented in two distinctly different ways. One group of subjects established an underlying scale or dimension (e.g., degree of lightness) and used the premises to order all three objects along that scale. For the example given in Table 14.5, a subject might order the geometric figures according to degree of lightness, triangle–circle–square. The subjects who used this representation were termed *abstract directional thinkers*. Another group of subjects, *concrete properties thinkers*, represented the information in the premises as properties of the objects. For instance, they thought of the lighter square as very bright and the darker triangle as very dark. Egan and Grimes-Farrow (1982) found that subjects consistently used the same types of representations for different relations, such as rougher–smoother and fatter–thinner.

In a second experiment, subjects were asked to give retrospective reports while drawing their mental representations of three-term series problems. In a third experiment, the subjects were given descriptions of the two types of representation and asked to choose the one that best described their method of solution. There was almost perfect agreement among these different types of data. An analysis of the pattern of solution errors revealed reliable and large differences between subjects choosing the two different representations. For each group, Egan and Grimes-Farrow (1982) were able to devise processing models that accounted for the pattern of errors remarkably well.

Using process data to measure the duration of component processes

In this section we illustrate how process data in conjuction with performance data can be used to measure the component processes of a task. We discuss how verbal reports and eye-movement recordings can provide data for decomposing the mental processes that influence the speed with which subjects respond in tasks.

Just and Carpenter (1976) made eye-movement recordings to assess the visual information used by subjects in their attempts to rotate three-dimensional objects mentally. As we noted earlier, analyses of eye movements can reveal what information is used in the performance of a task. Subjects were shown line drawings like those presented in a previous study by Shepard and Metzler (1971). An example of the stimuli appears in Figure 14.3. Shepard and Metzler instructed subjects to indicate as quickly as possible whether the rightmost object was the same object as the one on the left. Notice that the two drawings differ only in orientation. From their analyses of the subjects' reaction times, Shepard and Metzler found evidence for mental rotation. The subjects reported that they mentally rotated the object on the right to the same orientation as the one on the left so that they could make a direct match between the two figures in the mind's eye. These re-

Table 14.5. *Examples of verbal reports from two types of subjects in three-term series problems involving darker-lighter relations*

Type of thinkers	
Abstract directional	Concrete properties
"I set up a scale with the lightest on the far right and darkest on the far left and placed the figures on their appropriate spots." "I placed the figures in a line going up and down, darkest being on top."	"In my mind, I 'colored' in the object that was darkest." "I listened to the problem and tried to solve it mentally, at times picturing the objects colored in or not."

Source: Adapted from Egan and Grimes-Farrow (1982).

ports were corroborated by the reaction-time data, which showed that the farther an object had to be rotated, the greater was the reaction time.

In Just and Carpenter's study (1976) eye movements were collected to specify in greater detail what cognitive processes are used in mental rotation. The direction of gaze was recorded from the first presentation of two stimuli (see Figure 14.3) until the subject gave the response (same/different). Just and Carpenter determined from the direction of gaze which of the two figures the subject looked at and also what parts of the figures the subject fixated on. On the basis of their observations, they were able to break each figure into five parts: a joint connecting two arms, where each arm was broken up into a segment close to the joint (closed arm) and into a segment far away from the joint (open arm), as shown in Figure 14.4. Just and Carpenter reasoned that, in order to rotate one figure into another, it was necessary to identify the corresponding parts of the figures. When a subject looked at a part of one figure and then directly looked at the same part of the other figure, it was inferred that the subject had identified the correspondence. The subject would then look back and forth between corresponding parts of the figures; this phase was called transformation. In the final phase the subject would look, for example, at the joint and then other parts in one figure and then repeat the same scan paths for the other figure. During this last phase the subjects were thought to be confirming whether they had properly transformed the figures.

These three types of processes (search for correspondence, transformation, and confirmation) accounted for essentially all of the recorded eye fixations. Just and Carpenter (1976) decomposed the original reaction time into components associated with the different processing activities, as illustrated in Figure 14.5. They found that, when the angular displacement between the two figures was increased, the number of component processes that had to be performed also increased. It is interesting that these detailed

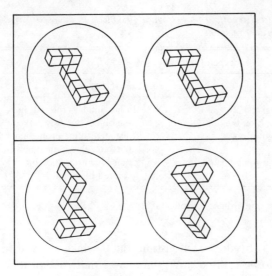

Figure 14.3. Pairs of figures that are the same. The figures on top are unrotated and the figures on the bottom differ by a rotation of 180 degrees. Adapted from Shepard and Metzler (1971).

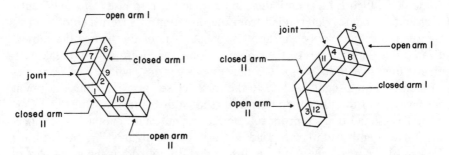

Figure 14.4. Labels for parts of a figure in different rotations. Adapted from Just and Carpenter (1976).

data led to quite different accounts of the way mental rotation is performed. On the basis of reaction times and the verbal reports alone, Shepard and Metzler were led to an explanation based on holistic imagery, whereas additional eye-movement data led Just and Carpenter to an explanation based on analytic decompostion of figures into their component parts.

Just and Carpenter (1985) have extended their analysis of eye movements in characterizing differences between subjects with high and low spatial ability. By means of eye movements, verbal reports, and reaction times, several investigators have found clear evidence for the use of strategies in solving spatial tasks (Barratt, 1953; French, 1965; Lohman & Kyllonen, 1983; Snow

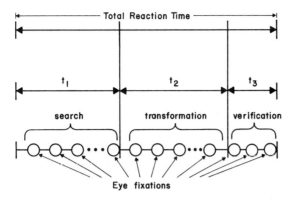

Figure 14.5. Schematic decomposition of total reaction time using criterial eye-fixation patterns for a mental rotation task.

& Lohman, 1984). Strategies used by subjects with high spatial ability are different from those used by subjects with low spatial ability.

Concluding remarks

Our attention in this chapter has been directed toward what we believe are crucial methodological issues for studies of thinking. We discussed the selection and design of tasks in order to study cognitive processes. We described several different types of observations that can be collected. Next, we proposed methods for instructing subjects and adapting the experimental situation so that the observations maximally reflect the characteristics of the cognitive processes. Finally, we discussed methods of analysis in which aggregation and averaging of data are used to identify general features of cognitive processes across subjects and tasks.

There is a legitimate concern with whether current methodology can deal with the complexity of the cognitive processes involved in thinking. Information-processing models of interesting behavior tend to be so complex that they are difficult to test empirically by traditional experimental methodology (Kintsch, Miller & Polson, 1984). Major efforts to test a particular model may fail. In fact, Newell (1973) has noted that extensive research rarely brings researchers to a consensus on the explanation of even simple tasks.

The strategies used by subjects in studies of thinking often change as the subjects learn more about the task, making research on thinking all the more difficult. The observations collected in these studies reflect *dynamic* processes. Many of the methods used in psychology, however, rely on statistical procedures that assume *static* measurement conditions. For instance, it is often assumed that subjects' behavior is not influenced by repeated measurements. But when subjects repeatedly generate answers to related tasks, they are actively learning, and in virtually all tasks there is improvement as a function of practice.

Research methods over the years have been adapted to deal with this problem. Following Ebbinghaus's lead, investigators assumed that their tasks reflected cognitive processes so basic that no learning could occur as long as the stimulus material was varied from trial to trial. When researchers later demonstrated general improvements in task performance, or training effects, there was a movement toward between-subject experimental designs. As we mentioned previously, these designs, while controlling for the effects of practice, may reveal little about the behavior of individual subjects. They are often uninformative because large differences among individuals make it unreasonable to assume that the behavior of all subjects within a group is alike. Other researchers have continued using within-subject designs and have been able to reduce practice effects by providing subjects with long practice periods before experimental testing. However, this extended practice on similar tasks reduces, or even eliminates, some of the sequential thought processes that may be particularly interesting to the investigator. For instance, subjects early in an experiment may be actively learning a problem-solving technique, whereas after extended practice they may be performing this technique by rote. How the technique is discovered by subjects may be of greater interest to the investigator than how it is applied after it is well learned.

In any study of thinking the investigator must gather sufficient information from observations to measure accurately critical aspects of the thought process. Standard methodology makes it possible to attain this goal because repeated measurements of observations on thinking performance are averaged over a long sequence of trials. When a cognitive process retains the same structure over trials, the average performance provides an accurate measure of it. In studies involving a series of related tasks, however, one almost invariably notices a reduction in reaction time and improved accuracy (Newell & Rosenbloom, 1981). The reduction in reaction time is particularly large in the beginning of the series but is still present to a smaller degree after thousands of tasks (trials). We believe that it is essential that these effects and the corresponding changes in cognitive processes be elucidated through direct research and become an integral part of our theoretical understanding of cognitive processes.

Because people's thought processes are both complex and likely to change with practice, we should gather as much information as possible each time a task is performed. By increasing the density of our observations we should be able to identify the cognitive processes used by subjects and the way these processes are modified by learning. Performance data, such as reaction time and accuracy, contain relatively little information and have to be supplemented by information-rich process data and postprocess data. Only by collecting all available data will we ever be able to account for cognitive processes at a very detailed level of description.

The collection of a large amount of data, especially process and post process data for individual subjects, creates problems of a different sort. To analyze these data fully is a major undertaking, and it is rarely possible to extend the analysis to 20 or more subjects, as is traditionally done in experiments generating performance data. Instead, analyses of a small number of individual subjects, occasionally only a single subject (case studies), are becoming increasingly common (Anzai & Simon, 1979; Ericsson, 1985; Pirolli & Anderson, 1985)

During the past two decades there has been a dramatic increase in research on thinking. Given the complexity and adaptability of thinking, it is particularly important that the methodology be developed to ensure a steady accumulation of knowledge. In this chapter we have described current methodology and outlined the progress that has been made in developing effective methods for the study of thinking.

References

Anderson, J. R., & Bower, G. H. (1973). *Human associative memory*. Washington, DC: Winston.

Anzai, Y., & Simon, H. A. (1979). The theory of learning by doing. *Psychological Review, 86,* 124–40.

Atkinson, R. C., & Shiffrin, R. M. (1968). Human memory: A proposed system and its control processes. In K. W. Spence & J. T. Spence (Eds.), *The psychology of learning and motivation: Advances in research and theory* (Vol. 2, pp. 89–195). New York: Academic Press.

Atwood, M. E., & Polson, P. G. (1976). A process model for water jug problems. *Cognitive Psychology, 8,* 191–216.

Barratt, E. S. (1953). An analysis of verbal reports of solving spatial problems as an aid in defining spatial factors. *Journal of Psychology, 36,* 17–25.

Bartlett, F. (1958). *Thinking*. New York: Basic.

Brewer, W. F. (1974). There is no convincing evidence for operant or classical conditioning in adult humans. In W. B. Weimer & D. S. Palermo (Eds.), *Cognition and symbolic processes*. Hillsdale, NJ: Erlbaum.

Chase, W. G. (1978). Elementary information processes. In W. K. Estes (Ed.), *Handbook of learning and cognitive processes* (Vol. 5, pp. 19–90). Hillsdale, NJ: Erlbaum.

Clark, H. H., & Chase, W. G. (1972). On the process of comparing sentences against pictures. *Cognitive Psychology, 3,* 472–547.

Dearborn, W. F. (1909). The general effects of special practice. *Psychological Bulletin, 6,* 44.

de Groot, A. (1978). *Thought and choice in chess*. (2nd ed.) The Hague: Mouton.

Dellarosa, D., Weimer, R., & Kintsch, W. (1985). *Children's recall of arithmetic word problems* (Tech. Rep. No. 147). Boulder: University of Colorado, Institute of Cognitive Science.

Donders, F. C. (1969). On the speed of mental processes. *Acta Psychologica, 30,* 412–31. (Translated by W. G. Koster from "Over de snelheid van psychische processen." *Onderzoekingen gedaan in het Physiologisch Laboratorium der Utrechtsche Hoogeschool,* 1868, Tweede reeks, *2,* 92–120.)

Duncker, K. R. (1945). On problem solving. *Psychological Monographs 38*, (5, Whole No. 270).

Ebbinghaus, H. (1964). *Memory: A contribution to experimental psychology* (H. A. Ruger & C. E. Bussenius, Trans.). New York: Dover. (Original work published, 1885.)

Ebert, E., & Meumann, E. (1904). Ueber einige Grundfragen der Psychologie der Uebungsphaenomene im Bereiche des Gedaechtnisses. *Archiv fuer gesamte Psychologie, 4,* 1–232.

Egan, D. E., & Grimes-Farrow, D. D. (1982). Differences in mental representations spontaneously adopted for reasoning. *Memory & Cognition, 10,* 297–307.

Ericsson, K. A. (1985). Memory skill. *Canadian Journal of Psychology, 39,* 188–231.

Ericsson, K. A., & Simon, H. A. (1980). Verbal reports as data. *Psychological Review, 87,* 215–51.

   (1984). *Protocol analysis: Verbal reports as data.* Cambridge, MA: MIT Press/Bradford.

Estes, W. K. (1976). The cognitive side of probability learning. *Psychological Review, 83,* 37–64.

French, J. W. (1965). The relationship of problem-solving styles to the factor composition of tests. *Educational and Psychological Measurement, 25,* 9–28.

Gilhooly, K. J. (1982). *Thinking: Directed, undirected and creative.* New York: Academic Press.

Ginsberg, H. (1983). *The development of mathematical learning.* New York: Academic Press.

Guyotte, M. J., & Sternberg, R. J. (1981). A transitive-chain theory of syllogistic reasoning. *Cognitive Psychology, 13,* 461–525.

Hamilton, J. M. E., & Sanford, A. J. (1978). The symbolic distance effect for alphabetic order judgements: A subjective report and reaction time analysis. *Quarterly Journal of Experimental Psychology, 30,* 33–43.

Hamilton, W. (1870). *Lectures on metaphysics and logic* (Vol. 1). Edinburgh: Blackwood.

Hayes, J. R., & Flower, L. S. (1980). Identifying the organization of writing processes. In L. W. Gregg & E. R. Steinberg (Eds.) *Cognitive processes in writing* (pp. 3–30). Hillsdale, NJ: Erlbaum.

Hayes, J. R., & Simon, H. A. (1977). Psychological differences among problem isomorphs. In N. J. Castellan, D. B. Pisoni, and G. R. Potts (Eds.), *Cognitive theory* (Vol. 2, pp. 21–41). Hillsdale, NJ: Erlbaum.

Humphrey, G. (1951). *Thinking: An introduction to its experimental psychology.* London: Methuen.

Hunt, E. (1978). Mechanics of verbal ability. *Psychological Review, 85,* 109–30.

Johnson-Laird, P. N., & Steedman, M. (1978). The psychology of syllogisms. *Cognitive Psychology, 10,* 64–99.

Jung, C. G. (1910). The association method. *American Journal of Psychology, 21,* 219–69.

Just, M. A., & Carpenter, P. A. (1976). Eye fixations and cognitive processes. *Cognitive Psychology, 15,* 151–96.

   (1985). Cognitive coordinate systems: Accounts of mental rotation and individual differences in spatial ability. *Psychological Review, 92,* 137–72.

Kahneman, D. (1973). *Attention and effort.* Englewood Cliffs, NJ: Prentice-Hall.

Kintsch, W., Miller, J. R., & Polson, P. G. (1984). *Method and tactics in Cognitive Science.* Hillsdale, NJ: Erlbaum.

Lashley, K. S. (1923). The behaviorist interpretation of consciousness II. *Psychological Review, 30,* 329–53.

Loftus, G. R. (1982). Picture memory methodology. In C. R. Puff (Ed.), *Handbook of research methods in human memory and cognition* (pp. 258–83). New York: Academic Press.

Lohman, D. F., & Kyllonen, P. C. (1983). Individual differences in solution strategy on spatial tasks. In R. F. Dillon & R. R. Schmeck (Eds.), *Individual differences in cognition* (Vol. 1). New York: Academic Press.

MacLeod, C. M., Hunt, E. B., & Mathews, N. N. (1978). Individual differences in the verification of sentence–picture relationships. *Journal of Verbal Learning and Verbal Behavior, 17,* 493–507.

Mathews, N. N., Hunt, E. B., & MacLeod, C. M. (1980). Strategy choice and strategy training in sentence–picture verification. *Journal of Verbal Learning and Verbal Behavior, 19,* 531–48.

McGuigan, F. J. (1978). *Cognitive psychophysiology: Principles of covert behavior.* Englewood Cliffs, NJ: Prentice-Hall.

Mill, J. (1878). *Analysis of the phenomena of the human mind* (2nd ed., Vol. 1). London: Longmans, Green. (Original work published, 1829.)

Montague, W. E. (1972). Elaborative strategies in verbal learning and memory. In G. H. Bower (Ed.), *The psychology of learning and motivation* (Vol. 6, pp. 225–302). New York: Academic Press.

Newell, A. (1973). You can't play 20 questions with nature and win: Projective comments on the papers of this symposium. In W. G. Chase (Ed.), *Visual information processing* (pp. 283–305). New York: Academic Press.

Newell, A., & Rosenbloom, P. S. (1981). Mechanisms of skill acquisition and the law of practice. In J. R. Anderson, (Ed.), *Cognitive skills and their acquisition* (pp. 1–55). Hillsdale, NJ: Erlbaum.

Newell, A., & Simon, H. A. (1972). *Human problem solving.* New York: Prentice-Hall.

Nisbett, R. E., & Ross. L. (1980). *Human inference: Strategies and shortcomings of social judgment.* Englewood Cliffs, NJ: Prenctice-Hall

Nisbett, R. E., & Wilson, T. D. (1977). Telling more than we can know: Verbal reports on mental processes. *Psychological Review, 84,* 231–59.

Pirolli, P. L., & Anderson, J. R. (1985). The role of learning from examples in the acquisition of recursive programming skills. *Canadian Journal of Psychology, 39,* 240–72.

Pope, K. S. (1978). How gender, solitude, and posture influence the stream of consciousness. In K. S. Pope & J. L. Singer (Eds.), *The stream of consciousness: Scientific investigations into the flow of human experience* (pp. 259–99). New York: Plenum.

Posner, M. I. (1978). *Chronometric explorations of mind.* Hillsdale, NJ: Erlbaum.

Puff, C. R. (1982). *Handbook of research methods in human memory and cognition.* New York: Academic Press.

Raynor, K. (Ed.). (1983). *Eye movements in reading.* New York: Academic Press.

Resnick, L. B. (1976). Task analysis in instructional design: Some cases from mathematics. In D. Klahr (Ed.), *Cognition and instruction* (pp. 51–80). Hillsdale, NJ: Erlbaum.

Riley, M. S. (1979, May). *The development of children's ability to solve arithmetic word problems.* Paper presented at the meeting of the American Educational Research Association, San Francisco.

Rosen, L. D., & Rosenkoetter, P. (1976). An eye fixation analysis of choice and judgment with multiattribute stimuli. *Memory & Cognition, 4,* 747–52.

Shepard, R. N., & Metzler, J. (1971). Mental rotation of three-dimensional objects. *Science, 171,* 701–3.

Smith, E. R., & Miller, F. S. (1978). Limits on the perception of cognitive processes: A reply to Nisbett and Wilson. *Psychological Review, 85,* 355–62.

Snow, R. E., & Lohman, D. F. (1984). Toward a theory of cognitive aptitude for learning from instruction. *Journal of Educational Psychology, 76,* 347–76.

Sternberg, R. J. (1977). *Intelligence, information, and analogical reasoning: The componential analysis of human abilities.* Hillsdale, NJ: Erlbaum.

   (1980). Representation and process in linear syllogistic reasoning. *Journal of Experimental Psychology: General, 109,* 119–59.

Sternberg, S. (1966). High speed scanning in human memory. *Science, 153,* 652–4.

   (1969). The discovery of processing stages: Extensions of Donder's method. *Acta Psychologica, 30,* 276–315.

Svenson, O. (1979). Process descriptions of decision making. *Organizational Behavior and Human Performance, 23,* 86–112.

Svenson, O., & Hedenborg, M. L. (1980). On children's heuristics for solving simple additions. *Scandinavian Journal of Educational Research, 24,* 93–104.

Svenson, O., & Sjoberg, K. (1983). Evolution of cognitive processes for solving simple additions during the first three school years. *Scandinavian Journal of Psychology, 24*, 117–24.

Watson, J. B. (1920). Is thinking merely the action of language mechanisms? *British Journal of Psychology, 11*, 87–104.

Wertheimer, M. (1945). *Productive thinking*. New York: Harper & Row.

White, P. (1980). Limitations on verbal reports of internal events: A refutation of Nisbett and Wilson and of Bem. *Psychological Review, 87*, 105–12.

Woodworth, R. S. (1938). *Experimental psychology*. New York: Holt.

15   A taxonomy of thinking

P. N. Johnson-Laird

Introduction

Imagine visiting a large group of islands and exploring each of them thoroughly. You learn how to find your way around each, yet you lack a complete understanding of the overall topography of the islands because you have no idea of the relations among them. You do not know how they were shaped into an archipelago. Indeed, you do not even know whether you have visited them all. When I tell you that the names of these islands are "Induction," "Deduction," "Problem solving," and so on, you will realize that I have in mind your predicament as a diligent reader of this book. Each of its chapters is a guide to some domain of thought, but there has so far been no account of the relations among these domains. Hence, you may wonder how many sorts of thinking there are and how they are related to one another.

To answer these questions it is helpful to bear in mind the distinction between the function of thinking and the underlying procedures that it relies on. The late David Marr (1982) referred to this distinction as one between the computational level (what the mind is doing) and the algorithmic level (how it is doing it). Many of the chapters in this book have described thought processes at the algorithmic level. My task in this final chapter is to establish the outlines of a taxonomy that will help you to fit the domains of thought into a single framework – a single map of the mind. To establish this taxonomy, I shall be concerned mainly with what the mind accomplishes at the computational level.

Thinking without a goal

The ability to think is crucial to human life, but it is difficult to study because we are not aware of how we do it. We can observe only its consequences in our conscious thoughts, in our behavior, and in our speech. It also occurs in such dazzling varieties that some cognitive scientists despair of our ever understanding it completely (see, e.g., Fodor, 1983). There is, at one extreme, the free flow of ideas in daydreams. James Joyce re-created this variety of thought in the final pages of his great novel *Ulysses*. Molly Bloom, the wife of the novel's protagonist, lies in bed thinking about her husband:

Yes because he never did a thing like that before as ask to get his breakfast in bed with a couple of eggs since the *City Arms* hotel when he used to be pretending to be laid up with a sick voice doing his highness to make himself interesting to that old faggot Mrs Riordan that he thought he had a great leg of and she never left us a farthing all for masses for herself and her soul greatest miser ever was actually afraid to lay out 4d for her methylated spirit telling me all her ailments she had too much old chat in her about politics and earthquakes and the end of the world let us have a bit of fun first . . .

Joyce chose not to punctuate Molly Bloom's soliloquy, perhaps to catch its fleeting, inchoate nature, but if you read it aloud, it makes excellent sense. The process generating such a daydream is rapid, involuntary, and, apart from its results, outside conscious awareness. You recall an episode, "she never left us a farthing [in her will]," and the memory triggers a judgment: "greatest miser ever," which, in turn, reminds you of something else: "was actually afraid to lay out 4d for her methylated spirit," and so on and on.

William James (1890), who may well have influenced Joyce's writing, likened the stream of consciousness to the trajectory of a bird − a sequence of alternating flights and perchings. Dreams depend on the same sort of thinking, but their narrative is often compelling (see Gerrig's remarks on narrative structure in Chapter 9). Indeed, more than one short story has been dreamed in its entirety (Brook, 1983). Perhaps the most important feature of this sort of thinking is that it has no goal. It is not directed toward solving any problem or reaching any conclusion.

There is a long tradition in psychology from Aristotle onward of explaining the flight of ideas in terms of associations: One thought triggers another in a chain of linked ideas, which often affect our emotions. A classic study of associations was carried out by the nineteenth-century English scientist Francis Galton (1883). He compiled lists of words, which he put away in a desk drawer and forgot. Later, he went through the list, making free associations to each word; that is, he read a word and responded with the first word that it called to mind. Sometimes his responses shocked him so much that in his report of the study he passed briefly over them, saying only that they revealed the otherwise "hidden plumbing" of the mind. (Molly Bloom was not so easily shocked.) In another classic study of free association, Carl Jung (1919) observed that it takes longer to respond to emotionally laden words than to emotionally neutral words. He was thereby able to unmask a thief from her slow responses to words relating to the details of the crime.

Goalless thinking is evidently important to our emotional lives, but it is also important theoretically because it illustrates a particular mechanism of thought. The traditional theory held that one thought A elicits another thought B because the two have somehow become linked, or associated, in memory. Of course, there may be associated with thought A a number of alternative thoughts, B, C, D, and so on, and the strength of the links may vary. Which thought emerges on any particular occasion, according to this theory, is a matter of chance, though it is biased according to the strength of the associations. The difficulty with this theory is that it is hard to imagine that all the links in the flight of ideas have been forged already. It may never have occurred to Molly Bloom before that Mrs. Riordan was "the greatest miser ever." Indeed, she may never have previously called to mind that Mrs. Riordan left her nothing in her will. There is always a first time for a memory to be recalled, and there is always a first time for a particular judgment to be made. Conversely, if the flight of ideas always depended on preexisting links, it would never lead to any novel thoughts. The notion of preformed links is perhaps feasible for associations between individual words (although even here it runs into difficulties; see Johnson-Laird, Herrmann, & Chaffin, 1984), but it is not feasible as a general account of the flight of ideas. I will return to the problem of creativity later. For the time being, the point to bear in mind is that thinking in certain circumstances may lack a goal; it may appear to be outside voluntary control and to have no particular destination. It throws up ideas that are related to one another but that, like clouds, have no overall structure.

Calculation and the "problem space"

Perhaps the antithesis of the flight of ideas is the thinking that occurs in mental arithmetic. If I ask you, "What is twenty times thirteen?" you deliberate in an explicit, voluntary, and consciously controlled way. You may say to yourself, for instance, "Two times thirteen is twenty-six" and "Ten times twenty-six is two hundred and sixty." You are not aware of the way you retrieve these arithmetical facts, and you are not aware of the way they are represented in your mind. You just happen to know them and can recall them as you need them. Likewise, your plan for dealing with the problem derives from a knowledge of how to multiply by 10, and it comes to mind almost without thought (see also the discussion of mental arithmetic in Chapters 10 and 14). Although some of the processes occur outside consciousness, you are nevertheless totally aware of the overall plan that you are following. You can choose how to do the calculation (or whether or not to carry it out at all), but once you have chosen a plan, you have no freedom about what to do to obtain the right answer. Your thinking has a single precise starting point, a single precise goal, and it unwinds like clockwork.

There was a time when psychologists believed that all behavior was controlled by external events. Karl Lashley (1951) pointed out that this hypothesis could not explain the rapid execution of skills, such as mental arithmetic, which call for an internal hierarchical organization. George Miller, Eugene Galanter, and Karl Pribram called these organizations "plans," and the publication of their book *Plans and the Structure of Behavior* (1960) sealed the demise of behaviorism. They defined a plan as "any hierarchical process in the organism that can control the order in which a sequence of operations is to be performed," and they demonstrated convincingly that planning is a major part of thought.

Allen Newell and Herbert Simon (1972), who pioneered the computational analysis of problem solving, provided a unifying framework for planning and thinking, which Lesgold has described in Chapter 7. In all cases of a problem, there is a *starting point* − the initial conditions − and a set of mental *operations* that must be carried out in an appropriate way so as to reach a *goal* − the solution to the problem. There is a "space" of all possible sequences of operations, and what has to be worked out is a sequence, if there is one, that forms a route through the space from initial state to goal:

state 1→ state 2→ . . . →goal

A successful plan generates a route that solves the problem.

Not all thinking depends on a goal, but the bulk of it does, and much of the taxonomy of thought can be based on characteristics of the problem space. Thus, mental arithmetic is deterministic; that is, at each point, the next step in the calculation is determined wholly by its current state. There is only one route through the problem space from one state to the next, and your knowledge enables you to follow it with little difficulty.

Nondeterminism

Perhaps most thinking lies between the two extremes of daydreaming and calculating − between the clouds and the clocks of the mind. Unlike a daydream it has a goal and thus a global structure, and unlike a calculation it does not unwind in a strictly determined way. When you are trying to solve the missionaries and cannibals problem (see Chapter 7), for example, you do not have a "sure-fire" procedure, like a procedure for multiplication. Different people tackle the problem in different ways; you yourself, if you could step backward in time and make another attempt in ignorance of the first, might take a different path. Nothing constrains you to one inevitable choice at each step in the problem space. Your choice is not deterministic.

In computational theory, a device that can yield different outcomes from the same input and internal state is known as "nondeterministic" (see Hopcroft & Ullman, 1979). Imagine, for instance, a computational device that generates sentences according to the grammar of English. According to one rule of English syntax, a verb phrase can consist of a transitive verb followed by a noun phrase, as in the sentence "John told a joke." According to another rule, a verb phrase can consist solely of an intransitive verb, as in the sentence "Mary laughed." Which rule should be used to produce a sentence? A device that followed some principle in making the choice would be deterministic; one that followed no principle would be nondeterministic. Real computers are deterministic, but they can easily be made to simulate nondeterministic behavior.

There are different ways to interpret nondeterminism. If you are trying to solve the missionaries and cannibals problem for the first time, then at many points in the problem space there will be several possible moves that could be made. Sometimes you may be guided by a hunch or an intuition or some miniscule aspect of your environment, in which case your choice will have been determined by some principle even though you may not have been aware of it. A causal explanation of how the choice was determined by, say, some fleeting memory of another puzzle would amount to a deterministic theory, but at present we have no such explanation. Hence, according to this interpretation, your thinking *is* deterministic, but our ignorance forces us to treat it as nondeterministic. On other occasions, however, you may make a purely arbitrary choice. Experiments have shown that people do not perform in a truly random way (e.g., Baddeley, 1966), but it does not follow that they have no machinery for making arbitrary choices. Indeed, the experimental results suggest that people can make arbitrary choices by means that are not available to introspection. The method is the mental equivalent of spinning a coin, albeit one that is biased and that does not yield independent results from one spin to the next. Still another interpretation of nondeterminism is that your choice depends on the state of your brain, your brain is a physical device assembled out of fundamental particles, and fundamental particles behave according to the indeterminacy of quantum mechanics. This last interpretation seems to be ruled out by the poor performance of people in tasks that call for random behavior. The other interpretations, however, seem plausible: There may be occasions when nondeterminism is a label for our ignorance and other occasions when it characterizes an arbitrary choice.

Types of search in the problem space

Thinking without a goal wanders around a hypothetical problem space defined by the set of possible mental operations that move from one thought to another. The traditional probabilistic account of associations assumes, in effect, that the mechanism is nondeterministic. The choice of the next step in the problem space is not completely determined by psychological factors. Any sort of thought directed toward a goal calls for a sequence of choices that leads from the initial state to the goal. Sometimes the goal is precise, and sometimes you have a procedure that enables you to proceed in the right direction without ever erring; that is, you have a successful deterministic plan. Sometimes, however, the task of finding your way to the solution may be difficult. Here, in theory, you could explore a single route at a time in a "depth-first" search, just as you do in trying to find a way through a maze. When you come to a choice of routes, you select one on the basis of whatever means are at your disposal. In trying to solve a problem, you might choose from your assessment of the potential values of the alternatives. Of course, if you had an absolutely certain method of assessing these values, there would be no difficulty: You would choose the best option at each point and thereby arrive at the destination without ever exploring any blind alleys. Your search would be governed by a deterministic plan.

Many problems, alas, are like the Hampton Court maze. You are forced to make a choice with only an uncertain guide to the value of any alternative. You must therefore simulate a nondeterministic procedure that would always yield the correct choice. "Solving a problem nondeterministically" is in these circumstances just a fancy way of saying "solving a problem by magic." A less magical simulation of nondeterminism is to proceed through the maze until you reach either the goal or a dead end. In the latter case, you can go back to the last point of choice and try a different tack. If you exhaust all the options at this point to no avail, you can go back another step, and so on. If you exhaust all possibilities at all choice points, the problem is insoluble. This procedure of working back through the choice points is called *backtracking*. Anyone who uses it must be as prudent as Theseus, who unwound a ball of thread given to him by Ariadne as he made his way into the Minotaur's labyrinth so that he could be sure of retracing his steps. It is also important to keep a record of each choice made at each choice point. "Those who know no history," it is said, "are doomed to repeat its mistakes." It is the same with simple backtracking, because it fails to take into account the *reason* that a particular choice failed. If you pick up a red hot poker with one hand, backtracking would lead you to try the other hand.

Another method of simulating nondeterminism is to pursue all possible routes in parallel. You start at the initial state, apply all feasible mental operations to it to yield a set of alternative second states, and then do the same to each of these states, and so on. Sooner or later, this so-called breadth-first search leads to the goal if there is at least one route to it.

There are still other methods of search, such as means-ends analysis, which the reader will find described in Chapter 7. But any plan for searching for a route may run into insuperable difficulties. The logician Alonzo Church (1936) proved that there can be no procedure that is guaranteed to determine the status of an argument in the predicate calculus of formal logic (see Chapter 5). If an argument in this calculus has a proof, there are procedures that are guaranteed to find the proof. But if an argument has no proof, there can be no procedure guaranteed to reveal this fact: Any procedure may get lost in the problem space of possibilities, wandering around for an eternity. Computer programs for proving theorems are accordingly designed to minimize the time taken to search for a route that constitutes a proof, because as they grind away there is no way of knowing whether they will ultimately yield a decision or go on computing forever. If a problem is equivalent to an argument in the predicate calculus, there is never any guarantee that one can discover that it is insoluble.

Even in domains that have a guaranteed search procedure, the number of routes to be explored will grow exponentially with each step of the search if there is more than one possible operation at each point. As in the game of chess, it will soon cease to be practicable to explore all possible routes. Hence, no matter what procedure is used, problems for which there is no deterministic procedure almost always require constraints of some sort to keep the search to a manageable size. Very often, the mark of an expert is precisely the ability to explore only fruitful paths. The expert has a knowledge of a domain − often a tacit knowledge − that constrains the search process (see Chapter 7).

So far, I have discussed the ways of finding a path in the problem space from the initial state to the goal, but I have said little about the mental operations that lead from one state to the next. The nature of these operations is, as we shall see, a major factor in distinguishing one sort of thinking from another.

Semantic information and deduction

Consider the following passage in a newspaper:

The victim was stabbed to death in a cinema. The suspect was on an express train to Edinburgh when the murder occurred.

You would probably conclude that the suspect was innocent. This example illustrates a number of phenomena that are typical of everyday reasoning.

First, the inference leads from several verbally expressed propositions to a single verbally expressible conclusion. Even when inferences are based on thoughts rather than words, these thoughts, as Rips argues in Chapter 5, are typically beliefs, that is, entities that may be true or false.

Second, your inference depends both on your understanding of the premises and on your general knowledge. You know, for example, that one person cannot be in two places at the same time and that there are no cinemas on express trains to Edinburgh. You use this knowledge to forge links in the inferential chain so rapidly and automatically that you are hardly aware of them. They play an important part in your comprehension of discourse and in your comprehension of events in the world. Cognitive scientists have proposed a variety of theories about the representation of knowledge in schemata, scripts, and other such structures (see Chapter 9).

Third, you drew an informative conclusion. The concept of semantic informativeness is important, particularly because it has often been overlooked by students of reasoning. Philosophers define semantic information in terms of the possible situations that a proposition eliminates from consideration. The more situations that a proposition eliminates, the more information it contains (see Bar-Hillel & Carnap, 1952; Johnson-Laird, 1983, chap. 2). For example, the assertion "It is freezing but there is no fog" excludes more situations than the assertion "It is freezing," because the former rules out the presence of fog, whereas the latter leaves the possibility open.

Whenever thinking leads from one state to another in a problem space, one can ask, Does the second state (the conclusion) contain more semantic information that the first state (the premises)? More precisely, does the conclusion rule out some additional situations over and above those ruled out by the premises? If not, the conclusion is a valid deduction. But if it does rule out some additional state of affairs, it is not a valid deduction. This definition is equivalent to Rips's definition: A valid deduction has a conclusion that is true in any state of affairs in which the premises are true. But the concept of semantic information, as we shall see, has some additional uses.

The reader should note that literally an infinite number of valid conclusions follow from any set of premises. Most of them are totally trivial. Consider the following inference:

It is freezing.
Therefore, it is freezing or it is foggy (or both).

It is deductively valid, but no sensible person would draw such a conclusion spontaneously. The conclusion contains *less* semantic information than the premises, and even when people reason validly, they do not throw semantic information away for no good reason. It follows that they must be guided by at least some principle altogether outside logic, because logic sanctions any valid inference including one with a conclusion containing less information than its premises. This consideration, of course, rules out any theory that bases all reasoning on logic alone, for example, the theory proposed by Inhelder and Piaget (1958).

There is a further observation to be made about your inference concerning the stabbing: It is not valid. The conclusion that the suspect is innocent, although plausible, is not necessarily true. Indeed, if you were challenged about it, you would test its validity. When Tony Anderson and I questioned our subjects about such conclusions in some unpublished experiments, they searched for alternatives and often produced scenarios in which the suspect is guilty. For example, he may have had an accomplice, he may have used a spring-loaded knife or a radio-controlled robot, or he may have used a post-hypnotic suggestion that the suspect stab himself during a certain climactic scene in the movie.

Deductive inference should depend on mental operations that do not increase semantic information. For a long time, these operations were assumed to be based on the formal rules of inference of a logical calculus. But as Rips describes in Chapter 5, there are some problems for this doctrine, notably that the content of premises can exert a marked effect on what inference is drawn. Likewise, as Holyoak and Nisbett observe in Chapter 3, the failure of a lengthy course on logic to improve inferential performance casts further doubt on purely formal theories.

Another school of cognitive scientists favors rules containing specific knowledge. Such systems have been developed in computer programs that function as "expert systems," that is, programs that capture aspects of human expertise and that enable the user of the program to obtain advice about such matters as medical diagnosis, the molecular structure of compounds, or the proper place to drill for oil. The programs rely on conditional rules with specific contents that have been extracted by interrogation of human experts. Although current expert systems differ strikingly from human experts – humans, for example, are rather better at making excuses for their mistakes, there are psychologists who propose that the mind contains content-specific rules of inference in the form of production systems (as outlined in Chapter 7). The conjecture explains the effects of content on reasoning, but it cannot be a complete explanation of human reasoning. It provides no machinery for general deductive ability. It swings too far away from formal procedures.

What we need is the best of both worlds: general inferential ability coupled with sensitivity to content. Another school of thought, which Rips describes, aims to meet this requirement. Its adherents argue that deductive reasoning depends on three processes: (a) imagining the state of affairs described by the premises, (b) using this "mental model" to formulate a conclusion about something that was not explicit in the premises, and (c) attempting to test the validity of the conclusion by searching for an alternative model of the premises in which it is false (see Johnson-Laird, 1983). The process of constructing a model based on the premises takes into account any relevant general knowledge; and the process of searching for alternative models is affected by the apparent truth or falsity of the premises. Although there is evidence supporting both these hypotheses, I will say no more about the possible mechanisms of deduction. The fundamental issue is whether they are, in essence, syntactic manipulations of strings of uninterpreted symbols or semantic manipulations of mental representations of situations. An analogous issue has arisen over language and thought. As Glucksberg points out in Chapter 8, it is now generally accepted that there can be thought without language. To most psychologists, in contrast, the controversy about deductive reasoning is a long way from being settled.

Induction

The discovery of penicillin began with a single observation. Sir Alexander Fleming noticed that areas of bacteria had been destroyed on a culture plate that had been sitting on his desk for a couple of weeks. In fact, a chain of coincidences had led to their destruction. "Chance," Pasteur is supposed to have said, "favors the prepared mind." Fleming was prepared. He knew that the bacteria were hardy, and so he reasoned that something must have destroyed them:

Events of this type do not normally happen.

An event of this type has happened.
Therefore, there is some agent that caused the event.

Making this inference depends on noticing something unusual, a factor that Holyoak and Nisbett note in Chapter 3, and it leads to an increase in semantic information: its conclusion rules out more states of affairs than its premises do. There are indeed systematic processes of reasoning that lead to such conclusions, and these processes are *inductions*. The invocation of a causal agent is an explanatory conjecture of the sort that the American philosopher C. S. Peirce (1931) called an "abduction." One cannot get something for nothing, and the price of trying to expand knowledge, (i.e., increasing semantic information) is the possibility that the step is unwarranted. The conclusion may be false even though its premises are true. Induction should come with a government health warning.

Let us suppose that, under the tutelage of a helpful doctor, you study some cases of smallpox. You note that each patient had prior contact with someone suffering from the disease. You reason thus:

Patient A was in contact with a case of smallpox and A has smallpox.
Patient B was in contact with a case of smallpox and B has smallpox.
. . .
Therefore, if anyone is in contact with a case of smallpox, he or she is likely to catch the disease.

The inference is an induction; it goes from a finite number of instances to a conclusion about every member of a class. It is an example of what Holyoak and Nisbett refer to as an "instance-based" generalization. The resulting conjecture about smallpox seems reasonable, but, to borrow an argument from Nelson Goodman (1955), the evidence also supports the following conclusion:

If anyone is in contact with a case of smallpox, then until the year 2001 he or she is likely to catch the disease and thereafter is likely to catch measles.

Obviously this inference is silly, but why? You might say, "Because we know that diseases no more change their spots than leopards do." But how do we know that? If you are not careful, you may reply, "Because all our observations support this claim." Alas, all our observations are equally consistent with the claim that smallpox will remain smallpox until the year 2001, when it will become measles.

One reaction to this problem is to reject induction altogether. Sir Karl Popper (1972) argues that science is based not on induction but on explanatory conjectures that are open to empirical falsification. And where do conjectures come from? Popper says it does not matter; they can come from anywhere. However, since not all conjectures are equally sensible, and since many of them appear to be based on systematic processes of thought, the problem does not go away. Induction cannot be swept under the cognitive carpet. Its basic operations have indeed been studied in the psychological laboratory, and inductive computer programs have been implemented in a variety of forms.

Although induction is a way of trying to solve a problem, it too can be treated as a problem in its own right. There is a problem space of possible inductive conjectures, and the goal is to move from the initial state of knowledge to the correct inductive hypothesis. In essence, it calls for a test-operate-test-exit (TOTE) procedure of the sort proposed by Miller et al. (1960). If a test reveals a problem to be solved, such as explaining an unusual event, an inductive operation leads to a hypothetical explanation. A rational individual, however, will not be satisfied with such a hypothesis until it has withstood empirical testing. If a test fails, the cycle may continue with further inductive operations. If the hypothesis withstands testing, it will be accepted, at least provisionally, as the solution to the problem. The concept of semantic information provides a framework for clarifying induction, and, as we shall see, it also suggests a general constraint that people may use in generating inductive hypotheses.

The formulation of inductive hypotheses

There are many potential inductive operations, and their basis can be traced back to John Stuart Mill's (1847) canons of induction (see Chapter 4), which in turn go back to Sir Francis Bacon's (1620/1889) formulation. They boil down to two main ideas. First, if positive instances of a phenomenon have only one characteristic in common, it may play a crucial role. Second, if positive and negative instances differ in only one characteristic, it is critical.

An inductive conjecture may be remote from the truth because it is not even based on appropriate notions (e.g., "smallpox is a punishment for blasphemy"). As Schustack points out in Chapter 4, the most difficult problem is to identify what is relevant. This problem is cracked when the relevant notions are among those available for formulating a hypothesis. The hypothesis should be general enough to include all positive instances of the phenomenon in question but specific enough to exclude all negative instances. There are accordingly, as Holyoak and Nisbett point out in Chapter 3, two main ways in which an inductive hypothesis may have to be revised. On the one hand, it may be too specific and exclude some positive instances: It must be generalized. On the other hand, it may be too general and include some negative instances: It must be specialized. Hence, induction calls for both generalization and its converse, specialization.

One form of generalization, which Holyoak and Nisbett describe, drops part of a conjunction. Thus, the conjecture:

If anyone is in contact with a case of smallpox *and* is elderly, he or she is likely to catch the disease

becomes:

If anyone is in contact with a case of smallpox, he or she is likely to catch the disease.

Another form of generalization adds a disjunction. Thus the previous hypothesis becomes:

If anyone is in contact with a case of smallpox *or* with infected clothes, he or she is likely to catch the disease.

When these changes proceed in the opposite direction, they produce more specific hypotheses.

There are two outstanding questions. First, what is the underlying nature of generalization (and specialization) and, second, how many distinct operations of generalization (and specialization) are there? The answers to both questions can be derived from the concept of semantic information.

The greater the number of possible states of affairs that a hypothesis eliminates from consideration, the greater is its semantic information. Generalization, which has been defined in several ways in the literature (as Holyoak and Nisbett remark), can be analyzed in a simple, uniform way. It is any operation that increases the semantic information of a hypothesis by ruling out at least some additional state of affairs. Specialization has the converse effect; it admits some additional state of affairs. In other words, specialization is a valid inference but one that reduces semantic information for good reason — for example, the step from:

If anyone is in contact with a case of smallpox *or* with infected clothes, he or she is likely to catch the disease.

to:

If anyone is in contact with a case of smallpox, he or she is likely to catch the disease.

The fact that a specialization is always a valid inference does not mean that it necessarily yields a true conclusion; the hypothesis that serves as its premise may be false. Moreover, even if the conclusion is true, it may be less than the whole truth. The premise above is a better explanation of the cause of smallpox than is the specialization.

Holyoak and Nisbett observe that there are many possible generalizations of any hypothesis. Indeed, unless the hypothesis has a very high semantic information content, the number of possible generalizations increases exponentially with the number of simple propositions that may be relevant to the formulation of a generalization (see Johnson-Laird, 1986). An important but unfortunate consequence of this fact is that any procedure based on eliminating putative hypotheses will be unable to examine them exhaustively in a reasonable amount of time. There are so many possible inductions that one cannot examine them all.

Although there are many possible generalizations, there is no need for a corresponding number of distinct inductive *operations*. Consider, for instance, the generalization that leads from two hypotheses of the form

If p and q, then s,
If p and r, then s,

to one of the form

If p, then s,

This operation is used in the computer model of human inductive reasoning that Holyoak and Nisbett and their colleagues have devised. But it does not require a separate operation of its own. Its premises validly imply

If p and (q or r), then s

and the generalization of this conjecture to

If p, then s

is just a case of dropping part of a conjunction. In fact, it turns out that only three operations are needed for any generalization in the ordinary predicate calculus (see Johnson-Laird, 1986). The first operation consists in conjoining the negation of the description of a situation to the original hypothesis. The second consists in moving from a finite number of observations to a universal claim, as in the earlier inference that contact with smallpox is sufficient for catching the disease. The third operation, yet to be exploited in any theory of induction or by any inductive program (as far as I know), is exemplified by the step from:

Any type of smallpox is cured by some drug.

to:

There is some drug that cures any type of smallpox.

Even though there are only three basic forms of generalization, it remains wholly impracticable to examine all their possible uses in generalizing a hypothesis. One moral to be drawn from this observation, and from Goodman's argument, which I presented earlier, is that induction cannot be a matter of manipulating symbols according to purely formal or syntactic rules. A hypothesis of a particular form may have one appropriate generalization in one domain and quite a different appropriate generalization in another domain. Another moral, which is drawn by Holyoak and Nisbett as well, is that the search for the appropriate generalization (within a vast problem space) must be constrained in some way. They describe a number of constraints to which I shall add a further candidate based on semantic information.

When human beings try to induce a novel hypothesis, they concentrate on positive exemplars of it (see the "confirmation" bias referred to in Chapter

4 and Peter Wason's 1977 study of the failure to examine disconfirming evidence). Thus, they concentrate on the people with smallpox rather than healthy individuals. In such circumstances, it is important not to formulate a hypothesis that contains too little semantic information. For example, in order to teach you to identify a particular disease, I show you a patient who has a fever, a rapid pulse, and a backache. You should therefore hypothesize that the disease has the following symptoms: fever, rapid pulse, and backache. This conjecture contains the largest amount of semantic information based directly on the evidence. If I now present a patient with a fever, backache, and a *slow* pulse, you will realize at once that your previous hypothesis eliminates too much. You will modify it to the maximally informative one based on the evidence: fever and backache. Suppose, however, that you had started off with the following conjecture: fever or rapid pulse or backache. It fits the facts, but it contains much less semantic information. Moreover, it remains unaffected by the evidence from the second patient. You will not home in on the real disease from positive exemplars alone, because your initial hypothesis will always accommodate them. Hence, when you are trying to formulate a hypothesis from positive instances, you must advance the most semantically informative hypothesis based on the data. It may rule out too much, but if so, sooner or later you will encounter a positive instance that allows you to correct it.

When children develop their taxonomies of the world, they appear to be guided by this principle. Frank Keil (1979) has shown that they organize their concepts in hierarchies, as in Figure 15.1. Overlapping arrangements like the one in Figure 15.2 are rare and sometimes arise from ambiguities. Keil derives the children's classifications from the pattern of their answers to such questions as: Does it make sense to say that a tree is an hour long? A child may have the following taxonomic rule:

If something is living, then it is a person.

An older child, however, distinguishes two classes:

If something is living, then it is a person or a plant (but not both).

This way of refining a taxonomy suggests that children are sensitive to semantic information. If a category is to be divided, the division that creates the most semantic information is one that yields two mutually exclusive subcategories; that is, no entity can belong to both. Perhaps it is this semantic principle that leads children to avoid overlapping taxonomies.

Knowledge as a constraint on inductive thinking

Some theorists, notably the linguist Noam Chomsky (1980), have suggested that there may be no general inductive procedures, only specific procedures based on innate knowledge of particular domains. The claim is debatable,

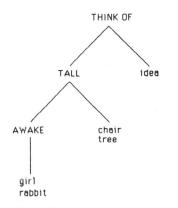

Figure 15.1. A tree representing the typical judgments of a five-year-old in Keil's study.

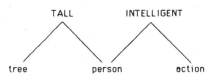

Figure 15.2. An artificial tree showing the sort of overlap that does not occur in children's judgments. The overlap occurs because of an ambiguity: An intelligent action does not possess intelligence as a person does.

but certainly a major constraint on induction is knowledge of a domain. Most of the inferences we make go beyond the information we are given and, like Fleming's inference about the destruction of the bacteria, they do so because they rely on our knowledge. We avoid any inductive conjecture that goes against our knowledge of the way the world works; we are biased toward conjectures that are compatible with our knowledge. It is no coincidence that knowledge is stressed as an important factor in so many chapters in this book: by Schustack, by Holyoak and Nisbett, by Perkins, by Sternberg, by Smith, Sera, and Guttuso, and in all the schemes for teaching thinking reviewed by Vye, Delclos, Burns, and Bransford.

The importance of knowledge is easily demonstrated by asking people to make judgments about matters on which they know little. For example, I attach a ball to a piece of string and spin it horizontally in a circle. The string snaps. What is the horizontal trajectory of the ball afterwards? People who do not know Newton's laws often say that it moves off in a spiral that gradually staightens out. They appeal to an almost medieval notion of impetus: something that a moving object is supposed to have (McCloskey, 1983). The correct answer, ignoring gravity, is that the ball moves in a straight line; the centripetal force pulling it toward the center of the circle ceases when the string breaks, and an object on which no forces are exerted moves uniformly in a straight line (or remains in a state of rest).

Knowledge of the variability of instances is critical when people make an inductive generalization. As Holyoak and Nisbett report in Chapter 3, a single exemplar suffices for most of us to conclude that a rare element conducts electricity, but a single instance of an obese member of an exotic tribe leads to no generalization. We know that people's properties vary much more widely than those of a chemical element.

A full grasp of variation calls for knowledge of the theory of probability. The theory is so different from its intuitive precursors that at least one commentator, Ian Hacking (1975), has remarked that anyone who had played dice in ancient times armed with the modern calculus of probabilities would soon have won the whole of Gaul. Numerous studies have shown that people make egregious errors of judgment because of their ignorance of the workings of probability (see Chapter 6). The burden of these findings is that the errors of the naive are reproduced at a sophisticated level by the experts. Amos Tversky and Daniel Kahneman have proposed an account of the phenomena, which assumes that people use various heuristics (rules of thumb) in order to estimate the probabilities of events and that they are particularly affected by the relative availability of information and by its seeming representativeness (see Chapter 6). Tversky and Kahneman's (1973) explanation dovetails neatly with the account of reasoning by mental models. They write:

Some events are perceived as so unique that past history does not seem relevant to the evaluation of their likelihood. In thinking of such events we often construct *scenarios*, i.e. stories that lead from the present situation to the target event. The plausibility of the scenarios that come to mind, or the difficulty of producing them, then serve as a clue to the likelihood of the event. If no reasonable scenario comes to mind, the event is deemed impossible or highly unlikely. If many scenarios come to mind, or if the one scenario that comes to mind is particularly compelling, the event in question appears probable. (p. 229)

Concepts and theories

A baby girl at 16 months hears the word *snow* used to refer to snow. Over the next months, as Melissa Bowerman (1977) has observed, the infant uses the word to refer to snow, the white tail of a horse, the white part of a toy boat, a white flannel bed pad, and a puddle of milk on the floor. She is forming the impression that *snow* refers to things that are white or to horizontal areas of whiteness, and she will gradually refine her concept so that it tallies with the adult one. The underlying procedure is inductive. We all continue to make inductions throughout our lives as we form impressions about classes of people, events, and the meanings of expressions.

Psychologists have often studied induction in terms of the means by which people acquire concepts. Following Mill and other Empiricist philosophers, they assumed until recently that a process of abstraction drops idiosyncratic details that differ from one exemplar to another and leaves behind only what they hold in common. But as Smith emphasizes in Chapter 2, this classical view of concepts does not hold for all concepts. Kenneth Smoke had this worry in the 1930s: "As one learns more about dogs, his concept of 'dog' becomes increasingly rich, not a closer approximation to some bare 'element' . . . . No learner of 'dog' ever found a 'common element' running through the stimulus patterns through which he learned" (Smoke, 1932).

Everyday concepts are not isolated, independent entities; they are related to one another. This idea goes back to the *structuralism* of the Swiss linguist Ferdinand de Saussure (1960). The perceptual boundaries of entities are set, in part, by the taxonomy in which they occur. Whether something is perceived as a dog depends on its similarity to typical dogs, typical cats, typical wolves, and so on. Granted the complex structures of certain domains, much of the development of knowledge, as Smith, Sera, and Gattuso argue in Chapter 13, depends on creating mental representations from which the appropriate relations among concepts can be recovered. It is natural to assume that these relations are represented explicitly, but this assumption should not be taken for granted. One of the interesting features of the current work on parallel distributed processing is that relations among concepts may not be explicitly represented at all, but may merely be an emergent property of an implicit representation that is distributed over many parallel processors (see Rumelhart, Smolensky, & McClelland, 1986).

Analogy

Lying behind the perceptual characteristics of concepts are schemata that relate form to function; and lying behind such schemata is a conceptual *core* – some kind of everyday "theory," that plays a role in the ordinary use of language that is analogous to the role of theories in scientific discourse (Miller & Johnson-Laird, 1976, Sec. 4.4.4). The development of a theory, however, may call for the discovery of the relevance of certain new ideas, or new combinations of existing concepts (see Smith's description of some of the principles governing conceptual combinations in Chapter 2). It is seldom merely a question of making inductive generalizations based on a given set of ideas.

New ideas come from mental operations (other than induction) that lead to an increase in semantic information. One such source is analogical thinking. When you realize that a problem (the target domain) is analogous to another more familiar topic (the source domain), you may be able to import new ideas into the target domain from the source domain; see, for example, Holyoak and Nisbett's account of the way an analogy can help you to solve the celebrated X-ray problem. Thus, analogies are important because they can provide the novel ideas necessary for the development of a new theory. (Generalization and specialization work only if the relevant ideas are already available.)

Could there be a purely formal theory of analogy? The answer appears to be negative for the same sort of reasons that formal theories of induction are impossible. Consider, for example, Rutherford's elucidation of the structure of an atom by analogy to the solar system. As Dedre Gentner (1983) has pointed out, this analogy maps the sun onto the nucleus of the atom and maps the planets onto the electrons. The properties of the sun, such as its color, are dropped, but the higher-order semantic relations are carried over. The sun's attraction of the planets causes them to revolve around it. Hence, it is inferred that the nucleus's attraction of the electrons causes them to revolve around it. If you ask people in what way a clock is analogous to the solar system, from my anecdotal observations, they are likely to respond: "Both involve a revolution: the hands of the clock go round just as the planets go round the sun." This answer and Rutherford's analogy depend on mappings from the same objects in the source domain:

Atom target		Source		Clock target
nucleus	←	sun	→	center
electrons	←	planets	→	hands

A purely formal theory would therefore lead to the transfer of the same information in both analogies. But unlike the case of atomic structure, the causal relation should not be carried over in the analogy with clocks: "The center's attraction of the hands causes them to revolve around it." This conclusion is obviously false, but matters of fact are precisely what formal theories must *not* depend on. Current theories of analogy accordingly rely on semantics and matters of fact (see the theories discussed in Chapters 3 and 10). Once again, knowledge is at the heart of the matter.

Creativity

Innovations in science and art often arise as a result of analogical thinking (see Hesse, 1966). Such analogies, however, call for genuinely creative thought. David Perkins argues in Chapter 11 that creativity calls for results that are both original and appropriate. I have similarly suggested that an act of creation yields a product that is novel (at least for the individual who created it) and that satisfies some existing criteria or constraints: One creates pictures, poems, stories, sonatas, theories, principles, games, and so on, and anything that lies outside the criteria of any domain is likely to be deemed uncategorizable rather than creative (Johnson-Laird, in press). Of course, the process does not occur in a vacuum; one cannot construct new ideas out of nothing. There must be mental elements that already exist −

concepts, images, principles, and so forth – that provide the raw materials for the process and the constraints on it. Yet there *are* new things under the sun; a combination, or modification, of existing elements can indeed be novel. Highly original works of art and science are constructed out of existing languages, such as English and mathematics. The criteria that I have referred to are not necessarily the sorts of explicit principles that are found in theoretical treatises on aesthetics and scientific method. They are any principles that an individual uses in order to constrain the processes by which elements are combined, modified, or refined within a particular domain. Most criteria will probably be implicit principles that are not available to introspection. Some of them may be common to many creators; they specify the genre or paradigm. Others may be unique to individuals; they constitute the idiosyncracies of individual style within the genre or paradigm. In short, the criteria are constraints on the mental operations available to the creator.

Unlike a reasoning problem, there is no clear and explicit starting point in the problem space for an act of creation. The creator possesses only the criteria of the domain, and although they place constraints on what can be created within that domain, they still allow an indefinite number of possibilities. If the criteria allowed only one possible continuation at each step in grappling with the task, the process would be trivial. There would be no choice about what to do next. Since creators almost always have a choice of continuations, it follows that the mechanisims of creation must be treated as nondeterministic.

This account is the beginning of a theory of creativity at the computational level. It tells us what a creative process has to do, namely, it must start with a set of criteria and make nondeterministic choices among the options they offer. Given these foundations, a striking conclusion can be derived: Only three general classes of procedure are capable of creativity. These classes have nothing to do with the details of creative mechanisms, though they place constraints on them, but rather concern the overall architecture of the creative process. They are as follows:

1. *Neo-Darwinian procedures.* They make arbitrary combinations of or changes in existing elements so as to generate a vast number of putative products. They then exploit the criteria of the domain so as to filter out those products that are not viable. Some theorists have argued that such procedures are the only mechanism for creativity (e.g., Skinner, 1953).
2. *Neo-Lamarckian procedures.* They form initial combinations of or changes in existing elements under the immediate guidance of the criteria of the domain. If a choice between equally viable alternatives arises, it is made arbitrarily. The choice has to be arbitrary, since by definition all the available criteria of the domain are used in the initial generation of ideas.
3. *Multistage procedures.* They make use of some criteria in the initial generative stage; they then use other criteria as filters. This procedure is perhaps the one that Perkins has in mind when he suggests that creativity is a pro-

cess of search and selection. Choices between equally viable alternatives may arise. Once again, certain of these choices must be made arbitrarily, since the complete set of criteria does not pinpoint a single unique product.

The mental criteria that a creator exploits can obviously differ in terms of their completeness. For certain domains, the criteria are complete. That is to say, the creator has sufficient criteria to guarantee that the result of the creative process will be at least viable. Completeness is thus a desirable property for all creation that occurs extempore, such as the making of artifacts in media that allow no second chances and the improvization of music, dance, poetry, and other forms of art. In such cases, the creator's mental operations define a problem space in which all routes lead to at least a satisfactory outcome. We can therefore think of the criteria as defining just the set of feasible routes, and it is natural to suppose that the creative procedure in this case will be neo-Lamarckian: a nondeterministic walk through a problem space that leads only to viable outcomes. Given the limitations of human processing capacity, the computational power of the procedure is likely to be weak, that is, to call on the minimal possible memory for the results of intermediate computations. I have examined jazz improvization as a test case of this sort of creativity and shown that it can be modeled in computer programs based on such procedures. Musicians improvizing in a particular genre have a tacit grasp of the criteria of the genre, which they can use to generate music spontaneously. If their grasp of the criteria is inadequate, they will produce unacceptable music and fail to find gainful employment as improvizers.

The creation of a poem, painting, or symphony is usually carried out within the conventions of an existing genre. Likewise, the creation of science normally occurs within the constraints of an existing paradigm (Kuhn, 1970). These sorts of creativity nearly always depend on a multistage procedure. There is no complete set of criteria that leads only to viable outcomes, but the initial generative stage can be partially constrained by some criteria. The result, however, almost always calls for further revision or elaboration, and this process may be governed by criteria that the creator is unable to exercise in the generative stage — we are all better critics than creators. This division of labor is exemplified by the cases that Perkins discusses. The problem space contains many routes that fail to terminate in an acceptable goal, but the creator is not striving to achieve a single unique goal; there are many acceptable goals.

In fact, the notion of problem spaces containing goals a priori is often merely a convenient fiction for creation. Unlike conventional problem solving, the process may not be goal driven in any realistic sense. Creators can start off with no very clear goal. They make a sequence of choices on the basis of often tacit criteria. They may not recognize their goal until after they have achieved it, or they may fail to achieve any worthwhile result.

However, a multistage procedure can call for considerable computational power, that is, memory for the intermediate results of computations. Thus, the creation of tonal chord sequences of the sort used in most Western music evidently calls for a considerable use of such memory (see, e.g., Johnson-Laird, in press; Steedman, 1982). Writing or a notation of some sort, of course, relieves the creator of the actual burden of remembering intermediate results, and in certain forms of art, such as sculpture and painting, the work itself provides such a record.

In the case of a major innovation in art or science, there are grounds for doubting whether there could ever exist criteria that always guarantee a successful outcome. On the one hand, there are too few instances of revolutions within a particular domain. On the other hand, it is hard to see what different innovations could possibly have in common. What criteria are common, for example, to both the invention of perspective and the invention of Cubism? What criteria are common to both the transition in physics to Newtonian mechanics and the transition to the special theory of relativity? By criteria here, I have in mind knowledge that would be effective in reducing the processes required to generate *all* successful revolutions within a particular domain. Indeed, it hardly has to be said that even the best of innovators may try out many bad ideas before discovering a good one.

Let us consider the invention of a profound analogy as a special case of this sort of creativity. By definition, the analogy does not depend on preexisting rules that establish mappings between the source and target domains. The innovation depends on the invention of such mappings. Establishing a mapping is a process that resembles the construction of a complex proposition that links an element in one domain with an element in the other. We can think of all domains of knowledge as constituting a vast epistemic space, which embraces knowledge of the solar system, of atoms, of waves, of clocks, of clouds, and so on. The task of creating a profound analogy consists initially in constructing a mapping from one domain to another. The more distant the two domains are from one another (before the construction of the analogy) the larger is the number of domains that might serve as the source, and the longer is the chain of links that will have to be established to form the mapping. Granted that at each point in the construction of a chain there are several possible continuations, the mapping is like the construction of a novel sentence − a sentence that captures the content of the mapping. Plainly, the number of possible sentences increases exponentially with the length of the sentence; and it soon ceases to be feasible to explore all possible mappings.

There are computer programs that have produced novel proofs of theorems, interesting mathematical conjectures, rediscoveries of scientific laws, and works of art (see Chapter 11). Their success depends on their operating in highly constrained domains, using a neo-Lamarckian procedure or assistance from the user (or both). Even a neo-Darwinian procedure will work if, like nature, one is prepared to use it over and over again in a cumulative way in billions of experiments every year for a period extending over millions of years and to countenance a high proportion of failures. The point of my argument is that there can be no feasible program that is *guaranteed* to make profound discoveries routinely by using analogies or any other procedure.

How, then, do those few exceptional individuals, whom we recognize as geniuses, succeed in making innovations? Is there perhaps some mental commodity, or "potency" to use Perkins's term, that leads to success – a higher degree of intelligence, a larger working memory, a more rapidly functioning brain, a larger number of associative connections, a higher degree of motivation, or an infinite capacity for taking pains? I suspect not. What evidence there is suggests that creativity is not merely a matter of some such property being enhanced; there are many highly intelligent and dedicated individuals (by any measure) who lack the spark of originality. My conjecture is that geniuses have mastered more constraints, but they have their knowledge in a form that can directly govern the generative stage of creation. Knowledge is the key – in this case knowledge of the specific domain, since, as I have argued, there are not likely to be any general criteria for innovation. But knowledge alone is not enough. To return to the inference about the murder in the cinema, everyone recognizes the ingenuity of the solution that the suspect used a posthypnotic suggestion that the victim stab himself. Yet very few people succeed in thinking of this solution for themselves. Conscious critical knowledge, which is relatively easy to acquire (and for educators to test), is impotent when it comes to the unconscious generation of ideas.

How knowledge comes to work in the generative stage of creativity is perhaps the most important mystery confronting students of thinking. One conjecture is that it does so only as a result of an individual's attempts to create. The only way to learn to be creative is by trying to create. If there is any truth in this conjecture, the pedagogical moral is that the best method of fostering creativity may be to encourage children to attempt to create within a particular domain as soon as they have acquired the rudiments of technique.

Free will, self-reflection, and metacognition

I have now discussed several types of thought. Is there any other sort? There is indeed one very important additional mechanism. A salient element of our conscious experience is self-reflection. We have the capacity to reflect upon what we are doing – our own process of thought becomes itself an object of thought at a higher level – and as a result of this self-reflection we may modify our performance. For example, if you are having some success in solving problems of a particular class but then you are stumped by a certain problem, you can ask yourself: "What was I doing when I succeeded with the earlier problems?" Or, to take an example from Chapter 5, if a problem reminds you of some other domain, you may say to yourself: "I should try to draw an analogy here." Such thoughts are based on your ability to scrutinize your own performance, that is, to raise yourself up one level to become a spectator of your own thoughts and behavior. This procedure may help you to reformulate how you should proceed at the lower level of actual performance.

You cannot inspect your own thought processes in complete detail. If you could, there would hardly be any need for books on the psychology of thinking. What you have access to is something like a *model* of your own abilities – an incomplete and perhaps partially erroneous representation of their major features (see Johnson-Laird, 1983, chap. 16). This ability of the mind to inspect models of its own performance and then in turn to use these models in thinking is the basis of all the so-called metacognitive skills that you possess. This account is one way in which Sternberg's idea of "meta-components" can be explicated (see Chapter 10). Hence you can think about how you remember things and take remedial steps to improve your memory (see Chapter 13 for some observations of the development of this ability in childhood). You can think about how you get on with people and work out a strategy for coping with difficult social situations. But self-reflection does not stop here. It, too, can be the object of itself: you can think about your own metacognitive thoughts. When you start to think about how you ordinarily deal with problems of a certain sort, you may realize what you are doing and think, "This is one of those problems that I can tackle by thinking about the way I have solved similar problems in the past, but whenever I use this ability, I tend to concentrate too much on previous successes." There does not appear to be any barrier that in principle prevents you from reflecting about such thoughts at a still higher level.

The ability to reflect at ever higher levels is essential to freedom of choice. When you follow a plan, you sometimes carry out a "cast iron" sequence of actions, that is, a deterministic sequence like that which underlies calculation. But often you observe the outcomes of your actions and, as a result, may modify the plan or even on occasion abandon it altogether. You usually have the freedom to choose among several options at various points in its execution, particularly if you are engaged in the creative exercise of your imagination.

The concept of freedom that I here invoke refers to freedom of will – the propensity that thinkers from Descartes (1637/1911–12) to Dostoyevsky (1864/1972) invariably cite in order to cast doubt on the feasibility of a science of the mind. Scientists often retort that free will is an illusion (e.g., Skinner, 1971); yet its existence is entirely compatible with the capacity for self-reflective thinking.

Suppose, for instance, that you are confronted with a choice between putting milk or lemon in your tea. Sometimes, you decide what you want almost automatically and without thinking about it. (If you are Richard Feyn-
mann, you may even choose both milk and lemon!) On other occasions you
may be unable to make up your mind. Sooner or later in this case, you will
say to yourself, "This is ridiculous; I'll have to choose one of them." And
you may then, as a result of this higher-order reflection, make an abitrary
decision. You may even ensure that it is arbitrary by recourse to external
means. You may spin a coin or, like the hero of Luke Rhinehart's novel *The
Diceman*, toss dice.

What gives you free will is the self-reflective ability to think about *how*
you will make a decision and thus to choose at a metalevel a method of
choice. At the lowest level, you can make a choice without thinking about it
at all. You just pour milk into your tea or put a slice of lemon into it:

Level 0:   Pour milk into your tea.

At the metalevel, you think about what to do and make a decision based,
say, on a simple preference (see Chapter 6):

Level 1:   By assessing preferences, you choose from:
Level 0:   Pouring milk into your tea.
           Putting a slice of lemon into your tea.

How did you arrive at this method of choice? You did not think about it
consciously. It was a tacitly selected method that came to mind as the right
way to proceed. Perhaps most choices are made this way. But the metalevel
method need not be tacitly chosen. You can confront the issue consciously
(at the meta-metalevel). And indeed if you do reflect about the matter, you
may assess different methods of choice and try to choose rationally from
among them:

Level 2:   Making a rational assessment, you choose from:
Level 1:   Assessing preferences   ⎤
           Taking your spouse's advice ⎬ to choose from:
           Spinning a coin   ⎟
Level 0:   Pouring milk into your tea   ⎦
           Putting a slice of lemon into your tea.

The method of decision at the highest level is, of course, always tacitly
selected − it just comes to mind. If it were chosen consciously, there would
be a still higher level at which that decision was made. In theory, there need
be no end to the hierarchy of decisions about decisions about decisions, but the
business of life demands that you do something rather than get lost in speculation about how to decide what to do. The buck must stop somewhere.

We have free will, not because we are ignorant of the roots of many of
our decisions, which we certainly are, but because our models of ourselves
enable us to choose how to choose, and among the range of options are

those arbitrary methods that free us from the constraints of an ecological niche or any rational calculation of self-interest.

Intentionality and self-reflection

Once you have decided what to do and how to do it, you can act intentionally to try to achieve your goal. There are computer programs that are goal driven, that is, that try to achieve a stated goal. Some cognitive scientists have argued that these programs have intentions. However, it seems more accurate to say that they act *as though* they had intentions. What is missing from them is self-knowledge. At the lowest level (like the computer programs), human beings can

Level 0: Construct a model of a possible future state of affairs.
          Compute what to do to try to bring about that state of affairs.
          Carry out this plan.

Unlike a computer program, human beings have access to a model of these abilities, and moreover they can use it by:

Level 1: Determining what to do by consulting a model of:
Level 0: Constructing a model of a possible future state of affairs.
          Computing what to do to try to bring about that state of affairs.
          Carrying out this plan.

In other words, people know that they can act to try to achieve some goal, and they can use this knowledge in determining what to do.

Once again, as the theory allows, people know that they can take into account their self-knowledge in making decisions. They can

Level 2: Determine what to do by consulting a model of:
Level 1: Determine what to do by consulting a model of:
Level 0: Construct a model of a possible future state of affairs.
          Compute what to do to try to bring about that state of affairs.
          Carry out this plan.

In other words, people know that they know that they can act to try to achieve some goal, and they can use this knowledge in determining what to do. Even this level is not necessarily the top of the hierarchy.

Of course, most of us recognize that the road to hell is paved with good intentions. We know that our having a particular intention, such as to give up smoking, is not necessarily sufficient to produce the appropriate actions. In the light of this knowledge, we sometimes take special steps to try to ensure an intended outcome.

When you are thinking about something, you can be so deeply engrossed in it that you forget all about your own condition. But you can perceive yourself as thinking about a problem – perhaps as a precursor to a metacognitive step. This state of self-awareness is phenomenologically distinct from ordinary perception and is perhaps the central riddle of human consciousness. What gives rise to self-awareness according to the present theory is the self-reflective mode of processing. Normal perception yields a model of the world; self-awareness depends on the mind constructing a model of itself constructing the model of the world. You perceive yourself perceiving the world or cogitating about it. Once again, the model representing perception is a radically incomplete one, but it is sufficient to create the subjective experience of self-awareness.

Conclusions

I have described a variety of types of basic thinking and above them all a higher-order type: self-reflection. Since we can carry out a calculation in the midst of a daydream, or daydream in the midst of a calculation, their names are merely convenient labels that reflect combinations of underlying distinctions. The taxonomy founded on these distinctions can be summarized in terms of the following questions:

Does a process of thought have a goal? If not, it is of the family of associative thinking, which includes the genera of dreams and daydreams. If it has a goal, it falls into the major family of thinking, which psychologists call problem solving. There are many genera here, and their classification continues:

Is the thought process deterministic? If it is, obviously it leads to a single precise goal and constitutes the genus of calculation. If it is not deterministic, then again there are many genera, and the classification continues:

Is there an explicit starting point? If not, the process is in the family of creative processes, of which there are three main species (neo-Darwinian, neo-Lamarckian, and multistage). If there is an explicit starting point, it is in the family of reasoning processes, and the classification continues:

Does the reasoning process increase semantic information? If so, it is a species of induction. If not, it is a species of deduction.

Figure 15.3 presents the outlines of this taxonomy, which can obviously be refined into many subspecies. The taxonomy omits self-reflection (metacognition), which depends on having access to a model of a thought process. All the genera of problem solving appear to be potential candidates for self-reflection. When thinking lacks a goal, however, matters are less clear. If you are daydreaming and start to reflect on the process, you can indeed influence its nature. Often, however, your metacognitive thoughts lead you to abandon the daydream and to enter into deliberations about some problem that emerges from it. If you are having a real dream and start to reflect on the process, the dream becomes what is sometimes known as "lucid": You are aware that you are dreaming. Most people find it difficult to influence the content of a lucid dream, but they can usually at least decide to wake

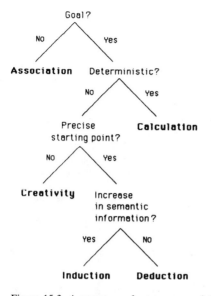

Figure 15.3. A summary of a taxonomy of thought (excluding self-reflection).

up. The essential point is that metacognition often changes the character of purely associative thinking. It either introduces a goal or brings it to a halt. It is hard to be an innocent witness of one's own thought processes.

Is the taxonomy complete? Perhaps. The underlying distinctions seem to be both fundamental and exhaustive, and they embrace all the varieties of thought that have been discussed in this book. A species of thinking that they failed to encompass would be a major discovery. It is clear, however, that thinking in practice may call for combinations of different genera.

The taxonomy derives primarily from an analysis at the computational level — an analysis in terms of what a thought process is computing. The reader may wonder whether it implies anything about the way thinking is carried out at the algorithmic level. In fact, one theme that has emerged in this chapter is that all the species of thought can be explained on the assumption that each is guided by knowledge and depends on representations of the world. There is only one domain — deductive reasoning — in which accounts based on the formal manipulation of uninterpreted symbols are still pursued by some theorists.

References

Bacon, F. (1889). *Novum organum* (T. Fowler, Ed.). New York: Oxford University Press. (Original work published 1620).

Baddeley, A. D. (1966). The capacity for generating information. *Quarterly Journal of Experimental Psychology, 18,* 119–29.

Bar-Hillel, Y., & Carnap, R. (1952). An outline of a theory of semantic information. In Y. Bar-Hillel, *Language and information.* Reading, MA: Addison-Wesley, 1964.

Bowerman, M. (1977). The acquisition of word meaning: An investigation of some current concepts. In P. N. Johnson-Laird & P. C. Wason (Eds.), *Thinking: Readings in cognitive science* (pp. 239–53). Cambridge University Press.

Brook, S. (1983). *The Oxford book of dreams.* New York: Oxford University Press.

Chomsky, N. (1980). *Rules and representations.* New York: Columbia University Press.

Church, A. (1936). A note on the Entscheidungsproblem. *Journal of Symbolic Logic, 1,* 40–1, 101–2. Reprinted in M. Davis (Ed.), *The Undecidable.* Hewlett, NY: Raven Press, 1965.

Descartes, R. (1911–12). *Discours de la méthode.* In *The philosophical works of Descartes* (E. T. S. Haldane & G. T. R. Ross, Trans.). Cambridge University Press. (Original work published 1637.)

Dostoyevsky, F. (1972). *Notes from the underground.* Harmondsworth: Penguin Books. (Original work published 1864.)

Fodor, J. A. (1983). *The modularity of mind: An essay on faculty psychology.* Cambridge, MA.: Bradford/MIT Press.

Galton, F. (1883). *Inquiries into human faculty and its development.* London: Macmillan.

Gentner, D. L. (1983). Structure-mapping: A theoretical framework for analogy. *Cognitive Psychology, 7,* 155–70.

Goodman, N. (1955). *Fact, fiction, and forecast* (2nd ed.). Cambridge, MA: Harvard University Press.

Hacking, I. (1975). *The emergence of probability.* Cambridge University Press.

Hesse, M. (1966). *Models and analogies in science.* Notre Dame, IN: Notre Dame University Press.

Hopcroft, J. E., & Ullman, J. D. (1979). *Introduction to automata theory, languages, and computation.* Reading, MA: Addison-Wesley.

Inhelder, B., & Piaget, J. (1958). *The growth of logical thinking from childhood to adolescence.* London: Routledge & Kegan Paul.

James, W. (1890). *The principles of psychology.* New York: Holt.

Johnson-Laird, P. N. (1983). *Mental Models: Towards a cognitive science of language, inference, and consciousness.* Cambridge University Press; Cambridge, MA: Harvard University Press.

  (1986). *Semantic information: A framework for induction* (Mimeo). Cambridge, Eng.: MRC Applied Psychology Unit.

  (in press). Freedom and constraint in creativity. In R. J. Sternberg (Ed.), *The Nature of Creativity.*

Johnson-Laird, P. N., Herrmann, D. J., & Chaffin, R. (1984). Only connections: A critique of semantic networks. *Psychological Review, 96,* 292–315.

Jung, C. G. (1919). *Studies in word association.* New York: Moffat Yard.

Keil, F. C. (1979). *Semantic and conceptual development: An ontological perspective.* Cambridge, MA: Harvard University Press.

Kuhn, T. S. (1970). *The structure of scientific revolutions* (2nd ed.). University of Chicago Press.

Lashley, K. S. (1951). The problem of serial order in behavior. In L. A. Jeffress (Ed.), *Cerebral mechanisms in behavior.* New York: Wiley.

Marr, D. (1982). *Vision: A computational investigation into the human representation and processing of visual information.* New York: Freeman.

McCloskey, M. (1983). Naive theories of motion. In D. Gentner & A. L. Stevens (Eds.), *Mental Models.* Hillsdale, NJ: Erlbaum.

Mill, J. S. (1847). *A system of logic Book* 3. London: Macmillan.

Miller, G. A., Galanter, E., & Pribram, K. (1960). *Plans and the structure of behavior.* New York: Holt, Rinehart & Winston.

Miller, G. A., & Johnson-Laird, P. N. (1976). *Language and perception*. Cambridge University Press; Cambridge, MA: Harvard University Press.

Newell, A., & Simon, H. A. (1972). *Human problem solving*. Englewood Cliffs, NJ: Prentice-Hall.

Peirce, C. S. (1931–58). *Collected papers* (8 vols.; C. Hartshorne, P. Weiss, & A. Burks, Eds.). Cambridge, MA: Harvard University Press.

Popper, K. R. (1972). Conjectural knowledge: My solution to the problem of induction. In *Objective knowledge: An evolutionary approach*. New York: Oxford University Press (Clarendon Press).

Rumelhart, D. E., Smolensky, P., & McClelland, J. L. (1986). PDP models of schemata and sequential thought processes. In J. L. McClelland, D. E. Rumelhart, & the PDP Research Group (Eds.), *Parallel distributed processing: Explorations in the microstructure of cognition: Vol. 2: Psychological and biological models*. Cambridge, MA: Bradford/MIT Press.

Saussure, F. de (1960). *Course in general linguistics*. London: Owen.

Skinner, B. F. (1953). *Science and human behavior*. New York: Macmillan.

(1971). *Beyond freedom and dignity*. New York: Knopf.

Smoke, K. L. (1932). An objective study of concept formation. *Psychological Monographs, 42* (Whole No. 191).

Steedman, M. J. (1982). A generative grammar for jazz chord sequences. *Music Perception, 2,* 52–77.

Tversky, A., & Kahneman, D. (1973). Availability: A heuristic for judging frequency and probability. *Cognitive Psychology, 4*, 207–32. Reprinted in D. Kahneman, P. Slovic, & A. Tversky (Eds.), *Judgement under uncertainty: Heuristics and biases*. Cambridge University Press, 1982.

Wason, P. C. (1977). 'On the failure to eliminate hypotheses . . .' – a second look. In P. N. Johnson-Laird & P. C. Wason (Eds.), *Thinking: Readings in cognitive science*. Cambridge University Press.

Author index

459

Subject index